Nutrition in the Community

Nutrition in the Community

Edited by

Donald S. McLaren

Professor of Clinical Nutrition and Director, Nutrition Research Program, School of Medicine, American University of Beirut, Beirut, Lebanon

Foreword by
CICELY D. WILLIAMS

JOHN WILEY & SONS
London · New York · Sydney · Toronto

Library of Congress Cataloging in Publication Data:
Main entry under title:

Nutrition in the community.

   Includes bibliographical references and index.
   1. Nutrition—Addresses, essays, lectures.
1. McLaren, Donald Stewart. [DNLM: 1. Nutrition.
2. Community Health services. QU145 N9753]

TX353.N87   641.1   75–32565
ISBN 0 471 58556 4

Text set in 11/12 pt. Photon Times, printed by photolithography,
and bound in Great Britain at The Pitman Press, Bath

Contributing Authors

Dr. Z. L. Awdeh *Nutrition Research Program, School of Medicine, American University of Beirut, Beirut, Lebanon.*

Dr. I. D. Beghin *Chief, Division of Applied Nutrition, Institutto de Nutricion de Centro America Y Panama, Carretera Roosevelt Zona 11 Guatemala, C.A.*

Dr. G. Briggs *Professor of Nutrition, Department of Nutritional Sciences, University of California, Berkeley, U.S.A.*

Dr. R. E. Brown *Department of Community Medicine, Mount Sinai School of Medicine, Fifth Avenue and 100th Street, New York 10029, U.S.A.*

Dr. R. Cook *Director, Caribbean Food and Nutrition Institute, Jamaica Centre, P.O. Box 140, Kingston 7, Jamaica, W.I.*

Dr. P. Dodd *Department of Sociology, American University of Beirut, Beirut, Lebanon.*

Dr. M. Gebre-Medhin *Director, Ethiopian Nutrition Institute, P.O. Box 5654, Addis Ababa, Ethiopia.*

Dr. H. Ghassemi *Associate Professor of Nutrition, School of Public Health, Teheran, Iran.*

Dr. J. P. Greaves *FAO/UNICEF Nutrition Officer, UNICEF House, 11 Jorbagh, New Delhi 11000, India.*

Dr. A. H. Hallab *Faculty of Agricultural Sciences, American University of Beirut, Beirut, Lebanon.*

Dr. D. M. Hegsted *Harvard University, School of Public Health, Department of Nutrition, Boston, Massachusetts 02115, U.S.A.*

Miss D. Hollingsworth *Director-General, British Nutrition Foundation Limited, London, England.*

Dr. D. B. Jelliffe *Professor of Public Health and Pediatrics, and Head, Division of Population, Family and International Health, University of California, Los Angeles, California 90024, U.S.A.*

Dr. A. A. Kanawati *Nutrition Research Program, School of Medicine, American University of Beirut, Beirut, Lebanon.*

Dr. J. I. Mann *Lecturer in Social Medicine, Department of Regius Professor of Medicine, Radcliffe Infirmary, Oxford, England.*

Dr. D. S. McLaren *Professor of Clinical Nutrition, Director, Nutrition Research Program, School of Medicine, American University of Beirut, Beirut, Lebanon.*

Dr. C. R. Pascual *56, R. Gonzales St., B. F. Homes Paranaque, Rizal, Philippines.*

Miss F. Patton *Community Dietitian, Area Health Authority, Camden/Islington, London, England.*

Dr. P. L. Pellett *Division of Nutrition, Department of Food Science, University of Massachusetts, Amherst, Massachusetts, U.S.A.*

Dr. N. W. Pirie *Rothamsted Experimental Station, Harpenden, Hertfordshire, England.*

Dr. W. N. Sawaya *Research Officer, Lebanese National Council for Scientific Research, Assistant Professor, Faculty of Agricultural Sciences, American University of Beirut, Beirut, Lebanon.*

Dr. Arnold E. Schaefer *Director, Swanson Center for Nutrition, Inc., Omaha, Nebraska, U.S.A.*

Dr. W. H. Sebrell *Professor Emeritus of Nutrition, Columbia University, Medical Director, Weight Watchers International Inc., New York 11023, U.S.A.*

Dr. E. L. Severinghaus *18319 Olympic New Drive, Edmonds, Washington 98020, U.S.A.*

Dr. P. D. Starr *Department of Sociology and Anthropology, American University of Beirut, Beirut, Lebanon.*

Dr. P. V. Sukhatme *Maharashtra Association for Cultivation of Science, Poona 4, India.*

Dr. M. C. Swaminathan *Adviser (Nutrition), Directorate General of Health Services, Ministry of Health and Family Planning, New Delhi 11, India.*

Dr. R. I. Tannous *Faculty of Agricultural Sciences, American University of Beirut, Beirut, Lebanon.*

Dr. C. E. Taylor *Professor and Chairman, Department of International Health, Johns Hopkins School of Public Health, Baltimore, U.S.A.*

E. M. Taylor *c/o Department of International Health, Johns Hopkins School of Public Health, Baltimore, U.S.A.*

Dr. R. W. D. Turner *Reader in Medicine, University of Edinburgh, Physician, Western General Hospital, Edinburgh, Scotland, U.K.*

H. D. Ullrich   *Executive Director, Society for Nutrition Education; Editor J. Nutrition Education, Berkeley, California 94704, U.S.A.*

Dr. Cicely D. Williams   *Visiting Professor, School of Public Health and Tropical Medicine, Tulane University, New Orleans, U.S.A.*

Dr. U. S. Yatkin   *Department of Psychology, American University of Beirut, Beirut, Lebanon.*

Preface

It is generally recognized that Nutrition is a subject that has relevance almost everywhere whilst not fitting in anywhere in particular. This has meant inevitably that it has not been well understood and in the academic world it has been sadly neglected, considering its acknowledged importance for the health and well-being of mankind.

Several years ago when I became involved in the teaching of students of public health, in addition to teaching in the medical school, I was amazed to find that the general texts on that subject contain only brief and antiquated accounts of Nutrition with virtually no attempt made to prepare the reader for activities in the community. While there are numerous publications, mostly from the United Nations agencies, that can be used in courses and seminars, there has been no single text to guide teachers and students alike.

This book, unlike so many of its kind appearing these days with multiple authorship, is not just a collection of disconnected essays. It has a distinct plan and provides a complete and balanced coverage of this very broad subject. General concepts and accounts of the state of the art give way to descriptions of the nature of the malnutrition problems facing the world today, in all their complexity. Then follows critical discussions of the various measures and approaches for control of malnutrition, the role of various agencies and finally some carefully chosen examples from around the world of country experiences.

It is a matter of considerable surprise and gratification to me that this not inconsiderable undertaking has been brought from conception to fruition in a space of only two years. The material is thus remarkably up-to-date for a work of this size and complexity of authorship. In order to do this I have had to lean quite hard at times on the contributors, most of whom are (and I hope will remain) my personal friends as well as being noted authorities in the field. I hope they will feel with me that the final result has justified all their efforts. If the reader learns as much from them as I have they should feel amply rewarded. Not only have they provided a great deal of new information but their views come through uninhibitedly. Nevertheless I detect no striking discord in the overall effect.

We are most fortunate to have the Foreword by my old colleague the greatly distinguished Dr Cicely Williams; the undisputed doyenne in the field. This incisive piece of writing is an integral part of the text, by no means to be brushed aside like most, as it sets the tone for all that is to come.

ix

It is a true pleasure to acknowledge the amicable assistance received throughout from John Wiley & Sons. Manoushag Kerteshian earns my gratitude once more for secretarial assistance.

DONALD S. McLAREN

Foreword

CICELY D. WILLIAMS

Whatever may be the affluence of the people, whatever the evolutions of the scientists, it is only when good, adequate, balanced and appropriate nutrition gets to individuals in the community that the money, skills and personnel devoted to this subject are doing a good job.

The affluent countries have achieved great advances in those areas that demand passive acceptance on the part of the people — water supply, waste and refuse disposal, reduced pollution and pest control. But when it comes to individual understanding and responsibility the position is depressing. Mass distribution of food is an indication of failure.

Nutrition in the community is a subject which is crying out for more attention from every type of worker. From the individual who wants to provide food for his own family and from his own backyard, to the politicians and scientists, who have spent millions in the last 30 years, from the humblest foetus to the greatest biochemist, food is essential.

All this expenditure of money and energy has done little to improve the world situation or individual competence. It is only within the past century that we have begun to appreciate the complexity of the subject but we have not yet discovered how important it is that it should be simplified and priorities graded and balanced.

There are two main concerns, one is the food and the other is the consumer, his physical, mental and social well-being. Much energy has gone into the first, and not nearly enough into the second. Biochemists have dominated the picture. Although they can analyse food and physique, they have failed to realize the mental and social aspects of feeding.

The meaning of the word 'community' must be clarified. 'Community medicine' is sometimes defined as health care of people in groups. Others take it to mean care of people in their environment, home or work, but outside of hospitals and institutional medicine. Concepts such as 'family medicine' and 'comprehensive care' are sometimes included in community health. 'Comprehensive medicine' or 'continuity of care' must supervise and support people throughout episodes of health and sickness, whether inside or outside institutions. Community nutrition must emphasize applied nutrition and in fact it is consumer-oriented. It cannot exclude individual nutrition or nutrition in institutions such as hospitals. Food sciences are essential but most of our knowledge of applied nutrition in communities derives from close observation of patients by clinicians and scientists as far as the consumer is concerned. The hospital is the power house for study of the causes leading to malnutrition. This power should be utilized. Through close observation and follow-up of individual cases we learn the natural history of the various types and degrees of malnutrition, acute or chronic. Without those studies cases merely become static textbook illustrations of advanced and picturesque conditions. The study of individual patients in depth and in longitude is the only reliable way of ensuring analysis and follow up — follow-up into the past to observe what has produced the disorder and into the future to identify the results and prevent recurrences.

'Community nutrition' is therefore the whole of the nutritional sciences applied to the consumer as groups or as individuals. It is the interface between food and people and probably some 90 per cent of all nutrition takes place in the home. Each culture has always had its special preferred food, food taboos and food habits.

About 400 B.C., Hippocrates stated 'The physician must know, and must be at great pains to know, what man is in relation to food and drink and habits generally, and the relation of each to each individual'.

The most usual and most dreaded impact of natural and man-made disasters is famine. The most vulnerable groups, children and women as usual, have been the greatest sufferers. This type of emergency can and must be met with food supplies. In these days of swift communication, aid and supplies are often generously provided. But distribution of those supplies is much less simple, and the resulting benefits may be slight.[1]

Too much attention has been given to food shortage, both at the mass and at the individual level. Too much attention has also been given to specific deficiencies such as protein lack or vitamin A deficiency while relatively little attention has been paid to mixed or marginal deficiencies and multiple causation. As a rule the wealthy and privileged have adequate quantities and access to large varieties of food. The poor and disadvantaged have a limited variety and uncertain quantities, like 'The wretched slave, who with body filled and vacant mind, gets him to rest crammed with distressful bread' (*Henry V*, Act 4, Sc. 1).

Even in an affluent, sophisticated and powerful country such as the U.S.A. there are abundant cases of malnutrition. Some, perhaps the majority, are due to over-nutrition. Cases of obesity, hypertension, cardiac emergencies and diabetes are found among the poor as well as the rich. Ignorance is more important than affluence. Among children there are numerous cases of marasmus and specific and non-specific cases of malnutrition which are due to the ignorance of doctors and other health workers, lack of follow-up for cases at risk, and lack of attention to behaviour problems.

Nutrition and malnutrition are processes and not points in time. In some cases the symptoms appear in a very acute form: Many are chronic. Only with close individual observation over long periods is it possible to say this or that child has or has not got beriberi or marasmus. Malnutrition can exist in any degree. It is not like measles.

Many factors, physical, mental and social, 'food and drink and habits generally' are concerned with the different types, stages, duration and manifestations of the nutritional state. Mass distribution of food supplements is an inadequate method of treatment.

Primary malnutrition is often described as that which is due to defective food intake in quantity or quality or both. Secondary malnutrition results from diarrhoea, malabsorption, worms, tuberculosis, dyspepsia, despair and many other causes. The latter are more common than the former, but both types may coexist.

Individual variations in ability to ingest, masticate, digest, absorb, metabolize, store and eliminate nutrients are often underestimated. Booyens and McCance[2] studied 36 healthy men and women. Three had basic metabolic rates more than 30 per cent below average, and one more than 24 per cent above. Many food dyscrasias are due to allergies which may be temporary. But allergies are relatively rare in undernourished populations. When there is a shortage of foodstuffs, some subjects react by increased efficiency of digestion, absorption and metabolism. In fact, many important aspects of nutrition are associated with habituation. These are physiological responses as well as emotional. It is on this account that the weaning process is one of the most critical periods.

Where there is much dependence on biochemical evaluation there must also be concern with factors related to haemoconcentration and haemodilution. Dehydration of the system, with oedema of extremities, may be found together at the same time in the same patient. Some cases of malnutrition develop oedema of the internal organs without external evidence of oedema. When a malnourished patient is put on a good diet he may begin to recover by losing weight.

Many developing areas have health services that reach only a small proportion, sometimes as little as 5 per cent, of the population. Children and adults may be admitted to hospitals, having never before had any sort of health care or supervision. Multiple pathology is then usual, especially in the more serious cases, and the total picture will vary according to the region.

In Singapore the registration of births and deaths has been relatively good for many years; in 1925 the Infant Mortality Rate (IMR) was about 280 per 1000 live births. By 1936 it was around 150. From 1925 maternal and child health centres were being established both in urban and rural areas but they were attracting only about 70 per cent of the relevant population. The muncipal authorities supervised babies up to one year only; they did little treatment but referred sick children to the dispensaries or the general hospital, while the majority of births took place at Kadang Kerbau Hospital.

The rural areas were supervised by the government and under the direction of an outstanding Health Matron, Miss I. M. M. Simmonds. Centres were well distributed and constantly expanding at the demand of the people. They conducted excellent ante-natal clinics and did a large proportion of house deliveries with well-trained, experienced and supervised midwives. Children were accepted for supervision and treatment up to and including school age. Adults were treated at rural dispensaries or at government hospitals. By 1940, the rural IMR was 90 compared with 130 in the town. Children's wards at the general hospital contained 120 beds for children under 6 and there was also a schoolchildren's ward. In the 120 beds there were 3000 admissions during 1936, with over 50 per cent death rate. Every effort was made to ensure good follow-up in the health centres, but this was of course much easier to achieve in the rural areas than in the city.

However, the hospital was able to identify the diseases from which children were suffering.[3] The majority suffered from multiple diseases and the 'Singapore syndrome' often consisted of beriberi, ascariasis, diarrhoea, scabies and terminal pneumonia. Rickets was exceedingly common and keratomalacia not uncommon, while non-specific 'secondary malnutrition' was a frequent cause of sickness and death. Unless care is taken to identify the disorders that are present, the causes of malnutrition will not be recognized, and the epidemiologists will be wasting their time. Good clinical diagnosis and treatment is the best method of good prevention.

Today the IMR in Singapore is 19, the Birthrate is 21.2. The housing is said to be the best in Asia. The vital statistics are very nearly as good as in the U.S.A., although the GNP is only about one quarter of that in America.[4] The 'Family Planning Society' started (after the Japanese occupation ended) in 1946. The government policy of Family Planning programmes began only in 1966. But the maternal and child care system on comprehensive lines has been well established, and as the post-war reduction in Infant Mortality Rate proceeded, so did reduction in the birthrate. Nutrition and fertility have been treated as integral parts of general progress.

The quality of the population is what matters. The quantity, be it dense or sparse, can look after itself if the quality is assured.

Table 1. Selected rates by country

Country	BR	IMR	Per cent deaths under 5 years
Algeria	40.9	86.3	57.9
Egypt	34.9	119.0	59.2
Guatemala	39.0	88.0	51.7
Hong Kong	19.0	18.5	17.5
Sweden	11.1	11.7	2.4

From Casazza, L. J. and Williams, C. D., 'Family Health versus Family Planning', *Lancet*, i, 712 (1973).

RECENT TENDENCIES

Tropical medicine throughout its history has concentrated on communicable and parasitic diseases. Today it appears that only the Liverpool School of Tropical Medicine has a Department of Tropical Child Health. Yet in many developing countries over 50 per cent of total deaths take place in the under fives compared with 2.5 per cent in Sweden.

Before World War II, there was relatively little attention given to nutrition except as rather rare specific vitamin or endocrine disorders. Since 1945, however, much time, attention and money have been devoted to nutrition and to food production, mainly in the form of:

(1) Mass feeding, or supplementary diet programmes.
(2) Surveys.
(3) Biochemical investigations.
(4) Food production — both to improve farming and to investigate new compounds to be modified and processed for food.

During the same period large funds have been devoted to communicable disease control programmes. These efforts have increased survival rate and longevity and have therefore produced rapid increases in population, without necessarily increasing education or responsibility.

The world-wide interest in economic affairs has concentrated on cash crops and industries, in order to produce economic stability. Consequently food production for local consumption has often been treated as of secondary importance. A third factor has been rapid development of education within newly independent countries. Medical schools have been established at great cost, while the training of medical assistants, nurses and midwives and even of illiterate aides has been reduced or even abolished. As many of the doctors trained at great expense have been unable to obtain work, or have elected to work overseas, the total expenditure on education and training of health personnel has often been damaging to the conduct of the service. In one African country there are now 48 methods of training available, creating inefficiency and confusion. When a new idea is introduced, instead of expanding the services, the tendency has been to create a whole new cadre of workers.

There are many aspects of nutrition that have worsened in the last 30 years in spite of the efforts of all concerned.

Finally, there have been recent climatic changes which were unpredictable. The uncertainty of the future makes it all the more urgent to reconsider the present situation and policies, especially relating to production and to economics.

To return to the recent tendencies in nutrition policies, these can be:

(1) *Mass feeding and supplementary food programme.* In times of crisis, these programmes may be invaluable, especially if distribution is well-organized. There are many instances when this is not the case. Milk given out in young-child clinics has damaged an excellent tradition of breast-feeding. It has resulted in many cases of diarrhoea and failure to thrive and delayed the development of a local milk industry. Reckless distribution of skimmed milk has actually increased the incidence of keratomalacia and blindness. Some modest struggling mother and child health clinics have been overwhelmed by the need to distribute powdered milk to hordes of demanding mothers, with no time to observe, diagnose, treat or advise. When the milk supply stops, the mothers stop coming. Demoralization by handout is now a common situation.

School milk programmes have sometimes been regarded as the basis of liberal philosophy by the inexperienced. Some children have no appetite for this sort of food. As one child said. 'The gutters were running white with lumps of it.' With a little more thought and trouble, milk powder can be mixed with maize meal or cassava flour and cooked and distributed with the cooperation of parents. But this has not been organized and people have become indifferent and dependent.

When the developed countries abounded in surplus food, it was easy for private or international organizations to ship supplies in the sincere belief that the situation was being saved. It is tragic that so much goodwill has often been so poorly directed. The habits of emergency action and 'if there is something we can do let us go ahead and do it' have done much to delay more thoughtful and constructive programmes for food production, nutrition education and training of personnel. They have often overlooked the need for diagnosis and care of the sick.

Policies that depend excessively on food handouts, food tickets and 'welfare' can do harm by indiscriminate distribution to the obese, the dyspeptic, and those with other forms of dyscrasia. Worst of all, they pauperize a country and initiative is replaced by greed and apathy.

(2) *Surveys* by nutrition teams, epidemiologists, demographers, anthropologists and others are now excessively popular. Some assessment is useful but evaluation is often out of all proportion to the action taken.

Surveys may identify the prevalence of certain disorders, but not the incidence. An acute disease (e.g. cholera, acute cardiac, beriberi, acute pneumonia) which can kill in days or hours, has little mathematical chance of being identified compared with chronic conditions such as pellagra, leprosy and tuberculosis.

Nutrition surveys may identify the nutritional state, but are often incompetent to recognize the many and various causes leading to the malnourished state.

Surveys that depend on height, weight, age ratios are useful, but it is often difficult to measure the height, the weight may be distorted by oedema, by enlarged spleen and liver, by a heavy load of ascaris or by a distended or overloaded abdomen. The age may be pure guesswork.

Anthropologists may have to spend some time in a community before they are trusted with sensitive information. Some communities will not divulge even such matters as numbers of children, alive or dead, until they have some degree of confidence in their interlocutors.

On the other hand, a health worker who has spent some time in an area and has given obvious help may be trusted with some basic answers to questions such as:

How many children have you had?
How many are now alive?
How big were they when they died?
Were any of them born dead?
Do you want any more?
Do you expect to have any more?

Well-kept records by health workers, any type of midwife, cooperating village elders, school teachers and policemen may provide much information.

(3) *Biochemistry*. Some scientists believe that biochemistry can pose all the questions and solve all the problems in the field of nutrition. Vast amounts of money, of personnel and of attention have been spent on institutes and projects

devoted in the main to biochemistry. In *Disaster in Bangladesh*,[1] Dr. Chen (p. xxiii) says 'Man is increasingly contributing his disasters' and one of these has been failure to observe other physical, mental and social conditions which relate to nutrition and malnutrition.

It is now recognized that the nutritional state helps to determine the reaction of the body to various assaults: viral, bacterial, parasitic as well as to purely physical and emotional stresses. Nutritional state also affects resistance to toxins. The 'vomiting sickness' of Jamaica which is sometimes ascribed to akee poisoning (*Blighia sapida*), a toxin-producing hypoglycaemia, appears to occur only in children who are disadvantaged or undernourished.[5]

(4) *Food Production.* The usual enthusiasm of the overdeveloped countries for 'crash progress' and 'mass impact' has achieved some progress in food production in some areas. But rarely have these efforts kept up with the increasing population. Even the U.S.A. is now experiencing a serious rise in prices and the threat of food shortage. The rich get richer and the poor get poorer. Perhaps this is due to all the emphasis on food intake, and relatively little attention to the varieties of malnutrition, the varieties of causation, and methods and content of nutrition education.

Part of Community Nutrition must be devoted not to mass production but to individual effort and economy in use of land, sea, and food. These are subjects that need to establish education and experience, and 'habits generally' in people. Without a totalitarian form of government there is no 'instant' agronomy that can be launched. It is in continuity of care and the comprehensive approach that success is likely.

FUTURE PLANNING

1. Evaluation

Swarms of planners, statisticians, administrators, sociopsychoanthropologists, geographers, demographers, financiers and data processors are now called in to assist, and often to suffocate, health programmes.

Gabaldon[6] describes in Latin America 'an accounting system of such complexity that the expenditure on administration is quite out of proportion to the costs of the programmes'. The position now is worse than it was in 1969.

To quote another example, AID/CDE *Status Report 1975, Demographic Survey Haute Volta and Nigeria*, p. 1, 'Disease surveillance can be defined as continuous monitoring and analysis of disease incidence and prevalence data'.[7] How can such figures be obtained except by trained and experienced medical personnel with vigilance and in great numbers? No amount of biostatistics and computers can replace good and regular observation. If the evaluators can do this, they can do medical diagnosis, care and treatment at the same time. On p. 8 of this publication it states that 'Information on causes of death was obtained for some 100 deaths in Upper Volta by questioning other family and household members'. In the table on p. 18, *no ages are given* but the following figures are produced: Enteric diseases, 25;

Malaria fever, 13; Old age, cardiac, cancer, 10; Pneumonia, bronchitis, 9; Measles, 2; Tetanus, 2; Other, 20; Unknown, 19: Total, 100.

This type of 'surveillance' is a waste of time and money and a mockery to serious international effort, but it is fashionable; just as fashionable as the emperor's new clothes.

The Massachusetts Institute of Technology has recently published a brochure on an 'International Nutrition Planning Program'. Page 5 describes 'Degree Programs Relating to International Nutrition' and states 'Courses likely to be common to students include Human Nutrition, Food Science and Technology, courses in Political Development and Comparative Politics, Micro Economic Theory, Economic Growth and Development and Statistics'. There are also courses in Urban Studies, Planning, Management, Anthropology and Engineering.

There is no mention of physicians, nurses, midwives or any medical or para-medical personnel. This sort of production is a grim travesty of concepts, human suffering, human need, intelligence and commonsense.

Until there is some more rational attitude towards assessment of needs and resources, and of policies, we should confine our efforts to providing modest medical care and supervision with training, experience, and support for health aides; with unpretentious observations, investigation and record keeping, but with relevant content and maximum extent. Follow-up through hospitals, health centres and homes is essential. Otherwise 'Community Nutrition' will become a monumental collection of Ph.D. theses and nothing else.

2. Training of Personnel

The training of physicians, nurses, midwives and all medical and health personnel in nutrition needs to be revised in order to be more realistic and practical and less encumbered with biochemistry. More attention should be given to the multifarious causes leading to the malnourished state, to the production, distribution, selection and presentation of locally available foods, to the need for education and continuing supervision in hospitals, health centres and homes. Treatment of nutrition cases in hospitals badly needs to be improved.[8,9]

The population most at risk is children and mothers. The organization of ante- and post-natal clinics must be revised. Ante-natal clinics should not just supervise or supplement the mother's diet, but should also prepare her for breast-feeding, for the practice of family planning, and ensure the supervision of older children. The toddler is always at risk, and the ante-natal clinic can do much to ensure that the mother retains her interest in the deposed baby and his diet.

Physicians, nurses, and all others in a supervisory position must learn to select, train and supervise other members of the staff — in wards, out-patient clinics and homes. Without this continuing interest so-called 'Well Baby' Clinics are apt to become a hollow routine of weighing, measuring and 'shots'. Anyhow, in some developing countries, few of them are 'well'.

Training of personnel must include knowledge of nutritional disorders, ability to diagnose especially those that are mixed, mild or marginal. Treatment can be categorized:

(a) Drugs or vitamins or fluids for serious cases by various routes.
(b) Diet according to need.
(c) Education of parents or guardian.
(d) Supplementary feeding and continuing supervision.

At present there is a tendency to call many diseases 'PCM' or 'avitaminosis' and to provide supplementary feeding programmes as a panacea. Workers with simpler forms of training must at least be able to suspect nutritional disorders and refer to clinics or hospitals. They must know about the local and popular foods, their values both nutritionally and financially, how to choose, prepare and present them. These workers must also be able to recognize the influence of environment, physical and mental, on the nutritional state, and be able to give relevant advice and support in the home. More attention to care of the sick will do much to lighten the case load in hospitals and also to improve the homes.[10]

Occasional seminars and short courses should be available. But above all the physician should be constantly willing and able to demonstrate patients and findings with the staff, and to encourage discussions. Curricula for other categories of staff can be modified according to their previous training, experience and function.

A sample curriculum for the training of physicians in nutrition follows. Practical experience is an essential part of all training.

Nutrition for physicians

School of Public Health
American University of Beirut
3 hr. a week for 1 semester

Introduction and history
Ecology of malnutrition
Food habits, tradition and culture
Food production, preservation, preparation, composition
Body composition, growth, development and activity
Diet evaluation

Common Types of Malnutrition
    Their geographical and social distribution
    Diagnosis, treatment, follow-up and prevention in home, health centres and hospitals.
    Special attention to mild and non-specific types and their aetiology, both from individual and collective aspects
Infant and child feeding
Milk and milk products
Diets in pregnancy and lactation
Special diets
Special feeding programmes:
    (a) in emergencies
    (b) in schools
    (c) in orphanages
    (d) supplementary feeding as a continuing policy

Nutrition investigations
    Individual care
    Longitudinal studies
    Surveys
Food hygiene and food poisoning
The mini environment — food protection and food production
Nutrition policies and organization — Legislation
Personnel in nutrition:
    Doctors, nurses, midwives \   Training — work supervision
    Nutritionists, dietitians, etc. /   Refresher courses
International and voluntary agencies
Literature and periodicals

24.3.65

---

3. Facilities for treatment and prevention of malnutrition

These must go together because *every* patient, client, or case should have as much treatment as may be needed and at the same time as much prevention as they can take.

Hospitals. Breast-feeding should be promoted by rooming-in and by flexible feeding programmes. Premature babies should, if possible, be breast-fed. In Baragwanath Hospital, Johannesburg, over 70 per cent of the prematures were sent home fully breast-fed and the survival rate was good.[11] Arrangements should be made for longer stay in hospital for juvenile mothers and their babies and for special risks. Early mixed feeding must be discouraged.

Diets of children in hospital must be related to local customs with modification and improvements. For instance, peanut soup is excellent, but should be made without pepper. Local forms of green leafy vegetables, legumes or youghourt can be emphasized. Mothers can learn how to beat an egg into the local maize or rice porridge. Mashed ripe banana can be mixed with milk powder dissolved in water. Out-patients can be an opportunity for demonstrating foods. However malnourished the child is, the total disease picture must be appreciated. Severe cases of kwashiorkor can be treated initially with small blood transfusions, or intraperitoneal infusions. Follow-up from hospitals for future checking or for transfer to a clinic should be organized.

Health Centres must give proper attention to nutrition teaching and demonstration. 'Family Health Centres' will ensure continuity of care — even though the most vulnerable groups are mothers and children (MCH) and the 'under fives' require much of the time and attention.

Nutrition Rehabilitation centres are best placed beside a hospital or health centre. They can admit ante- and post-natal cases in need or at risk as well as children.

Home Visits can be a valuable method of nutrition education and supervision. They can produce improvements in the back-yard garden as well as in the mini environment. They can also ensure proper use of water supply and latrine, encourage visits to clinics for women and children and for family planning. They are the best means of assessing the total family situation and of encouraging registration of births and deaths as well as home improvements. Care of the sick in the home needs to be developed as a major concern.

Supplementary Feeding Programmes may be of benefit but they should be used as a last line of defence except in emergencies.

Community Nutrition needs to develop an understanding of what can be done by mass methods and what can only be accomplished on a basis of care and support to families and to individuals. This applies both to the food and to the consumer. 'Public Health' must have regard for the concerns and for the needs of all people and must adjust health and nutrition services to meet those needs. Medical care is grossly inadequate in content and extent. It must be physical, mental and social, and only then will nutritional needs be understood.

Control of diseases, control of populations and food distribution are negative functions and can create dependence. Family health or mother and child health encourage comprehensive care and continuity of care and will not only help to cure diseases and prevent the preventable diseases, they will teach people what they can do for themselves. They will improve the standard of living and of responsibility. Whatever the type of health service, the availability of food and nutritional state of consumers must be considered.

As recently as 1975 the *P.A.G. Journal* states 'Although many causes have been identified, the ultimate pathway of all of them is inadequate and/or improper feeding.'[12] The old fallacy continues that it is always the food that needs correction. Perhaps when health workers have more to do with the community they will realize that factors other than food need attention.

A book which covers the various aspects of nutrition in the community is to be highly recommended. Its use should herald the era of a more realistic attitude towards nutrition problems.

REFERENCES

1. Chen, L. C. (Ed) *Disaster in Bangladesh*, Oxford University Press, N.Y., 1973.
2. Booyens, J. and R. A. McCance, *Lancet*, **i**, 225 (1957).
3. Williams, C. D. *J. Malaya Branch Brit. Med. Assoc.*, **2**, 113 (1938).
4. World Bank, *Health: Sector Policy Paper*, World Bank, 1975.
5. Williams, C. D. *J. Med. Women's Fed., London*, 43 (1954).
6. Gabaldon, A. *Lancet*, **i**, 739 (1969).
7. AID/CDE *Status Report, Demographic Survey Haute Volta and Nigeria*, 1975.
8. Cook, R. *J. Trop. Pediat.*, **17**, 15 (1971).
9. Ashworth, A. *Cajanus*, **15**, 238 (1975).
10. Williams, C. D. *Pediatrics*, **52**, 772 (1973).
11. Khan, E. *S. Afr. Med. J.*, **28**, 453 (1954).
12. Protein Advisory Group United Nations System, *P.A.G. Journal*, **5**, 1 (1975).

Contents

COUNTRY EXPERIENCES

SECTION I

Nutrition at the Community Level

CHAPTER 1

Concepts and Content of Nutrition

DONALD S. MCLAREN

Nutrition has proved to be difficult to define. Most dictionaries are unhelpful and often misleading; calling it a science, an analysis etc. Nutrition , like respiration, combustion, reproduction etc., is a process and it may be defined as '*The process by which the organism utilizes food*'. This phrase has the advantage of being sufficiently short to be readily committed to memory but for a fuller understanding of the nature and purpose of nutrition a more detailed description is required. *In nutrition food, or anything normally ingested by the organism is utilized by the processes of digestion, absorption, transport, storage, metabolism and elimination for purposes of maintenance of life, growth, normal functioning of organs and the production of energy.*

While nutrition is a process, *nutriture* is the corresponding state; it is equivalent to the more commonly used term *nutritional status*. Nutriture is *the state resulting from the balance between the supply of nutrients on the one hand and the expenditure of the organism on the other.* When the balance is within the normal range nutritional status is normal and the body's requirements are being met and not exceeded.

The relationship of nutrition to nutriture was likened by Sinclair[1] to a river flowing into a basin and forming a lake. Factors affecting the flow of the river determine the state of the lake.

It is indeed remarkable that the need has not previously been expressed for a term to describe the science or study of the process of nutrition. The failure to define terms and concepts in this area may well have contributed to the apparent lack of scientific progress so frequently complained about. In keeping with related disciplines the term 'nutrology' is proposed. The scientists and practitioners of nutrology would be known as 'nutrologists'. They would have their specializations and might therefore be known as Clinical, Animal, Biochemical Nutrologists, etc. Strictly speaking, this book would be entitled *Community Nutrology* but perhaps the reading public is not quite ready for that.

It has proved helpful to try to visualize the relationships of the various elements in the process of nutrition using the *Agent–Host–Environment* interaction of Greenberg[2] in the epidemiology of disease. Here the organism interacts with the causative agent of a disease which might be acting positively, as would be the case with a micro-organism, or negatively, as in deficiency of a vitamin. This interaction can be modified by the environment.

Figures 1 and 2 show the Agent–Host–Environment interaction as it applies to nutrition in health. The *environment* is *Food:* edible mixtures in the overall surrounding, which are ingested by the organism. A foodstuff, when treated, forms food. A *meal* is the sum of food ingested at one feeding. A *diet* is the sum of the daily or weekly meals, considered especially in relation to its quality and effects, and a *dietary* is a prescribed or adopted course of diet.

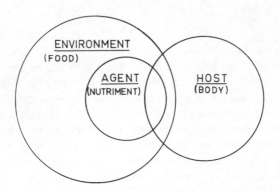

FIGURE 1. The Agent–Host–Environment interaction applied to nutrition (Figure 1A, *Nutrition and its Disorders*, D. S. McLaren, Churchill Livingstone 1972)

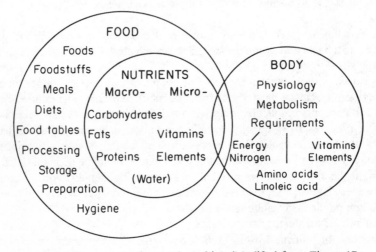

FIGURE 2. The content of normal nutrition (Modified from Figure 1B, *Nutrition and its Disorders*)

Within food lies the *agent* of nutrition, the active principle within the body, or *nutriment;* and this in turn comprises the *nutrients.*

Not everything in food nourishes, although it may have an effect, harmful or beneficial, on the body. For example toxins, either naturally occurring or added to alter the food in some way, may cause disease (see Chapter 12). Fibre, at least in monogastric animals, and other non-absorbable substances, do not nourish the body but influence absorption of nutriment and may play an important indirect role in nutritional and other diseases (Chapter 9). Retaining the *Agent–Host–Environment,* or *Nutrients–Host–Food* interaction concept, Figure 2 illustrates the content of normal nutrition. Only some of the aspects of food are mentioned here, the study of which may be considered to form food science.

Within the body of the host the physiological processes of digestion, absorption, transport, storage and excretion go on, together with innumerable processes of metabolism within the cells. The requirements for sources of energy and for each of the various nutrients are determined by the demands the organism makes as it seeks to maintain normal nutrition and health.

It is convenient to divide the nutrients into two categories, *micro-* and *macronutrients.* Micro-nutrients include vitamins and some elements. *Vitamins* are *chemical compounds occurring naturally in food and essential in small amounts for the health of the organism.* They can be divided into fat-soluble (A, D, E and K), and water-soluble vitamins (including thiamine, riboflavin, nicotinic acid, pyridoxine, folic acid and vitamin B_{12} of the B group and vitamin C). The former tend to be stored in the body and their precise mode of action is obscure. Except for vitamin B_{12}, water-soluble vitamins are little stored and they usually function as coenzymes.

Many *elements* are present in food and find their way into the body. Some, like calcium, phosphorus, potassium, sulphur, sodium, chlorine and magnesium, are essential for health and occur in the body in a concentration of more than 0.005 per cent. Others, like iron, iodine, copper, zinc, manganese, cobalt, molybdenum, selenium, chromium, nickel, tin, silicon, fluorine and vanadium, are also essential but occur in smaller concentration (less than 0.005 per cent) and are called *trace elements.* Other elements are suspected of being essential but final proof is lacking (e.g. barium, strontium). Finally elements for which no metabolic role has so far been demonstrated are absorbed occasionally (e.g. gold, silver, aluminium).

The macro-nutrients are the old 'proximate principles' (in the sense that they were the first arrived at in the process of analysis) and include carbohydrates, fats and proteins.

Micro- and macro-nutrients differ in a number of ways (see Table 1). Among the products of digestion of each of the classes of macro-nutrients, proteins, fats, and carbohydrates, there is a special group segregated by essentiality and dietary requirement. These products are amino acids, fatty acids and glycerol, glucose and other mono-saccharides.

Several amino acids (depending on the animal species) are called essential or indispensable as they either cannot be made at all or only in inadequate amounts by the body. For man these are lysine, tryptophan, methionine, phenylalanine, threonine, leucine, isoleucine, valine and histidine. For all but threonine and lysine the provision of the carbon skeletons is enough. There is no protein requirement as such. The requirement is for certain essential amino acids and a certain amount of non-essential nitrogen. Among fats certain polyunsaturated fatty acids are essential and must be part of the food. A dietary requirement for carbohydrate exists only under the artificial conditions in which protein is restricted and other precursors of glucose (carbohydrate and glycerol) are excluded.

Table 1. Micro- and macro-nutrients contrasted

Micro-nutrients	Macro-nutrients
1. Consumed in small amounts (< 1 g/day)	Large amounts (many g/day)
2. Absorbed unchanged[a]	Degraded by digestion
3. Essential, body cannot make them	No single carbohydrate, fat or protein as eaten is essential but products may be (see text)
4. Do not provide energy	Provide energy
5. Major function as coenzymes and catalysts	Enzymes are proteins
6. Structural function limited (calcium, phosphorus mainly)	Protein mainly structural, but also some lipid and carbohydrate

[a] Exceptions include carotenoids and folates.

Good nutrition (or nutriture) is a matter of balance, neither too much nor too little. *Malnutrition* is *disordered nutrition of any kind* and may be categorized in a number of ways (Table 2). Figure 3 illustrates how malnutrition of different causes and types occurs. Primary malnutrition arises from an abnormality in the nutriment (i.e. the agent) while secondary malnutrition is caused by a deficiency in the host. These disorders may be due to excess or deficiency, involve one or more different nutrients and be of varying degree, duration and outcome.

Table 2. Classification of Malnutrition

1. Cause:	primary (exogenous)
	secondary (endogenous)
2. Type:	excess, toxicity (overnutrition)
	deficiency (undernutrition)
3. Nutrient:	vitamins, elements, protein, energy sources
4. Degree:	(i) mild—moderate—severe or, alternatively,
	(ii) depleted stores—biochemical lesion—functional change—structural lesion
5. Duration:	acute, sub-acute, chronic
6. Outcome:	reversible, irreversible

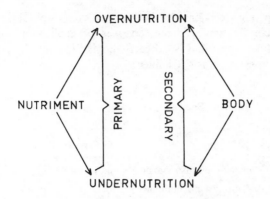

FIGURE 3. Causes and types of malnutrition
(Figure 6, *Nutrition and its Disorders*)

The *types of Undernutrition* (*Inanition*) are given in Table 3. The scheme is based on that proposed by Jackson in 1925 in his classic work *The Effects of Inanition and Malnutrition upon Growth and Structure*.[3] Complete Total Inanition is Starvation and Incomplete Total Inanition is Semi-Starvation, Underfeeding and 'Hunger'. Partial Inanition is equivalent to 'Hidden Hunger' and 'Misfeeding'. Many of these terms, especially those in quotation marks, have been used indiscriminantly in relation to the nutriture of the world's peoples.

Table 3. Types of Undernutrition

Aqueous Deficiency Inanition (no water, no food)

Total Inanitition (receiving water, food deficient in all nutriment)
      (i) Complete Total Inanition (no food)
     (ii) Incomplete Total Inanition (insufficient food)

Partial Inanition (deprivation of specific nutrients)
      (i) Complete Partial Inanition (diet devoid of a nutrient)
     (ii) Incomplete Partial Inanition (deficient in a nutrient)

Based on reference 3

Table 4 outlines the various ways in which secondary malnutrition occurs, giving a few examples from among many diseases which interfere with various steps in the utilization of nutriment.

This scheme is very similar to that given by Jolliffe in his text *Clinical Nutrition* and developed in more detail in his paper entitled *Conditional Malnutrition*[4] written 30 years ago. Recently Herbert has followed the same categories in his detailed application of the concept to the aetiology of deficiency of vitamin B_{12} and of folate.[5]

In addition to being involved aetiologically in disease processes, either primarily or secondarily, food may act in a harmful or helpful way in the body. The non-nutriment part of food may be beneficial to therapy, as in the case of the bland diet in treatment of peptic ulcer. Lack of dietary fibre such as cellulose may be at least partly responsible for some of the 'diseases of civilization'—atherosclerosis, diabetes mellitus, appendicitis, diverticulosis and cholecystitis—through predisposing to intestinal stasis (Chapter 9).

Table 4. Secondary or endogenous malnutrition

Defect in	Examples
Digestion	Pancreatic disease, intestinal surgery
Absorption	Malabsorption syndromes
Transport	A-β-lipoproteinaemia
Storage	Cirrhosis, haemochromatosis
Metabolism	Inborn errors (PKU, galactosaemia, etc.), vitamin dependency (B_6/B_{12}), ? obesity
Elimination	Trauma, renal failure, protein-losing enteropathy
Requirements (increased)	Pyrexia, injury, thyrotoxicosis

From McLaren, D. S. Nutrition and its Disorders. Churchill Livingstone, London 1972.

Toxins in food may cause disease. These include goitrogens, possible carcinogens such as aflatoxin, the unidentified toxin in fava beans of favism, various metals (e.g. mercury), food additives like monosodium glutamate and cyclamates, and many others (Chapter 12).

NUTRITION IN THE COMMUNITY

If we adopt an ecological approach we may picture man surrounded by several environments (Figure 4). The most intimate of these, as it actually enters, and in the case of food forms part of, his body is the biological environment. At different levels of experience there are physical and psycho-social environments. In the latter a number of factors can be identified as playing a role, prominent among which are education, culture and economics. While disease acts directly on man, the other factors tend to have their main effect on human nutriture through food. Thus the climate affects food production and preservation, culture determines beliefs and practices regarding food selection and preparation and education may further influence these, while economic factors largely determine the amount and to some extent the quality of food purchased.

Looked at in another way, food and the community in their interaction may be seen to have both quantitative and qualitative aspects. Food supply is quantitative while nutriment supply in relation to requirements is qualitative. In general, man eats diets that are qualitatively adequate but often not enough in amount. A diet which is qualitatively inadequate will be deficient in vitamins, minerals or protein while one quantitatively restricted will lack energy value. It is clearly of great practical importance in relation to policy-making and planning to decide which aspect predominates in a situation where malnutrition exists. It has been mistakes at this level in the past that have led to unfounded fears of a 'protein gap, crisis' etc. and the unnecessary pursuit of measures to produce protein sources to meet the non-existent problem (Chapters 3 and 16).

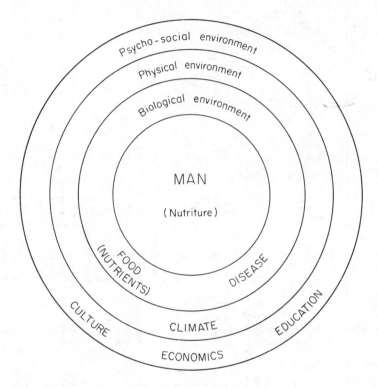

FIGURE 4. Man and his food

The community for its part may also be considered both qualitatively and quantitatively. Community quality in all respects would take into account not only various physical attributes, among which nutriture and health are prominent, but also mental and spiritual qualities. Quantitatively the community may be considered at the local, regional, national or global level and besides actual population size there are considerations of structure, particularly with regard to age distribution and trends of growth.

In essence it is the intention throughout this book to cover the various aspects of the agent–host–environment interaction in health and disease in the community

Table 5. A world view of nutritional disorders of the 1970s

Disorder	Related nutritional factors	Precipitating factors	Major clinical features	Consequences	Vulnerable groups	Geographic distribution	Numbers affected (very approx. any one time)	Control measures
I Undernutrition								
1. Protein–Energy Malnutrition				Impaired mental development	Infant, pre-school child	Developing countries	300 m	Total approach, education of mother, plan services
(a) **Early Stages**	Mild and moderate deficiency of all	Early weaning, infections	Stunting				200 m	
(b) **Marasmus**	Severe deficiency, mainly energy	Gastroenteritis, urbanization	Gross wasting	High mortality	Esp. infant	Slums (Asia, Latin America)	15 m	
(c) **Kwashiorkor**	Severe deficiency, mainly protein	Measles and gastroenteritis	Dermatosis, oedema, fatty liver, hypo-albuminaemia	High mortality	Esp. 2–4 years	Rural areas (Africa)	5 m	
2. Xerophthalmia	Carotene, vitamin A	Rice staple, measles, early weaning	Night blindness, xerosis of conjunctiva and cornea, keratomalacia	Blindness, high mortality	Pre-school	S. & E. Asia	100,000	Green vegetables, massive dose, fortification
3. Rickets, Osteomalacia	Calciferol (vitamin D)	Unfortified milk, sunlight lack	Bone softening, hypocalcaemia	Permanent deformities, obstructed labour	Infants, pre-school, pregnant, aged	Asians in U.K. Urban tropics	Several thousand	Massive doses, sunlight, fortification
4. Beriberi	Thiamine (vitamin B$_1$)	nonparboiled rice, alcoholism	Heart failure, neuropathy, encephalopathy	High mortality	Pregnancy, 2–5 months, adults	Parts of Asia cities of U.S.A.	Several thousand	Fortification
5. Pellagra	Nicotinic acid (niacin)	Maize (as porridge), jowar,	Dermatosis, diarrhoea, dementia		Adults	Parts of Africa, Middle East,	Rare	

6. Scurvy	Ascorbic acid (vitamin C)	Lack of fruit, excess cooking	Haemorrhages, impaired wound healing		Infants, old age	Desert	Very rare	
7. Folic acid	Folic acid	Excess cooking, pregnancy, drugs	Megaloblastic anaemia		Pre-school, pregnancy		Common	Dose
8. Vitamin B_{12} deficiency	Cobalamin (vitamin B_{12})	Veganism, genetic	Megaloblastic anaemia, sub-acute combined degeneration of the cord		Adults		Rare	
9. Iron deficiency	Iron	Prematurity, pregnancy, milk diet	Microcytic, hypochromic anaemia	Impaired work efficiency	Prematurity, pregnancy, child bearing, parasitism	Worldwide	Many millions	Enrichment, dose
10. Goitre	Iodine	Mountains (leached soil) ?goitrogens	Thyroid enlargement, deaf mutism in severe	Hypo-thyroidism, cancer in severe	Females	Hill areas, Americas, Middle East, Asia	Many millions	Iodized salt, oil injection
11. Fluorine deficiency	Fluorine	Low water content	Deutal caries		Starts in childhood	Parts of most countries	Many millions	Fluoridation to 1 p.p.m. of drinking water
II Overnutrition								
12. Obesity	Excess energy sources	Lack of exercise, overeating	Increased adiposity, poor risk	Reduced survival	Infancy for most, females	These are among the 'diseases of civilization' and seen throughout world among affluent communities	Up to 50 per cent in affected groups	Education re diet
13. Atherosclerosis	Excess lipid saturated, cholesterol, ?sucrose, ?lack of minerals, fibre	Smoking, hypertension, diabetes mellitus, stress	Coronary heart disease, stroke	High mortality, invalidism	Adult males 30–60 years		Many millions	Education re diet, smoking

Other vitamin deficiencies (E, K, riboflavin, pryidoxine) and other element deficiencies. (Calcium, electrolytes and trace elements) not of public health magnitude.

and to foster in the reader an ecological approach to nutritional matters which it is hoped will lead to the amelioration of the problems existing today, by the bringing about of a more balanced outlook leading eventually to balanced nutrition.

NUTRITION TODAY

Finally, to set the stage for what follows and to give an idea of the nature and the magnitude of the nutritional problems existing at the present time, I have drawn up in tabular form a very simplified account of our knowledge of nutritional disorders around the world (Table 5).

REFERENCES

1. Sinclair, H. M. *Vitamins and Hormones,* **6,** 101 (1948).
2. Greenberg, M. and Anna V. Matz, *Modern Concepts of Communicable Disease,* New York, Putnam, 1953.
3. Jackson, C. M. *The Effects of Inanition and Malnutrition upon Growth and Structure,* Philadelphia, Blackiston, 1925.
4. Jolliffe, N. *J. Amer. Med. Assoc.,* **122,** 299 (1943).
5. Herbert, V. *Amer. J. Clin. Nutr.,* **26,** 77 (1973).

CHAPTER 2

Characteristics of the Community

PETER C. DODD AND PAUL D. STARR

Although efforts to improve the health and well-being of people have taken place under a wide variety of circumstances, perhaps the most important settings for nutrition improvement programmes are 'communities'. Communities, as the term is used here, may range in size from less than one hundred to a few thousand people. Members of a community live and work together in a common geographical area, feel a sense of loyalty to the community, and share a limited number of common interests.

Until recently, most of the people in many countries lived in villages or small towns, places that could be readily defined as communities. The process of industrialization, however, has promoted the growth of cities and metropolitan areas where many inhabitants have found it more difficult to form definite communities. Even in large cities, however, social scientists have identified communities, often in the context of neighbourhoods or quarters.[1] Beyond the city centre, suburbs have developed a life-style of their own.[2] In these urban and suburban communities, people share common loyalties and patterns of living, develop friendships and common interests. Although much of the discussion in this chapter deals with rural communities, often of a traditional 'peasant' type, the general scheme of analysis can also be applied to urban and suburban communities.

It is the intention of this chapter to discuss briefly those characteristics of communities that are particularly important in programmes for the improvement of standards of nutrition, public health and social well-being. While all of the characteristics of communities described here may not be found in every society, or in every community within the same society, we have attempted to include those which are most common and most important for community-level workers seeking to plan, implement or evaluate programmes to improve standards of nutrition. This discussion will consider four basic areas of community life: socio-economic organization; the nature of social groups and relationships; local political processes and the role of community attitudes and values.

In many programmes, an understanding of the social life of a community may be as important as the technical aspects of a project. More effective methods of food production, storage or preparation are of little use by themselves unless they are accepted and successfully employed by local people on a continuing basis. It is therefore important for professional persons who attempt to influence community practices to be sensitive to the dynamics of community life just as they are familiar with technical requirements for improved nutrition.

In most countries, the small rural community or village is regarded with a certain ambivalence. While its inadequacies or 'backwardness' relative to urban areas are assumed, the village is also often viewed as embodying the 'soul' of the nation, possessing the traditional moral values. Village life is often idealized in popular poetry, songs and stories. The ideal features of community life are emphasized in many societies and become part of a common stereotype. Life in the village is seen as being direct, human and simple and having few complexities and disappointments. People familiar with urban areas often attempt to carry out village improvement schemes using these initial assumptions regarding the 'simple life'. These 'urbanites' may then discover that their assumptions are inappropriate and that they in fact know very little about such communities. This may occur when a project which has appeared to be in their eyes an obvious 'improvement' has been rejected or resisted by the 'irrational' villagers.

It is of vital importance for community-level workers to realize that attitudes and conduct which may appear to be 'irrational' in the view of outsiders may be quite appropriate given the circumstances in which many villagers find themselves. What may appear to be illogical beliefs and behaviour on the part of villagers may well be a quite rational adjustment to a difficult situation. Community improvement efforts require that professional workers take the perspective of the people who live in the community and understand the social, economic and political forces which shape their lives. By doing this, community workers may anticipate and avoid many problems and be better able to cope with unanticipated complications.

Programmes may also be made more effective if the worker regards the community as an entity in which problems cannot be dealt with in an isolated, piecemeal fashion. Most aspects of community life are interrelated with other features, being part of a complex web which encompasses a wide variety of activities. What may appear to be a relatively minor change in one activity can have a great effect on many other areas of life. In a particularly vivid example, Sharp[3] has described how the introduction of steel axes among Australian aborigines not only replaced traditional stone axes but significantly altered the religious, economic and political organization of that society. What appeared to be a minor change had wide-ranging social consequences, including the disruption of social patterns which had developed over several centuries. The same complex interrelationship may also concern accepted ways of producing, storing, preparing or consuming foods. This area of life frequently includes practices, norms and values which are related to religious rituals and ceremonies. These social patterns are usually very important to the people involved and are not easily modified.

SOCIO-ECONOMIC ORGANIZATION

In many societies, rural agriculturalists not only comprise the vast majority of the population but also produce surpluses which support the other sectors of the society and provide the basis for economic development. Their ability to change is limited by the human, technological and natural resources available to them, as well as by the attitudes and values present in their community. An understanding of the situation in which such groups live requires the consideration of the economic forces which impinge upon them as well as the internal dynamics of community life.

While rural communities in the Third World may produce much of their own food and other necessities, small settlements usually depend on larger towns in which to sell their surplus or to buy items which they themselves cannot produce. Marketing may take a variety of forms, generally ranging from the direct exchange of goods and services between producer-consumers to the transfer of goods and services to a central point where they are later redirected by economically dominant groups for distribution. The economies of most Third World communities involve some combination of these types of exchange.

Few communities are totally self-sufficient; most are involved in multi-dimensional relationships which include economic, religious, social and political activities within a network of several communities in the surrounding area. Usually the larger the community, the more often it serves as a source of diffusion for innovations in fashion, religion, technology and other new ideas. Through the process of economic exchange and the necessity of coming into contact with others from outside areas during such activities, many persons are drawn out of their home community. Religious festivals, pilgrimages and the desire for entertainment not available at home also provide opportunities for increased contact with outsiders. With the growth of literacy, the advent of mass media and the improvement of transportation facilities, the isolation so typical of rural areas only a few years ago has been significantly reduced. Such changes, described by some social scientists to be of revolutionary proportions, have brought several innovations into villages more rapidly than has any previous means of communication.

Broadcasting services, publications and posters have introduced and promoted many new ideas and continue to offer great potential for programmes which require informing or stimulating the interest of large masses of people.

Although prosperous communities may have power to change their situation, poor communities usually have little control over the conditions which govern their lives. Occupying the lower socio-economic positions in the society in which they live, the vast majority of community dwellers find that it is not within their power to change the economic system, the class structure, or the political system. Basic decisions affecting them are often made in cities or large towns far outside their home community and are infrequently explained to them. Government decision-making is ordinarily accomplished by centralized bureaucracies. Economic forces, such as price fluctuations for basic commodities, are beyond the influence of the community. Initiative in the community is usually permitted in limited spheres of activity and even then produces little reward.

Based on his observations in several parts of the world, Foster[4] has noted, with some pessimism, that:

The orders, the levys, the restrictions, the taxes that are imposed from the outside have for (the peasant) the same quality of change and capriciousness as do the visitations of the supernatural world. And the peasant feels much the same toward both the authorities of the city and the supernatural ... but in neither can he expect by his own action to have any effective control.

When economic surpluses are produced and marketed, they typically provide for only modest returns, leaving families with scarce resources which must be carefully managed to provide for bare essentials.

In several societies, a family which prospers is expected to share its increased wealth with distant kin or non-kin who belong to the same community, leaving it with little real reward for increased effort, a practice described by some social scientists as one which suppresses the will to achieve. Even if the individual wishes to improve his standard of life, such social commitments require the expenditure of acquired resources which could otherwise be reinvested for increased production. Few are able to resist the expectations which others have of them as a member of a community. Such circumstances contribute to the lack of interest or the resistance a group may have toward an innovation either proposed from within a community or promoted from the outside. Any innovation which affects existing economic practices must be demonstrated to be beneficial, not threatening to cut down production or to require the increased use of scarce labour, money, materials or other resources. This also indicates that unless resources from outside are to be applied to a programme, existing resources by themselves may very well impose a limit on what could possibly be accomplished by adopting new practices. Even if resources are sufficient in objective terms, it is also important to consider the ways in which they are perceived and are employed within the social context of the community.

One additional point is important. Although one may often find some sort of resistance to proposed changes in a community, such problems appear to have been frequently exaggerated in studies of directed change. While several types of problems are discussed in this chapter, it should be emphasized that communities are often quite receptive to change, particularly if they can be shown that real benefits are to be secured without threatening their limited resources or valued patterns of social life.

SOCIAL GROUPS AND RELATIONSHIPS

Almost all communities are composed of smaller social units which are characterized by certain kinds of social relationships. An understanding of the nature of these smaller units is required in development efforts and should be of primary interest to change agents during every phase of their effort. Rather than viewing his efforts as concerning independent individuals, the community worker should consider his programme as relating to persons who are members of groups, participating in many different types of social relationships. The worker should be aware of forms of communication and association, as well as distinctions in social status.

As in all societies, social relationships in the community tend to be regulated according to group memberships, either real or imagined. The members of one's circle of companions are regarded as an 'in-group'. Other people, even some of those who may live in the same area, are viewed as belonging to 'out-groups'. Individuals typically share the perspective of their in-group, or those who occupy a common status in the community. The rules and shared perspectives of the in-group usually exert a strong influence on group members. Conformity to the rules is customary and automatic in most social situations.

Every individual, however, belongs to a number of groups. The rules and perspectives of his groups may occasionally come into conflict with each other, creating a difficult situation for him. He may have to deviate from one set of rules in order to conform to another. An example is that of the rural school teacher who sees himself as a member of the urban 'modern' middle class while at the same time adopting the view of a traditional group within his community.[5] Differences in the viewpoints of these two groups may result in a sense of conflict for the individual. One might also have *negative reference groups,* those which provide an individual with an example of ways one should *not* live. 'City people' may serve as a negative reference group for rural people who cling tightly to traditional ways of doing things. Differences in reference groups often account for differences in individuals' perceptions of and receptivity to new ideals and activities.

Groups within communities often have a history of conflict or competition. Such conflicts may be based on economic or political rivalries, sometimes reinforced by ethnic differences. Unless the community worker is aware of these conflicts, he may become identified with one group and gain the hostility of the others. The community worker who comes in with the support of government authorities, for example, is often regarded with suspicion by community groups that are opposed to the government.

Not all communities are full of group conflict and rivalry. All communities, however, do have networks of *social relationships* between individual members of the community. A knowledge of these social relationships is invaluable to the community worker seeking to introduce change.

In general, there are six forms of these social relationships: kinship, patron–client, ethnicity, fictive kinship, voluntary associations and friendship.

Kinship is by far the most common form of social relationship. It is based on one of two bonds: descent (blood-tie) or marriage. Kinship ties usually involve deep affection, include many aspects of the individual's life, and endure for many years. The family is the social group based on kinship ties, although kinship relations may take many other forms as well. A useful distinction is that between nuclear and extended families. A nuclear family is composed of husband, wife and their non-adult children. While this is the most common unit in industrialized societies, extended families are also found. The extended family may include persons from an older generation, such as the parents of the wife or the husband; it may include adult brothers and sisters of the husband and wife; or it may include other relatives, such as uncles and aunts. The residential unit is called the household and may number as many as twenty or thirty people in non-industrialized communities.

Kinship ties provide the basis for support and allegiance which members of a household expect from each other. The system of kinship permits members of the community to determine the limits of rights and obligations, as when a father is held responsible for the actions of his non-adult children, or a mother is expected to look after the health of her children. Similarly, kinship groupings provide the community with a mechanism for social integration, through extended families or family alliances.

Although most family relationships are affectionate, they may also contain elements of conflict. Certain tensions potentially exist within all family groups, particularly between successive generations of extended families who may have quite different perceptions of the world. Additionally, there are inevitable problems of succession, as when aging parents must yield decision-making and production roles to their children. There may also be conflicts based on differential perceptions of male and female roles or among siblings competing to assume authority or control of property.

Although there may be substantial self-sufficiency within family groups or production units, members of other families may be called upon for some type of cooperative activity or support. Ties among different family members take a variety of forms, ranging from the holding of joint property and a continual sharing of activity to occasional visits and an exchange of gifts.

Community members frequently become involved in *patron–client relationships* to protect, maintain or promote their interests. Patrons usually are wealthy persons, large landowners or religious or political leaders, with some potential power to aid their clients, the ordinary people in the community, in the conduct of their affairs within the community as well as those involving the larger society. Patrons frequently serve as go-betweens in the relationships concerning ordinary community dwellers and government authorities. They may also serve as mediators in disputes among those within their clientele. Such relationships can also be based upon fictive kinship ties.

Fictive kinship, the establishment of kinship-type relations among persons who are not related by blood ties, is also a frequent method by which individuals and groups seek to maintain or improve their position in a community. These relationships may involve the use of special 'kinship' terminology, particular forms of address such as 'brother', 'son', 'godfather' or 'uncle' and certain patterns of mutual conduct which indicate such relationships. Fictive kinship is similar to actual kinship based on blood ties. It is sometimes formally created by a ritual act, as in a baptism ceremony where a godfather swears to aid in bringing up a child. Once established, it usually lasts for the lifetime of the participants.[6] Such relationships also include those in which individuals are ritually joined together as hypothetical equals, such as 'brothers'.

Voluntary associations also provide the basis for social groupings in a community, usually in conjunction with other forms. These include religious or temple associations, local political parties, youth clubs, money-lending circles, burial societies, craftsmen's guilds, agricultural associations and other groups of individuals held together by a recognized set of rules, with the aim of achieving a specific set of purposes. These rules may be set forth in a written constitution or they may be a set of practices which have developed over many years. Leaders of these voluntary associations may be important to the community worker concerned with nutrition, since they may be able to influence large numbers of community members. One of the characteristics of industrialized societies is that voluntary associations tend to take the place of kinship groupings. In these societies, many voluntary associations have purposes specifically concerned with improvement of health.

Many social relationships are based on common *ethnicity,* an affiliation with an ethnic group possessing a special language and culture. Sometimes the ethnic group has its own religious or political system and calls forth intense loyalty from its members. Ethnicity is not the same as nationality, since a nation may include many different ethnic groups. Relationships between different ethnic groups may not be harmonious; often there is a long history of tension and conflict. When a community includes members of several ethnic groups, the professional worker must be alert to the possible areas of tension. These may well include differences in food habits, since strong beliefs are often attached to the use or prohibition of particular foods. Some religions, for example, forbid the eating of pork, and members of these religious groups report that they find the smell of pigs' meat both noticeable and offensive to them.

Friendship, while it is based on feelings of affection and mutual intimacy, has none of the formal qualities of other types of social relationships. Friendships are freely chosen, not prescribed. In this respect they differ from kin and ethnic group relationships. An individual may have friendships with a wide variety of persons, forming a network of relationships that is intricate and widespread. Friendships may cut across other social ties, binding persons of different families, ethnic groups and communities. Within a community, news and information often spreads through friendship networks.

There are, therefore, a wide variety of social relationships within any given community. These relationships may occur in various combinations, as when two family members also belong to the same voluntary association. Some relationships have priority in one area of life and little influence in others. Health problems, for instance, are often handled through family relationships, whereas patron–client relationships are more likely to be concerned with politics or economics.

LOCAL POLITICAL PROCESSES

The nature and types of leadership are important factors which in some way influence all efforts to bring about change. Some communities have leadership roles fairly well-defined while others have no leadership or leadership structure. Some persons may be regarded as leaders in one sense, perhaps as spokesman for affairs concerning the local community and government bureaucracies, but not in others, such as those dealing with methods of farming or health care. Dube[7] has observed in his study of Indian villages that no person held a monopoly of leadership in all areas of community affairs, but several were regarded as leaders in separate domains. Regardless of the specific circumstances, there is usually a distinction between 'formal' and 'informal' leaders. 'Formal leaders' are those, either elected or appointed, who occupy specific positions or offices and are responsible for certain functions which are typically specified in legal codes or government directives. 'Informal leaders' are those who are regarded with high esteem and whose guidance is sought on certain matters even though they may not have 'official' status.[8]

Some experienced community development workers feel that many community problems are basically due to the lack of effective indigenous leadership. They contend that development can only proceed with success through the mobilization of dynamic local groups, representatives of the community. These local groups must recognize, plan and implement ways of enhancing life within their domain, sometimes in conjunction with outside institutions.

Communities are frequently divided by factionalism among different component groups, making the job of mobilizing local resources or gaining some consensus an extremely challenging task. As Erasmus[9a] has indicated, it is a frequent misconception that people are naturally cooperative or that they will automatically take collective action if they are only shown the need for it.

Local government officials may lack power. Individuals with wealth and prestige in a local community often exert more authority than those who hold political offices or titles recognized by the state. Depending on the requirements of a particular undertaking, little may be accomplished in a community without the approval and support of these non-governmental leaders. Even specific directives ordering the implementation of changes from the central government may only be implemented with the consent of such influentials. Failure to recognize this and failure to acquire the approval of such persons may lead to overt or covert resistance, the formation or mobilization of various factions, or the creation of other types of barriers to the implementation of change. Community decision-making very often consists of informal consultation among local influentials. Formal meetings, if any are held, may be the public acting-out of decisions previously made. Many community development specialists have stated their view that the cooperation and approval of local influentials is of primary importance in many programmes and that action workers should initiate their activities with them.

Some efforts at improving community well-being may be viewed as threatening the security of certain individuals or groups. Traditional healers or local midwives, for example, often feel threatened by modern medical programmes or services. In some instances this problem has been solved by incorporating traditional healers into modern programmes and making them the local contact persons for implementing agencies. Changes in economic practices, such as those affecting the distribution of land, water, farm animals or other resources, the availability of farm equipment, insecticides or fertilizers, or the establishment of consumer or producer cooperatives may be strongly resisted by those in the community who feel that existing arrangements benefit them more than the proposed changes. These persons, often landlords, merchants or local specialists, may possess much influence over local affairs. If proposed changes are perceived as benefiting the community as a whole and also as benefiting those with such vested interests, they may, on the other hand, enthusiastically work for or use their influence to help accomplish such ends. Many successful projects have worked through local interest groups, such as merchants, to increase the diffusion of improved production methods, household technology, drugs, food supplements, insecticides, fertilizers and other beneficial innovations. In any programme which requires local sponsorship, community workers should consider the possibility of working with and through those who provide the goods and services relevant to the target activity.

ATTITUDES AND VALUES

Many ways of doing things in communities can be understood as a rational adjustment to a difficult circumstance. In places where community members have been taken advantage of by merchants, civil servants and others from the outside world, it is quite natural that they should be sceptical of programmes designed by outsiders to improve their situation. Fatalism, the view that whatever happens in one's life is due to fate or the will of God, is a common and reasonable adjustment to poverty and powerlessness. Under conditions in which there are limited productivity and resources, rudimentary technology, high disease and death rates, little political influence and the promise of little change, a more optimistic perspective is not encouraged.

Peasants and other rural people often envision the outside world as an unknown place, unpredictable and filled with potential danger. Do community members, faced with the dangerous unknown, join in common action or do they also fear each other? There is conflicting evidence on this important question.

Wolf[10] has indicated some ways in which communities have developed local mechanisms for sharing resources in time of need and in order to meet the misfortunes which may strike one group at one time and another group later, in a sort of indigenous social security system. Others have described villages in several different parts of the Third World in which the inhabitants are so envious and suspicious of one another that they cooperate on a very limited basis.[4, 11] Accounts of life in small settlements frequently portray them as pervaded by feuding, mutual hostility on the part of various factions, malicious gossip and tension in interpersonal relations which make it difficult for people to cooperate for their common welfare.

In attempting to account for such attitudes, Foster[4] has suggested that some villagers possess an 'image of limited good' in which they view their community as having a set amount of resources and rewards which cannot be increased but for which all are competing. If one family or individual gets ahead and prospers, their success is viewed as being at the expense of others. Efforts at altering existing arrangements for changing accepted ways of doing things are regarded with suspicion as attempts to take advantage of others and reduce their share of the limited good.

A provocative study by Banfield[11] came to similar conclusions about the lack of cooperation primarily due to the world view held by community residents. Basing his observations on a Southern Italian village, he has described 'amoral familism', the practice of avoiding cooperative activities while striving to maximize the material, short-run advantage of the nuclear family and to assume all others will do likewise, as being a major barrier to social progress. Because the world appears to be such an uncertain and fearful place, those who stand outside the small family circle are seen as potential competitors and enemies.

While such descriptions will not apply to all communities, they do indicate that the values held by a group provide the basis for much of their conduct and that an understanding of the view of the world held by residents can be of vital importance to any improvement effort.

Community members are often aware that they hold a disadvantaged position in comparison with others and that they are also often held in low esteem by urban or more 'advanced' people, but they usually retain pride in certain aspects of their way of life. They may feel that while they lack economic and other resources, they are more moral or follow a more genuine form of religion or way of life. They may take the view that their life style embodies the purest form of folk art, handicrafts, music, dancing, cuisine, marriage, or family life. These beliefs may significantly influence the evolution of a development programme. In one instance, for example, a superior variety of white maize was rejected after most farmers in a Latin American village started cultivating it. They claimed that the colour and flavour of the ground meal was not of the type that made a good *tortilla,* or flat corn wafer, a basic food and also an important indicator, in their culture, of a good cook and homemaker.[9b] In this instance, a scientifically sound innovation was rejected when it came into conflict with the local value system.

There is, therefore, strong evidence that people in traditional communities value their culture, their technology and their social structure, and they may not welcome attempts to change existing ways of doing things. This does not mean, however, that they are satisfied with *all* aspects of their culture. The community worker, with patience, can discover areas of dissatisfaction in which to start people thinking about innovations, about ways of changing to more satisfying patterns of action. He can utilize his knowledge of community attitudes and values in constructing a new and positive programme of action.

CONCLUSION

Professional workers concerned with the improvement of the nutrition of individual human beings must recognize the importance of the social setting in which people live, especially the importance of the community. Members of a community influence each other in many ways. The channels of influence may be used to block innovations and attempts to introduce change, or they may be used to facilitate innovations, depending on the skill and patience of the community workers. Economic organization, group allegiances, local politics, individual values and attitudes, may all have a vital effect on programmes designed to improve health conditions in the community.

REFERENCES

1. Gans, H. J. *The Urban Villagers: Group and Class in the Life of Italian-Americans,* New York, The Free Press of Glencoe, 1962.
2. Whyte, W. H. *The Organization Man,* New York, Simon and Schuster, 1956.
3. Sharp, L. Steel axes for Stone Age Australians, in *Human Problems in Technological Change,* Spicer, E. H. *(Ed.) New York, Russel Sage Foundation, 1952.*
4. Foster, G. M. *Traditional Cultures and the Impact of Technological Change,* New York, Harper and Row, 1962.
5. Gubser, P. *Politics and Social Change in Kerak, Jordan,* Oxford University Press, 1973.
6. Potter, J. M., M. N. Diaz and G. M. Foster (Eds.), *Peasant Society: A Reader,* Boston, Little, Brown and Co, 1967.
7. Dube, S. C. *India's Changing Villages: Human Factors in Community Development,* London, Routledge and Kegan Paul, 1958.
8. Hunter, F. *Community Power Structure,* Chapel Hill, N.C., University of North Carolina Press, 1953.
9. Erasmus, C. J. *Man Takes Control,* Minneapolis, University of Minnesota Press, (a) p. 89, (b) p. 61.
10. Wolf, E. R. *Peasants,* Englewood Cliffs, N.J., Prentice-Hall, 1966.
11. Banfield, E. C. *The Moral Basis of a Backward Society,* New York, The Free Press, 1958.

SUGGESTED READING

Arensberg, C. and A. H. Niehoff *Introducing Social Change,* Chicago, Aldine, 1964.
Batten, T. R. *Communities and Their Development* (rev. ed.), London, Oxford University Press, 1967.
Bennis, W. G., K. D. Benne and R. Chin (Eds.) *The Planning of Change* (2nd edn.), New York, Holt, Rinehart and Winston, 1969.
Goodenough, W. H. *Cooperation in Change,* New York, Russell Sage Foundation, 1963.
Lenski, G. and J. Lenski *Human Societies,* New York, McGraw-Hill, 1974.
Lionberger, H. F. *Adoption of New Ideas and Practices,* Ames, Iowa, Iowa State University Press, 1960.
Mead, M. (Ed.) *Cultural Patterns and Technical Change,* Paris, UNESCO, 1953.
Neihoff, A. H. (Ed.) *A Casebook of Social Change,* Chicago, Aldine, 1966.
Paul, B. D. and W. B. Miller (Eds.) *Health, Culture and Community,* New York, Russell Sage Foundation, 1955.
Peattie, L. R. *The View from the Barrio,* Ann Arbor; University of Michigan Press, 1968.
Rogers, E. M. *Diffusion of Innovations,* New York, Free Press, 1962.
Rogers, E. M. *Modernization Among Peasants: The Impact of Communication,* New York, Holt, Rinehart and Winston, 1969.
Ward, R. J. (Ed.) *The Challenge of Development,* Chicago, Aldine, 1967.

CHAPTER 3

Historical Perspective of Nutrition in the Community

Donald S. McLaren

The role of food and nutrition in history has been recounted on a number of occasions and the reader is referred to several of these works at the end of the chapter.[1-3] The subject is clearly an enormous one and superficial treatment in the present context would hardly serve any useful purpose.

There would seem to be three major topics that could be approached in an historical context with the purpose of trying to gain a better understanding of the forces at work influencing nutrition in a community context. The first of these may be formulated as a question: 'Has man been subject to nutritional disorders throughout his existence and if not then what were the forces that caused them to emerge?' Easy to ask, perhaps impossible to answer in the face of the dearth of evidence but nevertheless worth attempting. The second topic is of considerable interest in relation to the approach to the formulating of policies and planning of programmes in nutrition and will be outlined by Dr. Ghassemi later (Chapter 13). It concerns the way in which the focus of interest in nutrition has shifted from the patient to the laboratory, from the laboratory to the hospital, and from the hospital to the community. The third topic concerns some lessons that might be learned from past experience, ancient and not so ancient. Unfortunately it is too often true but perhaps overly pessimistic that 'history teaches us that history teaches us nothing'. In any case, to learn from the past something of benefit for the present and the future must surely be seen as a major purpose of history.

HOW ANCIENT ARE NUTRITIONAL DISORDERS?

During the millions of years that elapsed while true man was evolving from hominids, food collection was the only means of obtaining nourishment. As for large apes and gorillas today, the sources in the earliest stages were leaves, fruits, berries, roots, nuts and bark. After the appearance of the first true man *H. erectus* one million or possibly more years ago extremes of climate probably led to cave dwelling, hunting for covering with skins and food. 40,000 years ago, in the middle of the first Ice Age, Cro-Magnan man *H. sapiens* appeared in Europe using tools. The cultivation of crops probably dates from the beginning of the Neolithic Age which occurred in parts of the Middle East and Asia as early as 9000 B.C. but due to climatic differences did not reach the temperate zone of Europe until 4000 B.C. and Northern Europe only by 1500 B.C. Excavations at Catal Hüyük in Turkey dated about 6500 B.C. show that Neolithic man besides growing wheat also cultivated barley, peas, vetches, almonds, crucifers, and pistachios for vegetable oil and probably hackberries for wine. The plough was probably developed in S.W. Asia and China about 4000 B.C., first drawn by man and later by oxen.

With an abundance of a wide variety of foodstuffs, animal as well as plant, in the developing centres of civilization in relation to the relatively small and scattered numbers of people it seems unlikely that nutritional disorders were at all common. Universal breast-feeding and exposure to sunlight would have been protective for young children. Only in times of drought (as described in the book of Genesis) would mass starvation have threatened whole populations.

Although most of the classical nutritional deficiency diseases have a rather characteristic clinical picture and should therefore be readily identifiable from ancient medical records there is little to indicate that most of them occurred in antiquity, let alone that they were of any public health significance.

Goitre was probably endemic in mountainous parts of Europe in Roman times. Pellagra does not appear to have emerged in southern Europe until the middle of the 18th century. Reliable accounts of epidemics of scurvy date no earlier than the 15th century, coincident with the commencement of long sea voyages of exploration. Beriberi may have an earlier history than most other deficiency diseases as it is reliably described in a Chinese work about 200 B.C. and in several Chinese and Japanese writings in the early centuries of the Christian era. In his historical introduction to 'Rickets, osteomalacia and tetany' Hess has found little evidence of the disease in classical times apart from the account of Soranus of Ephesus who practised medicine in Rome during the 1st and 2nd centuries A.D. Its occurrence in the greatest city of the day is probably significant. There are no clear accounts of xerophthalmia before those of the last century and the frequently quoted reference in the Eber's papyrus of ancient Egypt to the use of liver for eye disease should in no way be taken as evidence that there was vitamin A deficiency at that time or that the ancients knew the liver to be effective. The liver, as the seat of the soul, was used in many prescriptions quite arbitrarily. It is equally fanciful to see in the Psalms the description of a child with kwashiorkor.

It is probable that the transition from hunting and gathering to cultivation brought about an increase in both fertility and mortality with the net effect of only a slight increase in population growth.[4] Village life, by bringing comparatively large numbers together, may have provided opportunity for the spread of infectious diseases, and greater contamination of food and water. Agriculturalists would also be vulnerable to crop failure. Deficiency diseases and famine are unlikely to have stricken man before he began to come together in this way. For them to occur on any sizeable scale a considerable degree of specialization and sophistication was probably necessary.

Early descriptions of deficiency diseases have the common feature of occurring under unusual situations: of famine, war and confinement (siege, sea voyages, imprisonment). Generalized malnutrition of the protein–energy malnutrition type occupies a rather special position. The infant and pre-school child are primarily affected and the form taken by the disorder is influenced by social and environmental factors. Marasmus, the predominant form at present, has probably been predominant throughout history. Earliest known descriptions date from about the *16th century* but it is not evident that it was ever a massive scourge as it is at present. Today it predominates in the urbanizing societies undergoing rapid social change in developing countries. It is the nutritional hallmark of the urban avalanche. It is doubtful if the cities of antiquity were large enough, sufficiently overcrowded, or the population under the kind of economic stress or ill-advised government and commercial pressure for breast-feeding to have been abandoned; an almost *sine qua non* for it to occur. Kwashiorkor is much more characteristic of rural communities, or new slum dwellers who have not yet abandoned their dietary habits and infant feeding practices. Prolonged breast-feeding into the second or third years is usual and supplementation takes place with a protein-poor staple such as starchy roots. In the conditions of life of earlier times it is very doubtful if any group of people subsisted in this way, as perhaps 100 million or so do today, mostly in parts of Africa, Oceania and South America. It seems more likely that such poor basic diet was only accepted by those who were driven by some outside pressure, often probably invaders and colonizers. The introduction of new infections may have been critical and any influence that may have cut down the care the mother gave the child would have been harmful, resulting in the 'deposed child' situation characteristic of kwashiorkor. Among many primitive peoples it has been customary for men to have more than one wife. Under these circumstances after the birth of a child the father may not resume intercourse with the mother for a prolonged period. In the Koran such a period of two years is specified for the full care of the child. However, the influence of alien cultures, such as the European, where monogamy has been mandatory would have tended to disrupt this pattern and the Christianizing of people in Africa and elsewhere may well have been the origin of kwashiorkor. In Europe during the early part of this century the same disease there named Mehlnährschaden or starch dystrophy, occurred as a result of artificial infant foods poorly formulated with very low protein and high starch content.

In summary, there is very little if any evidence that man in antiquity suffered to any extent from nutritional disorders, apart from famine. It was probably only as life became more complex and 'unnatural' that special situations of privation arose and that the grossly unbalanced diets needed to produce the disorders mentioned emerged.

Albrink[5] has argued that the survival of early man depended in part on his ability to store excess energy after a successful kill, to be called on in time of food shortage. Man is therefore endowed liberally with many mechanisms which favour fat mobilization but is ill-equipped for massive fat storage and relies almost entirely on a single hormone, insulin, for fat synthesis. The prehistoric role of adipose tissue has been reversed by the modern sedentary way of life and affluence and the adipose tissue is more frequently called upon to store fat than to mobilize it, and when its limits are exceeded obesity results.

It is also very unlikely that other 'disorders of civilization' were common in the distant past. Low physical activity, diets high in saturated fat and sugar, and low in fibre content and habits of smoking and drinking were neither then, any more than they are today, features of the way of life of primitive man, whereas they are frequent accompaniments of such 'diseases of civilization' as atherosclerosis and coronary heart disease, diverticulosis and other stasis conditions of the gut and circulation, cholelithiasis and diabetes mellitus (Chapter 9).

SOME LESSONS FROM HISTORY

Vitamin A, carotene and xerophthalmia

'Hikam' was the name given to a blinding disease of children of epidemic proportions in Japan at the turn of the century. It occurred when a child was suddenly transferred from breast milk to a diet poor in fat, consisting of barley, flour and vegetables but no cow's milk or meat. Cod liver oil was curative and it was clearly xerophthalmia. It remained a problem until after the Second World War, when it disappeared with the economic development without any specific measures being taken. At the present time programmes of repeated massive doses of vitamin A are being implemented in several rice-dependent countries of South or East Asia but so far it is only where economic development has been dramatic (Japan, Taiwan, Hong Kong and Singapore) that the disease has disappeared.

Xerophthalmia is a disease that really gives the lie to the common belief that nutritional deficiencies are due to food shortage. Provitamin A carotenoids occur in abundance in the green leaves that on all sides greet the visitor to the typical village in the monsoon tropics. The curse is that rice, the staple food in these areas, is devoid of carotene and the people do not realize the importance of the green leaves. No other cereal cooks as softly as rice or produces satiety so easily; a combination especially dangerous to the young child. Thus there is poverty in the midst of plenty. It seems that there are some little-used strains of rice containing some pigments, but these may not be provitamin in activity and a coloured rice might not prove acceptable. When xerophthalmia occurs elsewhere it indicates the real 'bottom of the barrel', nutritionally speaking, and under these conditions its emergence (as in Johannesburg or the Luapula valley of Zambia) indicates a rapidly deteriorating situation, not necessarily economic but perhaps cultural-social. It may equally readily disappear under these circumstances.

Xerophthalmia has had a special tendency to be iatrogenic, or man-made. The first outbreak that occurred after 'fat-soluble vitamin A' had been recognized experimentally to cure eye diseases induced in rats by feeding a deficient diet, was in Denmark during the First World War.[6] Butter was sold to Germany at a high price and oleomargarine was substituted. The poor could obtain only separated milk or buttermilk, almost free from fat. Besides this the diet of these children consisted of oatmeal gruel and barley soup. Eighty per cent of the several hundred cases of xerophthalmia were in infants. When butter was rationed in 1918 as a result of the German blockade and everyone, including children, was entitled to 0.25 kg per week xerophthalmia diminished. As a matter of fact, there is not so much difference between that and the way xerophthalmia has blinded many thousands of children every year in Indonesia for at least the past 50 years. The Dutch established red palm oil plantations on Sumatra and this very rich source of provitamin has been exported to Europe to colour and fortify margarine.

A further instance of man-induced xerophthalmia has been through the introduction of milk from which vitamin A has been removed by processing. This was first recorded for condensed milk in Singapore and Djakarta before the Second World War. In the first city xerophthalmia virtually disappeared during the early years of the war when condensed milk was unavailable. After the war, when the surplus skim milk from the United States began to be distributed to malnourished children little attention was paid to its nutritional value apart from its being a good protein source. Cod liver oil capsules were also supplied sometimes but these were rarely given to the children properly. Outbreaks of xerophthalmia from skim milk have continued to recur in recent years in Indonesia, Brazil (where it is called 'can blindness') in the war in Bangladesh, and in Taiwan, where it had disappeared.

Ethiopia was the stage for another kind of lesson from vitamin A. The ICNND Nutrition Survey there in 1958 revealed, among other things, a high incidence of Bitot's spots among school children in Addis Ababa.[7] A United Nations expert had carried out a survey previously in the country, obtained similar findings, and had recommended to the government a countrywide distribution of vitamin A capsules. The ICNND group decided to investigate the matter further and recommended that pending their results there should be no intervention. Carefully controlled vitamin A dosing was commenced in the schools and six months later I returned with an ophthalmologist, Dr. David Paton, who was then at the NIH. We carried out slit-lamp microscopy, conjunctival biopsy, plasma vitamin A determinations, and dark adaptometry. All tests were normal and the Bitot's spots persisted. They were probably related to ultraviolet light exposure at the high altitude, irritation from dust, smoke in the homes, and mild eye infection; certainly not due to vitamin A deficiency. Our supposition was further backed up by the absence of xerophthalmia in the much more susceptible pre-school age.

Before I went to India in 1949 as a medical missionary I remember being told what excellent opportunities I would have to do research on little-understood diseases. I did not have to be there long to realize how busy such a hospital can be and how primitive the facilities. However, I was soon confronted with numerous cases of duodenal ulceration and liver failure with unfamiliar characteristics and aetiologies still obscure. After becoming very familiar with the people and their customs in a tribal area of Orissa over several years I did observe that keratomalacia was common in the young children of the plains Oriyas and rare among the hill tribe Khonds.[8] Both consumed rice as a staple and clinical signs of nutritional deficiency were similar among members of the two groups. This suggested that some factor(s) limited to the very young Oriya child was responsible.

The clue slowly emerged, after painstaking enquiry, that the Khond children were protected by a tribal tabu forbidding intercourse for two years after a baby was born, while the Oriya had no such practice and keratomalacia frequently presented in a child who had been forcibly weaned and 'deposed' when the mother knew she was pregnant again. This little piece of nutritional-anthropological investigation, with many similarities to the story of Cicely Williams' work on kwashiorkor, stands as a salutory reminder of the difference between nutrition the process and nutriture the state. All the food balance sheets and biochemical tests in the world will not answer this kind of question.

Beriberi

This disease due to thiamine deficiency is another good example of a nutritional disorder whose emergence and spread has been closely related to technological innovation and the sociological consequences thereof.

By the 19th century thousands of cases were being described from Japan and other parts of the Orient where the introduction of mills to pound the rice had led to greater destruction of the grain than in home pounding.

In the pre-revolution cities of the rice-eating areas of China beriberi was rife. The close relationship between thiamine requirement and energy expenditure was demonstrated there by such observations as the finding that wrist drop affected the right hand of Shanghai tram drivers using this arm almost exclusively, and the occurrence of overt cases in certain families of affected districts, always in the homes that were dirtiest, had the most bed bugs and where the occupants got the least sleep.[9]

Today, more frank cases of beriberi of all clinical types can probably be observed in some of the great cities of the richest country on earth (the United States of America) and among the Bantu of the most affluent country of Africa (Republic of South Africa). Alcoholism is the common factor largely responsible, whether it is the cheap wine of the Boston 'wino' or the Kaffir beer in the government beer hall in the African township.

An example of just how inflexible and unrealistic hospital statistics can be is provided by the reporting of beriberi from the Philippines. Long after the disease has ceased to occur other than sporadically it is still high on the list of causes of infant death; largely because the earlier propaganda for its importance was so effective.

Pellagra

Most physicians would answer 'yes' to the question 'Can most cases of pellagra be attributed to prolonged subsistence on a diet low in nicotinic acid (niacin)?' and they would be wrong. The usual diet, maize or corn, is not especially low in this vitamin. Perhaps the area of the world with the highest endemicity at the present time is Andhra Pradesh, in central India, and the staple is 'jowar' or millet. Tryptophan, a precursor of nicotinic acid in the body, is absent from the main protein of maize and its metabolism is probably interfered with by an excess of leucine in jowar. Lime treatment in the preparation of 'tortillas' in Central America releases the vitamin from a bound form in maize.

There is thus in pellagra a good deal more than meets the eye. Until Goldberger, in a series of classical human experiments, proved it to be a deficiency disease pellagra was regarded as infectious in origin. How the disease finally disappeared from the Southern United States is an interesting and not altogether clear story. The physician who attributed this to the discovery of nicotinic acid would be wrong again. The vitamin was discovered in 1937 but the case rate and mortality had begun to decline sharply years before. In the United States, mainly from the south, in 1928 7000 deaths were attributed to pellagra and in Georgia alone there were 20,000 cases. The economy was at its worst in 1930 but despite this there was a sharp decline in pellagra, starting with that year and continuing for several years. Mortality was at its peak in 1930 and between 1932 and 1934 cases fell by 58 per cent. By the mid-1940s the disease had virtually disappeared.

Davies[10] and Roe[11] have pieced together the evidence for the part played by various factors in the story. The economy of the southern states was based on cotton and the whole area had been almost bankrupt for years. In the prevailing sharecropping system tenant farmers mortgaged their future crop yields and if crops failed or prices fell they could not repay the loans. Cotton operatives bought their rations from factory commissaries. Stocks were very limited and usually consisted of the three Ms: meal (cornmeal), meat (salt pork and lard) and molasses. In better times wheatmeal, rice and dried beans were available.

The sudden decline in pellagra in the early 1930s Davies attributes to the break up of the cash crop monoculture on the advice of the agricultural extension service agents who persuaded people to grow a variety of pulses, fruits and vegetables when cotton became almost unsaleable in the Depression. However, the sharecropping system recurred once the economy improved and the decline of pellagra was halted. In the late 1930s, despite the availability of cheap nicotinic acid and free yeast, the poor food habits, ignorance and inertia among the people prevented eradication. Only the entry of the United States into the Second World War, with increased employment, food rationing and enrichment of bread and other cereals brought about the final phase.

Rickets

The discovery in recent years of active forms of vitamin D that give it the characteristic of a hormone rather than of a vitamin has been rightly hailed as marking a new epoch in the knowledge of vitamin D and of its functional disorders. Nevertheless, in this context it can hardly compete in importance with the discovery of the aetiology and treatment of rickets by one man more than 100 years ago. Armand Trousseau showed that rickets resulted from an inadequate diet and a sunless climate, that osteomalacia is the adult form and that both conditions could be cured by fish liver oil, preferably accompanied by exposure to sunlight. He called attention to the experimental production of rickets by Guerin in puppies and the cure by mother's milk and sunlight. His teacher Bretonneau had cured rickets with cod liver oil and Trousseau extended its use to osteomalacia and even postulated it was acting as a fat containing unknown food components. He tested many other oils and fats. Jean Mayer has recounted[12] how the work of this celebrated Paris physician was completely discredited by 1900 and most physicians then thought the disease was infectious like tuberculosis. Subsequent historical accounts have often ommitted any reference to Trousseau. Mayer suggests that it may have been the fact that Trousseau's findings were isolated and unsupported by general concepts of deficiency disease that they were swept aside in the enthusiasm for Pasteur's germ theory of disease. This cautionary tale has a salutory lesson for its readers.

The Protein Myth

As the 'newer knowledge of nutrition', to quote the title of a famous book by E. V. McCollum, spread in the first decades of this century it does not seem to have occurred to anyone that disease could arise from deficiency of protein. Just as the 'germ theory' had swamped Trousseau's observations so did the 'vitamin era' dominate thought later on. When Cicely Williams was appointed the first woman Medical Officer to the Gold Coast and suggested that the common childhood disorder there, known as 'kwashiorkor' in the local language, was 'a deficiency disease' and 'some amino acid and protein deficiency cannot be excluded', she had difficulty in getting her paper published and elsewhere the disease was repeatedly attributed to vitamin deficiency.

This classical description of disease, one of the most important contributions ever to tropical medicine, has been duly acknowledged with many honours bestowed upon Dr. Williams, who is happily still with us to write the Foreword of this book. Nevertheless, it was from this historic discovery that a disastrous series of events was due to stem; what I have elsewhere described as 'The Great Protein Fiasco',[13] and what may also be regarded as the Protein Myth. A myth is defined as 'a fictitious narrative, embodying some popular idea'. Here I am concerned to show how a (partly) fictitious narrative was built around a popular but only partly correct idea.

By the 1950s kwashiorkor had become a new and interesting diagnosis throughout the tropics and doctors were looking for cases to report from all over the world. WHO published a report on 'Kwashiorkor in Africa' and at conferences the term 'protein malnutrition' was being freely used. The surplus skim milk from the United States was a fortuitous answer to prolems of treatment. As the source of this dried up attention was turned to producing 'protein-rich food mixtures' from local vegetable sources. This soon became big business for manufacturer and scientist alike. Laboratory tests to detect protein deficiency early proliferated and amino acid supplementation was advocated. A special committee, the Protein Advisory Group of the United Nations, had been formed to advise on solving the protein 'problem' especially by promoting protein foods. Evidently the horse was not being whipped hard enough, for soon there were frantic cries to 'close the protein gap' and 'combat the impending protein crisis'.

Despite the firmness with which vested interests had become entrenched on this issue and the strength of the stranglehold which they had established, there had now and again been voices raised against this one-sided view. These concerned doubts about the high levels at which human protein requirements had been set (now lowered—see Chapter 5), the evidence from food balance sheets that showed energy rather than protein deficit on a national and community basis (see also Chapter 5) and, most important in the present context, the growing evidence that marasmus was much more common on a worldwide basis than kwashiorkor, with definite indications that it was rapidly replacing kwashiorkor even in the latter's few strongholds of Africa, the Caribbean and parts of South East Asia. As these voices began to get a hearing and further evidence accumulated in their support the short-sighted measures adopted to combat the 'protein problem' began to fail. What had been known to those close to the problem all along slowly became evident to even the most biased. Kwashiorkor and protein deficiency were a part, and that diminishing, of a whole spectrum of nutritional disorders of young children, with energy shortage predominating and in which the basic causes were socio-economic and not dietary.

It is not without significance that there was no mention of a 'protein crisis' at the recent world Food Conference in Rome. It should also be noted that the subject often recurs in this book but the various contributors speak with one voice against the emphasis that was for too long placed on protein shortage. Although, from the scientific point of view, present attitudes are to be welcomed the fact remains that untold harm has been done and the damage resulting to the cause of combating malnutrition is incalculable.

How did this situation come about? Much of the blame has to be placed on the United Nations Agencies concerned. These organizations are in a unique position to take a world view of problems, but they and their advisors failed conspicuously to understand the true nature of childhood malnutrition.

The Role of Nutrition in Degenerative Disorders

We live at a time in history when forces are not only becoming polarized as never before but when more of mankind are aware of what is happening. Conspicuous among these forces is the ever-widening gap between the haves and the have nots. Poverty and its frequent accompaniments of ignorance, disease, misery and hunger are well enough known but it is often unthinkingly assumed that affluence inevitably brings in its train knowledge, health, happiness and satiety. However, Nature does not seem to work on the principle that 'the more you have of a good thing the better *ad infinitum*'. Rather the secret of life lies in balance rather than lack or excess, comprise for the good of others as well as oneself, and adaptation to things as they are rather than wishful thinking for the unattainable.

It is easy to make the mistake of believing that malnutrition is a problem exclusive to the poor. Rather is it difficult to find a people anywhere in the world amongst whom malnutrition does not exist in one form or another. The dilemma is put rather cleverly in the following 'fable'.[14]

Once upon a time there was a very poor country where nobody had enough to eat, and the average expectation of life was 24 years. There was also a very rich country where everybody had plenty to eat, and the average expectation of life was 64 years. In the very rich country, people used to save up milk and butter and cream and eggs and send them to the very poor country where they were distributed, especially to the children who would otherwise have had none. In this way the expectation of life in the very poor country was raised from 24 to 27 years. Meanwhile the expectation of life in the very rich country was rising too and went up from 64 to 67 years, and everyone who did not die of cancer of the lung from smoking too many cigarettes died of coronary thrombosis. Then someone discovered that coronary thrombosis was due to eating and drinking too much milk and butter and cream and eggs in the very rich country. So they sent all these materials to the very poor country, so that the expectation of life in the very poor country might be raised high enough for them to start dying of coronary thrombosis so that they, too, could stop eating and drinking milk and butter and cream and eggs.

This is hardly the place to elaborate on the part played by diet in atherosclerosis and other degenerative disorders so common among the affluent. Epidemiological and public health aspects are fully covered in subsequent chapters (8, 9, 19 and 20). As the authors of these chapters make abundantly clear, the present-day problems of overnutrition and undernutrition are extremely complex and have in common the fact that many nutrition and non-nutritional factors play a part. In fact they are all merely symptomatic of a certain way of life. This is equally true of the marasmic infant in the overcrowded, unhygienic, poverty-ridden slum hut or of the middle-aged sedentary business executive in his spacious suburban villa. It also follows that diet is only part of the picture in both cases and that a complete change of life-style is necessary for both if they are to survive.

There is a great deal of hobby-horse riding at the present time, with the incrimination of single factors such as saturated fat, sugar, lack of fibre or softness of the water. The need is for a global approach to be made towards the investigation of the causes and adoption of measures for prevention of the degenerative disorders.

REFERENCES

1. McCollum, E. V. *A History of Nutrition,* Boston, Houghton Mifflin, 1957.
2. Pyke, M. *Food and Society,* London, John Murray, 1968.
3. Walters, A. H. *Ecology, Food and Civilization,* London, C. Knight, 1973.
4. Coale, A. J. *Sci. Amer.,* **231,** 40 (1974).
5. Albrink, M. J. Overnutrition and the Fat Cell. In *Duncan's Diseases of Metabolism* 6th edition, P. K. Bondy (Ed.), Philadelphia, W. B. Saunders, 1969.
6. Blegvad, O. *Amer. J. Opthal.,* **7,** 89 (1924).
7. Paton, D. and D. S. McLaren. *Amer. J. Opthalm.,* **50,** 568 (1960).
8. McLaren, D. S. *J. Trop. Pediat.,* **2,** 135 (1956).
9. Platt, B. S. *Fed. Proc. 17,* Part II, Suppl. No. 2, p. 8 (1958).
10. Davies, J. N. P. *Lancet,* **1,** 195 (1964).
11. Roe, D. A. *A Plague of Corn. The Social History of Pellagra,* Cornell University Press, Ithaca and London, 1973.
12. Mayer, J. *Nutr. Revs.,* **15,** 321 (1957).
13. McLaren, D. S. *Lancet,* **2,** 93 (1974).
14. Anon. *Lancet,* **1,** 635 (1956).

CHAPTER 4

Population and Food Supply

DONALD S. MCLAREN

There are few people who would not acknowledge that the rapid growth of world population in recent years, with the consequent strain placed upon food supplies, constitutes one of the major challenges to the survival of mankind at the present time.

Population control and family planning on the one hand, and the production and distribution of food on the other, each comprise vast areas of human endeavour lying largely outside the scope of the present work. A study of these closely related fields is made especially difficult by the host of factors at work, the rapidity with which changes are taking place, the inacurracy of many data, the great geographical differences that exist, and finally the important, but often imponderable, part played by politics.

With the requirements of the public health worker in mind, an attempt has been made to show how population and food supply interact, with some attention being given to possible future trends. The interaction is two-way; while population size influences food supply, an inadequacy of food has an effect on reproductive function.

In the Population—Food equation there is a distinct sequence with the production of food being a response to population needs. Consequently it appears logical to consider food in relation to previously established population needs.

POPULATION

There are qualitative as well as quantitative aspects to be considered. It is evident that at any time there is enough food to feed the population in existence at that time. The crucial questions concern how well the population will be fed at the time and what part food shortage will have played in mortality until that time. Assessment of the food situation in terms of nutrient requirements and food availability will be dealt with in Chapter 5.

The quantitative aspects of population in relation to food supply are generally well-known and agreed upon.[1] The world population is estimated to have been 250 million at the time of Christ. It has doubled since then, successively in 1600, 1800,

1930 and 1975 to top 4 billion some time during that last year. Low and high projections range between 5.5 and 7.0 billion for the year 2000. The greatest rates of population growth are occurring in the developing countries of Asia, Latin America and Africa (about 2.4 per cent per annum) compared with only 1 per cent for the developed countries. It is in the densely populated underdeveloped regions that per capita income is lowest. In relative terms on a global basis this means for example that Asia (minus Japan) has 54 per cent of the world's population and only 6.6 per cent of the wealth. Comparable figures for Africa are 9 per cent and 1.8 per cent, while for North America they are 6.2 per cent and 34.5 per cent respectively and for Western Europe 9.1 per cent and 25.6 per cent.

There is a prevailing air of pessimism about the achievements to date of population control programmes and this was expressed in the World Population Conference held in Bucharest in 1974. In developing countries dramatic reductions in birth rates have in general been confined to small and/or sophisticated countries like South Korea, Mauritius, Taiwan, Singapore. However, the effect of earlier mass abortions in Japan and evident success in China must not be ignored. In India 10 million sterilizations and over 2 million IUD insertions have failed to have a major impact, probably because the campaign has not been accompanied by social and economic development that could provide the necessary motivation for limitation of family size. In other words, so long as 6.5 children have to be born to ensure a 95 per cent chance of having the insurance of a son to look after one in old age voluntary limitation of family size will not occur. Whether people in fact think about procreation in this way is doubtful but it has been shown that with increase in life expectancy the birth rate falls steadily.

From the nutritional point of view there is not only a great difference between the average person in a developed and in a developing country, but also between the urban and the rural dweller in the same region. In the developed countries the urban dweller is more sedentary and more likely to suffer from overnutrition. In developing countries the rush to the cities, which has been picturesquely termed the 'urban avalanche',[2] carries special problems of susceptibility to malnutrition and the infections which often predispose, especially among the very young. Everywhere the urbanization trends are increasing but at a greater rate in the developing regions. It has been estimated[3] that urban populations on the average are increasing at twice the rate of the general world population. However, the rate of increase is more than three times greater in the cities of the developing countries than it is in those of the developed countries. This, of course, means relatively more children in the future in the cities of the developing countries and an even greater problem of malnutrition there (Chapter 8).

National population policy has emerged into the open only recently as the overriding determinant of trends in the immediate future. Many nations in the Bucharest Conference demanded that the affluent West redistribute its wealth rather than advocating birth control for others. China espoused this cause, called the Western proposal for curbing population growth an imperialist plot; and omitted reference to their own massive birth-control programme. Brazil, with 100 million, now supports population growth, ostensibly to develop its vast land mass, while neighbouring Argentina thinks twice about its own policy to make birth control readily available. Most African states have no policy on population. The most dramatic recent reductions in birth rate have come about in those countries where there has been no population policy as such but where an educated public has been enabled to choose voluntary control through liberalized laws on abortion and moral attitudes; in the United States and the United Kingdom for example. By contrast, it has been estimated by the International Planned Parenthood Federation that two-thirds of the world's population, admittedly all in developing countries, has no knowledge of any effective method of contraception.

FOOD SUPPLY

1. Food production

To produce food there are only four basic requirements: (i) the living organism, whether seed or animal, (ii) a medium for it to grow in, usually soil but often water, (iii) suitable climatic conditions, and finally (iv) man to cultivate it. The sciences of agriculture and food are concerned with these matters and the way in which they have been influenced by man. The degree of sophistication of man's influence on each of these elements varies greatly. In the past, advances have mainly been confined to improvement in methods of cultivation and to some extent of the medium, by fertilizers for example, but only in recent years, with our knowledge of genetics, have seeds and animals been improved and new, unconventional sources of nutriment, such as those discussed in Chapter 14, been sought. Very little has been done to control climate, and wind, rain, heat and cold still have the final say as to whether or not the world will be short of food. Recent evidence suggests that cooling of the polar ice caps, now occurring, creates droughts, early frosts and heavy rains and that the world may be entering a period of disastrous weather.

What food production will be at any particular time or place is detemined by a variety of forces that operate on these basic elements mentioned above and which arise out of the complexities of the societies into which man has organized himself. These forces may be broadly categorized as (i) political (national, international), (ii) cultural and (iii) economic. Not only are they themselves closely interrelated but their influence on the elements of food production is highly complex.

2. Food distribution

These same forces arising out of human society can be seen at work in determining the distribution of food once it has been produced. In considering food distribution we are interested in the patterns of growth and of consumption of foodstuffs in and within different communities, their trends, past, present and future and the way in which political, cultural and economic factors influence them. Movements of food, whether under the influence of trade or aid between countries and stockpiling of food are recognized to be important elements in food distribution. Maldistribution within the family, with young children being especially vulnerable, is a phenomenon well-documented by medical and social scientists but often ignored by economists.

In this connection a warning has to be sounded against the misuse of statistics recently evident at the World Food Conference in Rome and elsewhere. It is stated that about 10 million people will probably die of starvation this year, mostly children under the age of 5 years old. This figure can be accounted for by the estimates made by Bengoa[4] of about 100 million malnourished children in the world at any one time, resulting in at least 10 per cent deaths in one year. This problem is separate from that of population and food shortage, it is steadily increasing all the time, does not depend on food shortage simply, but is related to poverty, ignorance and disease.[5]

With these introductory remarks a number of topics will be touched upon to illustrate the forces at work in the present situation and the prospect for the immediate future.

It is important to realize that the world food situation has taken a sudden and serious turn for the worse in the last year or two. In 1969 the statement was made[6] 'There has been no major famine since the Bengal famine of 1948. There is no known previous famine-free period of equal length. The present is no time for despair'. In the subsequent five years the estimated world population has passed 4 billion, more rapidly than most predictions suggested, the Sahelian famine persists across Africa for the second year and mass starvation threatens most of Bangladesh and parts of India. In the same period the vast reserves of grain in the United States have been used up. Some 8–9 million tons of food were sent in several years to India in the 1960s to avert famine there. It is estimated that throughout the world there is no more than three weeks' supply of grain stored away, the lowest level for 20 years and about one-fifth of the level in the 1960s. In the United States the level is the lowest for forty years. The United States has been supplying about 40 per cent of the world's wheat export, 50 per cent of the animal feed grains, and is the biggest exporter of rice. But in 1974 all of these and maize and soya beans were down because of droughts earlier in the year. Ninety per cent of U.S. grain exports is controlled by seven giant grain companies. The Secretary of Agriculture was reported as saying recently that the United States had about $1000 million for food relief in the current year. About $900 million were spent in 1973 at a time when the U.S. government owned no food and had to go into the market and buy it. Until these last years the U.S. direct food aid programme had been running between $1.5 and 2.0 billion annually since its inception. Thus there has been an actual cut by between 30 and 50 per cent, taking no account of devaluation of the dollar or the sharp increase in food prices. However, now the trend is from aid to trade, grain prices are at record levels but even so exports are up from $8 billion to $21 billion over the past three years and even India is a net cash customer. It may be worthwhile to summarize the situation as Brown saw it in 1963 so that the contrast with the present (1974–5) may be better understood.[7] At that time grain output per capita was rising considerably in developed regions but fell in developing regions, and this trend, accentuating the gap between the well-off and the poor, has continued. Starchy food provided only 24 per cent of total energy intake in North

America but 74 per cent in Asia, while livestock produce ranged from only 4 per cent in Asia to 35 per cent in Oceania. These figures are similar today. All regions had raised grain yields per acre since before the 1939–45 war, most in North America to 927 kg and lowest in Africa at 318 kg. With the word population bound to increase at more or less the same rate it was recognized that there were two ways to achieve the necessary expansion of food output which had to be at a faster rate than ever before in history. These are expanding the cultivated area and increasing yields. Until 1950 output was increased mainly by expanding the cultivated area, from 1950 until the early 1960s four-fifths of the population increase resulted from increased yields.

Looking back from 1975 it is possible to see that increased yields were further attained through such measures as the 'green revolution' but that now a crucial turning point has been reached when this is not being maintained through the necessary inputs.

Two adverse factors have to be held largely responsible for the present very depressing situation. The first of these is the evident failure of the 'green revolution' to meet the most optimistic expectations. The new strains of wheat, rice and other crops have succeeded under optimal conditions but the necessary inputs, particularly water, fertilizer and mechanization, have not been sufficiently forthcoming. Moreover, the benefit has in general not reached down to the poorest who were most in need of it.

The second factor is the energy crisis, precipitated, at least in part, by the Middle East oil embargo and the consequent phenomenal inflation by which the oil-less developing countries have been hardest hit. As the effects of the energy crisis are increasingly felt in the West more and more restrictive measures are taken by governments to protect the home farmers, much of the value of whose produce is in terms of animal products, about ten times less efficient use of crops than direct human consumption. Furthermore there is gross overconsumption of food in countries like the United States. It has been computed that the amount of food being eaten by 210 million Americans could feed more than seven times that number of Asians on their average diet. The overriding influence of political forces can also be seen in attitudes towards food supply, as for population control. Governments have been reticent in admitting the existence and magnitude of famine among their populations. After the war over Bangladesh in 1971 the United States drastically reduced its aid in food and technicians to India, the inputs to sustain the progress made in the green revolution were not forthcoming and food production has seriously fallen. The non-participation of Russia in FAO, its massive purchases of grain from the United States, and its refusal to publish carryover figures make coordination of a world food bank virtually impossible.

NUTRITURE AND FERTILITY

One often hears the blame for the food shortage being laid on the people of the developing countries, and as 90 per cent of the predicted growth to the end of the century will take place in those countries this is perhaps fair comment, although apportioning blame is hardly anyone's prerogative. These largely undernourished people appear to be remarkably fertile but we know that severely malnourished animals are sterile. We have already seen how malnutrition in early life is the most important cause of the high rate of infant and young child mortality and in an indirect way appears to have the effect of keeping the birth rate high in an effort to obtain the security provided by surviving sons. What effect does malnutrition have directly on fertility?

Sex ratio of populations

In most affluent countries the F/M ratio (females per 1000 males) is above 1000 while in developing countries it is below 1000 (Table 1). India has one of the lowest at 941 and has fallen progressively by about 40 points in this century.[8] Most significant in relation to fertility is the F/M ratio during the child-bearing period. Throughout all ages during this period the ratio is higher in the U.K. and the U.S.A. than it is in India. This is probably due to the neglect of girls in such countries as India and is accentuated by a higher maternal mortality, much of which is related to malnutrition (Figure 1).

Table 1. Sex ratio of populations

Country	Sex Ratio
U.S.A.	1031
U.K.	1056
France	1050
Japan	1036
Philippines	983
Israel	943
Pakistan	900
Thailand	996
India	941

Source: U.N. Demographic Yearbook, 1965

Age of menarche

The onset of menarche appears to occur at constant weight rather than a constant age. This seems to be about 45 kg and appears to have held true over the past century.[9] It therefore occurs earlier in better nourished populations, also earlier in obese girls. In anorexia nervosa amenorrhoea sets in when the weight drops below this threshold. The depressing effect on fertility will be definite but probably not great.

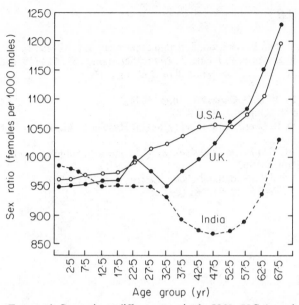

FIGURE 1. Sex ratio at different ages in the U.K., U.S.A. and India. Sources: U.N. Demographic Yearbook, 1965 and Census of India, 1963, Paper No. 2

Foetal wastage

Abortions, miscarriages and stillbirths are all said to be considerably higher in populations subject to undernutrition but there are few well-conducted comparative studies.

Lactation

The relative infertility associated with successful lactation is generally recognized. Prolonged breast-feeding, still practised in rural areas of developing countries, although breaking down under the influence of urbanization, is much to be encouraged as a constraint on fertility where more effective measures are not practised fully for a variety of reasons. It is probable that nursing would prolong amenorrhoea more effectively in a population where the mean weight is close to the critical level of 45 kg, because of the severe energy drain of pregnancy and lactation, than in a well-nourished group. This point does not seem to have been investigated.

That undernutrition does lower the fertility of a population is suggested by comparisons of fertility rates for undernourished communities at the present time and similar data for communities from the past who were well-nourished but before family planning was widely adopted. The rate, for example, is nearly 100 per cent greater for French Canada in the early 18th century than for present-day India.

42

REFERENCES

1. Freedman, R. and B. Berelson. *Scientific American,* **231,** 31 (1974).
2. Jelliffe, D. B. and E. F. P. Jelliffe. *J. Amer. Diet. Assoc.,* **57,** 114 (1970).
3. Notenstein, F. W. in *Overcoming World Hunger,* Hardin, C. M. (Ed.), Prentice–Hall, N.J., 1969, p. 9.
4. Bengoa, J. M. *W.H.O. Chronicle,* **28,** 3 (1974).
5. McLaren, D. S. *Lancet,* **2,** 93 (1974).
6. Paarlberg, D. In *Overcoming World Hunger,* Hardin, C. M. (Ed.), Prentice–Hall, N.J., 1969, p. 41.
7. Brown, L. R. *Man, Land and Food,* U.S. Department of Agriculture, Economic Research Service, 1963.
8. Gopalan, C. and A. Nadamuni Naidu. *Lancet,* **2,** 1077 (1972).
9. Frische, R. E. *Pediatrics,* **50,** 445 (1972).

CHAPTER 5

Assessment of Food and Nutrition Situation

P. V. SUKHATME

A simple method of assessing the food and nutrition situation is to compare the gross availability of food expressed as energy and nutrient supply per capita with the corresponding requirements. Gross availability is derived by what is called the food balance sheet method. Given the production P of each of the several foods grown in the country, the stocks S_1 and S_2 in the beginning and end of the year, the imports I and exports E in the course of the year and the amounts spent on manufacturing inedible foods (M), waste (W), seed (S) and feed (F), the method is to calculate for each of the several foods the gross availability given by

$$P + S_1 + I - S_2 - E - M - W - S - F$$

Gross availability so calculated is then converted in terms of energy and nutrients using food composition tables and summed over all foods to give energy and nutrient supply per capita.

If food were distributed according to physiological needs, the method could tell us how far a country or community is in short supply. In practice, however, the rich take all that they need and more, and the poor only what they can afford. Consequently the method, humourously called the 'method of meaningless mean' by Miller, is of limited value, since a much larger proportion of the population than indicated by the overall gap between what is available and what is required fails to meet its energy and nutrient needs, i.e. is undernourished and malnourished. In this situation, the balance sheet method must be supplemented by data of dietary surveys to provide information on the distribution of intake among individuals. In this chapter, we shall describe how to evaluate such dietary data for energy and protein needs, starting with an account of the sources and limitations of the statistics of intake and requirements for energy and protein.

FOOD AND NUTRIENT INTAKE

Household dietary surveys provide the primary source of information on food consumption. Used in conjunction with the data on food composition, they give the statistics of nutrient intake.

There are two basic methods of collecting data on food consumption: (i) estimation by recall and (ii) measurement of food *as eaten*. In the recall method households are asked to estimate by recall the names, together with a description, of each of the various foods consumed at each meal (and between meals) together with their quantities. The information is noted in chronological order for each individual member of the household. In the second method, the food is required to be measured *as eaten* either by means of direct weighing and/or in terms of household measures like a cup or spoon. In using either method it is desirable that information on food consumption should be supplemented by weighing of raw ingredients and of the final products prepared for consumption from them.

A food consumption survey is a difficult undertaking. There are two principal difficulties. The first concerns the selection of the sample of households. If a statistically valid procedure of estimation is to be used the sample households should be randomly selected. However, experience shows that many of the households included in the sample do not like to take the trouble of systematically recording or weighing the quantities of foods they consume. The sample is thus reduced to those households which are willing to cooperate. The second difficulty concerns the measurement of food eaten. Households generally do not know the quantities of foods consumed by them in the course of the day. The difficulty is particularly great in the rural areas of the developing countries where people largely use the foods grown by them on their farms. Moreover, it is common experience that people have little idea of the units used in expressing quantities for statistical purposes. The method of weighing foods with the assistance of trained investigators helps to provide accurate information, but other biases may appear in the process. Thus, the very presence of an investigator may introduce what is known as the prestige bias, with households either consuming food in quantities which are considerably in excess of the normal or changing the pattern of their consumption in favour of the more expensive foods. This may particularly apply in the first few days. In any case, the normal course of life in households is disturbed, with a consequential effect on the representative character of the data, though the effect of this disturbance is likely to be mitigated as the investigator comes to know the households better, through the extension of the period of observation to a week or longer as necessary. Information about expenditure on different food items is somewhat easier to collect than information on quantities, but the method is applicable to purchased items only and, further, information of this kind is of limited use for assessing the food consumption levels.

The length of time for which information on food consumption should be recorded for each selected household presents a further difficulty. The shorter the length of time the greater is likely to be the willingness of households to cooperate. This consideration has led many studies to adopt a period of 1 day, usually the past 24 hours, for recording information on food consumption. On the other hand, the variation in consumption from day to day is so large that a single day's intake can hardly be taken to represent the usual intake of an individual. For this reason a period of 7 consecutive days of a week is used on the ground that 7 days usually constitute a cycle of eating and work. The International Biological Programme recommends a period of 3 consecutive days at least twice a year. The longer the period of observation, the greater is likely to be the stability of the estimated intake. But it is wrong to assume that intra-individual variation can be reduced in this way to a point where it can be assumed to be negligible. Analysis of available data shows that within individuals variation remains large, even when the length of time is as great as a week and the resulting variation is comparable in magnitude to the estimated true variance between individuals. It is as important in food consumption surveys to estimate accurately the intra-individual variation as to estimate inter-individual variation if the information is to serve the purpose of assessing the nutritional status of the individuals. On the other hand, collection of information on consumption for all items and for all members of a household every day for a whole week, whether by means of recall or weighing methods, however desirable, may make far greater demands on the time of the households than they can afford and thus jeopardize the success of the survey altogether, particularly if surveys have to be conducted over several years. Because of their increased costs, such household surveys are usually conducted on small samples and mostly confined to poor segments of the population residing in small areas. Over a period of years, however, such surveys may provide a valuable record for a continuing evaluation of the nutritional status of the population.

Altogether, it is exceedingly difficult to collect accurate data on food consumption through household surveys. The difficulty is increased when we come to convert the foods consumed into energy and nutrient intakes. An accurate way of determining nutrient content is to analyse duplicate portions of everything eaten, but this is a costly method and not always practicable in developing countries. An alternative method is to use food composition tables. However, the food tables used should be applicable to the situation under study. Weighing of raw ingredients selected for cooking and of the final products prepared for consumption can be of great help in this but it is not easy to get the households to carry out this weighing as part of the survey routine. Yet another alternative is to use information on average recipes which correspond with those of foods consumed in the households. Such average recipes and their analyses are available in the publications issued by national organizations. However, variation in foods cooked and eaten in different households is so large that the use of average recipes to calculate nutrient content is known to introduce appreciable errors in estimating individual intakes. As food tables become more and more comprehensive to include analysis of a larger and larger number of different foods, and with increasing care given to the description of food eaten in the household, errors in the use of food tables are expected to be reduced. But there is little doubt that, at present, in most of the developing countries these errors can be great.

The need to analyse diets as eaten to determine protein quality is even more critical but is again impracticable. Of necessity we have to be guided by analyses of typical diets to provide factors for converting dietary protein into their equivalents as egg or milk protein, in terms of which protein needs are worked out. The broad guiding principles are that diets of the developing countries have a protein value of 70–80 per cent relative to egg and those of the developed countries a value of 80–90 per cent.

..e, the accuracy of observation on intake depends upon many fac-
..uich it is usually difficult to exercise adequate control. Unlike
..ts such as height and weight, nutrient intake involves measuring a large
. foods eaten in the course of the day and determining their nutrient con-
.ch height and weight, techniques of acceptable accuracy are available to
v.   .t assumptions that errors of measurement are negligible. Such an assumption, is however, not warranted in the case of nutrient intake. When to this we add
the difficulty that intake may vary from day to day in the same individual with variation often equal to that between individuals, the errors in data become large and
their interpretation difficult. It is clearly desirable to provide for pilot surveys before
embarking on a household diet survey, and it is also desirable that continuous
supervision and checking should be made a part of the survey procedures in order to
keep the errors under control.

Table 1. Recommended intakes of Nutrients

Age	Body weight	Energy		Protein	Vitamin A	Vitamin D
	kilo-grams	kilo-calories	mega-joules	grams	micro-grams	micro-grams
Children						
<1	7.3	820	3.4	14	300	10.0
1–3	13.4	1 360	5.7	16	250	10.0
4–6	20.2	1 830	7.6	20	300	10.0
7–9	28.1	2 190	9.2	25	400	2.5
Male adolescents						
10–12	36.9	2 600	10.9	30	575	2.5
13–15	51.3	2 900	12.1	37	725	2.5
16–19	62.9	3 070	12.8	38	750	2.5
Female adolescents						
10–12	38.0	2 350	9.8	29	575	2.5
13–15	49.9	2 490	10.4	31	725	2.5
16–19	54.4	2 310	9.7	30	750	2.5
Adult man (moderately active)	65.0	3 000	12.6	37	750	2.5
Adult woman (moderately active)	55.0	2 200	9.2	29	750	2.5
Pregnancy (later half)		+350	+1.5	38	750	10.0
Lactation (first 6 months)		+550	+2.3	46	1 200	10.0

[1] For women whose iron intake throughout life has been at the level recommended in this table, the daily intake of women of childbearing age. For women whose iron status is not satisfactory at the beginning of pregnancy, the not be met without supplementation.

NUTRIENT REQUIREMENTS

The primary sources of information for statistics of energy and nutrient requirements are FAO/WHO reports (Table 1). National reports are also available in the case of a few countries. Estimates of the requirements for energy and nutrients given in the international reports are prepared by Expert Committees on Nutrition, convened by FAO/WHO, and are based on a review of published research data of the past 50 years. The first comprehensive review, containing recommendations for energy, appeared in 1957 (FAO/WHO);[1] the second publication appeared in 1965,[2] while the latest appeared in 1973.[3] In the 1973 report the words 'calorie needs' are substituted by 'energy needs' and estimates are given in terms both of kilo calories as well as in joules. In this chapter we shall use the words 'energy' and 'calories' interchangeably.

Thiamine	Ribo-flavine	Niacin	Folic acid	Vitamin B_{12}	Ascorbic Acid	Calcium	Iron
milli-grams	milli-grams	milli-grams	micro-grams	micro-grams	milli-grams	grams	milli-grams
0.3	0.5	5.4	60	0.3	20	0.5–0.6	5–10
0.5	0.8	9.0	100	0.9	20	0.4–0.5	5–10
0.7	1.1	12.1	100	1.5	20	0.4–0.5	5–10
0.9	1.3	14.5	100	1.5	20	0.4–0.5	5–10
1.0	1.6	17.2	100	2.0	20	0.6–0.7	5–10
1.2	1.7	19.1	200	2.0	30	0.6–0.7	9–18
1.2	1.8	20.3	200	2.0	30	0.5–0.6	5–9
0.9	1.4	15.5	100	2.0	20	0.6–0.7	5–10
1.0	1.5	16.4	200	2.0	30	0.6–0.7	12–24
0.9	1.4	15.2	200	2.0	30	0.5–0.6	14–28
1.2	1.8	19.8	200	2.0	30	0.4–0.5	5–9
0.9	1.3	14.5	200	2.0	30	0.4–0.5	14–28
+0.1	+0.2	+2.3	400	3.0	30	1.0–1.2	(1)
+0.2	+0.4	+3.7	300	2.5	30	1.0–1.2	(1)

iron during pregnancy and lactation should be the same as that recommended for nonpregnant, nonlactating requirement is increased, and in the extreme situation of women with no iron stores, the requirement can probably

Energy and protein needs are defined separately for each of the several age and sex groups. Calorie needs are based on measurement of energy intake and/or expenditure in healthy active subjects. Needs for protein represent amounts observed to ensure a satisfactory rate of growth of children and to maintain body weight and nitrogen equilibrium in healthy adults. Both energy and protein needs are simply expressed as rates per kilogram of body weight in the latest FAO/WHO report. Used in conjunction with information on reference body weight and activity, the rates provide the means for calculating the requirements of individuals for satisfactory growth and maintenance of health.

For energy, the requirements are defined as average per capita needs of specified age and sex groups. It is recognized that individuals within a group may need energy at a rate which may be above or below the recommended average. But the principal concern is with establishing averages and not with variation within age and sex groups. Excessive intake is as bad as inadequate intake, which is the reason why energy needs are stated that way. The magnitude of individual variability is placed at 15 per cent.

Unlike energy, requirements for protein are based on the consideration of an individual as well as of the group. The earlier report on protein requirements by FAO/WHO (1965) defined the needs at three levels, namely, average, average + 20 per cent and average − 20 per cent. The upper level is placed at a distance of twice the standard deviation above the average need and is expected to cover the requirements of all but a small proportion of the population. In other words, the probability that a healthy individual will have a requirement exceeding the upper level will be very small. The lower level is placed at twice the standard deviation below the average and represents the level below which protein deficiency may be expected to occur in all but a few individuals. In other words, the probability that a healthy individual will have a protein need below the lower level will be very small. The magnitude of individual variability was placed at 10 per cent.

The 1973 report has given up the practice of defining protein needs at three levels. Instead, the requirements are now defined at the upper level only, namely, average + twice the standard deviation $(m + 2\sigma)$. The estimate of σ has been revised upwards to 15 per cent of the mean. The requirement so defined was previously called the recommended intake and is now called the 'safe level of intake'. To facilitate interpretation of the term, a principle is stated in the report to the effect that as the intake falls below the safe level, the risk of dietary deficiency increases. It is emphasized that for this reason an individual should aim to eat at or above the level represented by $m + 2\sigma$.

By way of example, Table 2 gives the new recommended levels for energy and protein as they apply to the pre-school child and adult living in India. Protein requirements are shown in terms of egg as well as dietary protein. Available data show that net protein utilization (n.p.u.) of the average cereal/pulse diet relative to egg is approximately two-thirds in the case of children and 90 per cent in the case of adults. However, we shall ignore this difference and assume a uniform value of two-thirds for n.p.u. The recommended levels of dietary protein thus calculated will slightly overestimate adult need but will be on the safe side. They are shown in the table. It will be seen that the cereal/pulse diet, on average, will have to provide 48 g of dietary protein to meet the recommended adult requirement and about 22–23 g to meet the requirement of a child aged 1–3 years.

Table 2. Recommended levels of nutrient intake for pre-school child and adult in India (FAO/WHO, 1973)

Age (years)	Weight (kg)	Energy/kg Kcal	Energy/kg MJ	Total energy Kcal	Total energy MJ	Protein as egg (g/kg)	Total protein as egg (g)	Protein/ energy concentration (%)	Dietary protein of n.p.u. relative to egg = 67 (g)
1–3	12	100	0.42	1200	5.0	1.25	15	5.0	22.5
Adult	55	46	0.19	2550	10.63	0.57	32	5.0	48.0

Three points need to be made about the statement on requirements. Recommended levels of protein for adults are much lower than those previously used. In part this is due to the protein quality of diet relative to egg being higher in adults than previously assumed. Clearly, protein needs are much lower compared to what people eat in rich countries. The explanation appears to be that people with high and rising incomes must find it difficult not to eat more, especially tasty animal foods, when they can afford to do so.

The second point concerns the belief that a child needs much more protein relative to his energy needs compared to an adult. This is, however, not borne out on current evidence. The table shows that if a diet has 5 per cent of its energy from good-quality protein such as in egg, the individuals need for protein will be met regardless of whether the individual is a pre-school child or an adult man, provided the individual eats enough to meet his energy needs. It nevertheless is true that the dietary protein is less efficiently utilized by a child than by an adult so that relative to energy a child will undoubtedly need more dietary protein than an adult. However, as long as a diet has an equivalent of 5 per cent of its energy from good quality protein such as in egg, the child's needs will usually be met, infants excepted. Even human milk contains only 6–7 per cent of energy from protein and is an ideal infant food.

The third point is that the requirements for protein are valid only when energy needs are met. If this is not ensured, the body will use protein to meet its needs of energy.

At this stage, we may pause and think over the interpretation to be placed on the meaning of recommended intake. Defined as the average plus twice the standard deviation of individual requirement (i.e. $m + 2\sigma$), it represents a level at the upper end of the distribution of individual's requirement and means that most individuals will have their requirements less than $m + 2\sigma$. It follows that an individual eating below $m + 2\sigma$ might not necessarily be malnourished, but may run the risk of developing protein deficiency. In practice this is unlikely since requirement is not constant in an individual; but varies over time. Available evidence shows that by far the greater contribution to the variation of an individual's requirement is made by variation in requirement over time in the same individual (σw) and not by the intrinsic differences between individuals (σb). The variation over time in the same individual is called intra-individual variability and the intrinsic variation between individuals of the same age-sex group is called the inter-individual variability. The two are related as $\sigma^2 = \sigma^2 b + \sigma_w^2$.

It might be thought that by averaging the daily requirement over a longer period like three days or five, intra variance relative to variance of individual requirement can be reduced to a point where it can be considered as negligible. The evidence available does not support this expectation. Rather, it shows that requirement is distributed over time with stationary variance. The precise manner in which requirement for any day is regulated is not known, but the cyclical character of requirement is evident with output increasing sharply over one or two days and diminishing gradually over four to eight day intervals. This pattern is found in all healthy men. Statistical analysis of this pattern confirms the stationary character of the variance[4]. This means that the daily requirement of an individual in health will vary around his average requirement most of the time within critical limits set by the value of the intra-individual standard deviation and the chosen level of significances. If we should adopt 0.5 per cent level of significance and further assume that $\sigma_b^2 = \sigma_w^2$, then the critical limits based thereon can be shown to be approximately $m - 2\sigma$ and $m + 2\sigma$. It follows that we will rarely go wrong in classifying an individual as protein deficient when the intake falls below the lower limit of $m - 2\sigma$.

To sum up, while we should counsel individuals to eat at levels approaching $m + 2\sigma$, the appropriate cut off point to adopt for purposes of estimating the incidence of protein deficiency in the community will be $m - 2\sigma$. Likewise, while counselling individuals to avoid excessive or inadequate energy intake, we cannot regard him as undernourished (or overnourished) unless intake was so low (or so high) as to be outside the critical limits set by the intra-variation over time in healthy individuals. A student of public health has always a two fold task in keeping under review the nutrition situation in the community, (a) to counsel individuals approaching him on the desired level of intake and (b) to assess nutrition in the community. It is important that he should clearly distinguish between the two situations, one requiring the use of recommended intake and the other calling for $m - 2\sigma$ as the cut off point to estimate the incidence of protein deficiency in the community.

NUTRITIONAL STATUS

We are now in a position to evaluate the dietary data to assess the nutritional status of the community. This can be done by comparing the energy and protein intakes with the respective requirements. Such a comparison at the macro-level is given in Table 3, for India. It will be seen that the energy supply falls short of needs by a small margin, but that there is no protein gap at the national level. Far from any gap there is an excess to the tune of 50 per cent. We must conclude that unless protein intake is very unevenly distributed, it must be rare to find that protein deficiency will occur as a result of low protein intake.

Table 3. Energy and protein supply compared with respective requirements. (Macro-comparison on per capita basis)

Year	Energy			Protein (g)			
	Supply	Require-ment	% gap	Supply	Require-ment	Recom-mended	% Supply require-ment
1971	Kcal 2000	2200	10	50	30	36	166
	MJ 8.36	9.2					

Yet protein deficiency does occur. This is confirmed by the data of numerous clinical nutrition surveys which show that an appreciable proportion of children suffer from states of protein malnutrition ranging from retardation in growth to signs of severe protein deficiency such as nutritional oedema and reduced serum albumin. If protein malnutrition does occur and is widespread it must be due either to abnormal losses such as occur during infections or to low energy intake. It would thus appear that protein malnutrition is the indirect result of low energy intake. The deficit is small but its significance in the context of protein malnutrition cannot be overstressed. Unless a diet provides the energy cost of synthesizing and retaining protein a person must lose protein.

Ordinarily, in a healthy active population with each person meeting his requirement of protein, most people can be expected to have their protein intake per nutrition unit higher than the critical limit given by $m - 2\sigma$. It follows that in any observed distribution the proportion of individuals with intake per nutrition unit below 20 g can be taken to provide an upper limit to the estimate of the proportion of individuals with diets inadequate in protein. By way of example, we have given in Table 4 the distribution of households in Maharashtra, India, by protein intake per nutrition unit. It will be seen that only about 5 per cent of the nutrition units have protein intake below the critical limit. The data in Table 3 thus confirm the expectation that the incidence of simple protein deficiency in the population is small. However, the evaluation of data in this way does not bring out the role of energy in causing protein deficiency. This is brought out by classifying intake data according as diets are deficient or not in energy, protein or both as in Table 5. The dividing lines in this table are placed at critical limits for energy and protein. It will be seen that individual units that are protein-deficient are also energy-deficient and that when energy needs are met protein needs are also met. In other words, the concentration and quality of protein in the diets as eaten in Maharashtra (India) are more than adequate to meet protein needs. However, even this way of evaluating diets

Table 4. Distribution of households by protein intake per nutrition unit in Maharashtra (in terms of egg protein g per day)

	1971	
	Urban %	Rural %
0–5	—	—
5–10	—	—
10–15	0.8	0.5
15–20	1.6	3.5
20–25	8.0	6.0
25–30	16.0	15.4
30–35	19.6	14.9
35–40	16.2	15.2
40–45	12.0	10.5
45–50	8.4	9.3
50–55	6.2	7.0
55–60	4.6	5.4
60–65	2.6	3.7
65–70	1.8	2.8
70–75	0.8	2.3
75–80	0.4	0.7
80–85	0.2	1.2
85–90	0.4	0.5
90–95	—	—
95–100	0.2	0.2
100 and over	0.2	0.9
	100.0	100.0
N	500	429
$\bar{u}$	38.5	41.5
S.D.	14.3	15.8
% C.V.	38	38
% Incidence[a]	5	6

Source: National Sample Survey of India, Round 26, July 1971 to June 1972.

[a] Calculated from original values.

does not explain in full the discrepancy between the incidence of simple protein deficiency as evaluated from the data and as observed in clinical nutrition surveys. For this we must turn to the known fact that on any given level of protein intake the nitrogen balance is determined by the energy intake. In particular it has been observed that when the energy intake falls short of the energy needs for maintenance of body heat (Cm) protein in the diet is partially diverted to meet the energy needs, thereby causing protein deficiency. Calculations show that this is also the value of the critical limit for energy intake and represents the cost of synthesizing and retaining protein. This interrelationship of energy and protein intake is well brought out in Table 5. It shows that some 35 per cent of the nutrition units fail to meet the energy cost of synthesizing and retaining protein. Clearly the limiting factor in the Indian diets is not protein but energy to metabolize the protein people actually do eat. In effect protein malnutrition is the indirect result of poverty, as can

Table 5. Classification of households in Maharashtra according to whether the diets are deficient (D) or not (N) in energy and protein.

	Urban			Rural		
	PD	NPD	Sub-total	PD	NPD	Sub-total
CD	5	32	37	4	30	34
NCD	0	63	63	0	66	66
Sub-total	5	95	100	4	96	100

Source: National Sample Survey of India, Round 26.

be seen from Table 6. As income increases the energy intake also increases. Likewise, the level and quality of protein intake are also influenced by rising incomes. However, unlike energy the level of protein intake for the lowest income class is seen to be already adequate to meet man's needs. While it is common knowledge that malnutrition is precipitated by a number of factors (Chapter 7) the data leave little doubt that it is primarily caused by the lack of purchasing capacity of the masses and all that that stands for in terms of the capacity to buy health services, including adequate sanitation, personal hygiene, etc. In the ultimate analysis, justification and effectiveness of a nutrition programme must be judged by the ability of the programme to improve the incomes of the masses and not by humanitarian considerations to which appeal is often made in prevailing upon the developing countries to institute such programmes.

It needs to be added that in two respects the method of evaluating the nutritional status from dietary data indicated in this chapter differs from the method commonly adopted. First, we have taken into account the interrelationship of protein with the rest of the diet. Second, we have refrained from assuming that intra-individual variability is zero as this is not supported by experimental data. How deviations from these assumptions may lead to oversimplistic models and gross exaggeration of the dimensions of the problem is seen in the quotation below:[5]

I well remember the occasion when that distinguished statistician Sir Arthur Bowley, noting that the mean level of calories consumed by the British population in the Spartan period of the early post-war years coincided almost exactly with the accepted calorie requirements concluded (to the consternation of officials in the Ministry concerned) that some 50 per cent of the population must be undernourished. His argument was that if intake x, and requirement y are each normally distributed with the same mean then the difference can be considered to be normally distributed around zero with a given standard

Table 6. Daily per capita energy and protein supply by expenditure level, Maharashtra State, India, 1971

Item		18	18–24	24–34	34–44	44–54	54–64	64–74	74 plus	Average
					Monthly per capita expenditure in Rupees					
					Urban					
Total energy	Kcal	1380	1430	1620	1870	2060	2210	2210	2760[a]	2080
	MJ	5.77	5.98	6.77	7.82	8.61	9.24	9.24	11.54	8.69
Total proteins (g)		42	42	49	56	60	64	66	80	61
Animal proteins (g)		1.3	2.2	5.1	5.5	6.6	8.2	10.4	14.2	7.9
Number of households		11	27	94	90	73	56	38	111	500
					Rural					
Total energy	Kcal	1360	1530	1850	2330	2480	2890	3060	3490	2160
	MJ	5.68	6.40	7.73	9.74	10.37	12.08	12.79	14.59	9.03
Total proteins (g)		40	45	56	70	75	87	89	106	65
Animal proteins (g)		3.6	4.0	5.3	7.5	8.8	10.2	10.6	15.4	7.1
Number of households		27	67	126	78	56	24	19	29	426

(Source: National Sample Survey of India, Round 26.

[a] These values are unduly high partly due to the exclusion from the household size of guests and labourers taking meals.

deviation. It followed that the probability of y exceeding x or that a person is undernourished is $\frac{1}{2}$.

The suggestion that half the people of Great Britain were either losing body weight or were forced to reduce their physical activity for want of adequate food or both would always have serious policy implications, which no government would accept without having the factual data to support them. There is nothing surprising, therefore, if the officials of the Ministry concerned were taken aback by the assessment made by Bowley and thought fit to reject it. This was, however, 50 years ago when the concept of requirement had hardly developed to a point to understand its full implications; but to adopt the same method today for assessing the incidence in the developing countries, when it was discarded as inapplicable to the conditions in Great Britain, clearly brings an element of political nutrition which ought to be kept out of all objective assessments.

REFERENCES

1. FAO *Calorie Requirements* (Nutritional Studies No. 15), Rome, 1957.
1a. *Handbook of Human Nutritional Requirements 1974*, WHO Monograph Series No. 61, World Health Organisation, Geneva.
2. FAO/WHO *Protein Requirements*. Nutrition Meeting Report Series No. 37, FAO, Rome, 1965.
3. FAO/WHO *Requirements for Protein and Energy,* No. 522, Geneva, 1973.
4. Sukhatme, P. V. The Protein Problem: Its Size and Nature, *J. Roy. Statist. Soc.,* A. **137,** part 2, 166 (1974).
5. Wright, N. C. Book Review 'Feeding India's Growing Millions', *Population Studies,* **19,** 201 (1965).

CHAPTER 6

Assessment of Nutritional Status in the Community

ABDALLAH A. KANAWATI

Over the years many different approaches and methods have been used to assess human and sometimes animal growth and nutriture. For example, by pinching the skin to estimate the fullness of the subcutaneous fat stores, or by weighing the subject and comparing the result with the mean of normal subjects of similar age or with a known standard of that specific age. Systemic nutriture assessment as complete as it is now was developed only when some specific medical and biochemical tests became available. Anthropometry was probably first applied to nutrition when Liharzik[1] produced the first tables of child weight and height in mid-19th century Vienna.

Since 1932 the problem of assessment of the nutritional status has attracted attention internationally. At that date the Health Organization of the League of Nations called for a meeting in Berlin to discuss the baselines for clinical and physical examination applied for assessment of the individual's nutriture. The first Joint FAO/WHO Expert Committee on Nutrition (1949) indicated the need for nutritional assessment, including dietary assessment, for planning national nutrition policies. In the same year FAO published a booklet entitled *Dietary Surveys; Their Technique and Interpretation*. Recently the Joint Committee (1963) published a manual on *Medical Assessment of the Nutritional Status*[2] which was revised three years later.[3]

On a national basis The Inter-departmental Committee on Nutrition for National Defense (later Development) (ICNND) of the United States of America published in 1957 its first manual for a complete survey, and this body has carried out rather detailed surveys along these lines in many developing countries. More recently a 10-State survey and follow-up in the United States were completed (Chapter 31). It is generally agreed that none of these manuals and methods is perfect and that there is a great need for further investigation and revision.

Assessing the nutritional status of a community involves two constituent elements; man's needs and food intake. For normal nutritional status it is agreed that these two elements should be balanced and that both extremes of under- and overnutrition are considered abnormal. To complete the picture another complementary element has to be studied, namely the environmental, social and cultural factors that are involved in balancing the other elements (see Chapter 1). In other words, a total approach should be made in order to know who is short of what, by how much, and why?

Assessment of nutritional status is now being accepted as the first step in planning and programming nutritional activities (see Chapter 13). It should be a continuous process aimed at evaluating and extending such activities to the most needy communities whenever resources will permit.

Certain important problems affect the assessment process. The objectives of a study are sometimes not made sufficiently clear to be able to answer the planners and the decision-makers. Most studies have concentrated on the nature and scope of the problem and less attention has been directed to the root causes. There is often lack of trained personnel and financial resources. Instruments, methodology and clinical definitions are often not fully standardized. The studied sample is sometimes small and may not be representative of the whole population. Such studies are expensive and time-consuming, and by the time the data are collected, tabulated and analysed conditions are likely to have changed. Last but not least, normal nutritional status itself has not been fully defined, and whether optimum nutriture should be recognized by size of the adult, by rate of growth, by length of life or by resistance to infection is still uncertain.

Causal analysis of the nutritional status of a community depends on various kinds of information (see Table 1). Each kind has its own shortcomings, but taken together they are capable of presenting a reasonable and reliable picture. Background data of a general nature include age, sex, ethnic group and religion. Socio-economic data and geographic distribution of the population are usually collected from previously available sources and do not fall within the scope of a cross-sectional nutrition survey. They are of value in the selection of the area or population groups and for planning nutritional programmes. Methods that are especially related to assessment of the food situation are covered in Chapter 5. Those directly or indirectly concerned with human nutriture (Table 1, nos. 6–10) are discussed here.

VITAL STATISTICS

Malnutrition tends to be an accompaniment of poverty and ignorance and affects specific age groups, particularly young children. Data collection on mortality and morbidity of these vulnerable groups is a satisfactory method of gaining greater understanding of health problems in a given population.

Mortality data are in some areas unavailable and in others incomplete or unreliable. Frequently births and deaths, especially deaths in early life, are not registered. Death certificates if completed by a physician are usually done so without autopsy. In some countries death certification may not be an obligatory formality and in others it is occasionally completed by non-medical authorities. Nevertheless numerous data are available to show that mortality rates of certain age groups, e.g. infant mortality rate[4] and 1–4 year-old mortality rate were higher in developing countries than those in industrialized countries[5] (see Table 2). But none of these studies was precise. The only comprehensive study on childhood mortality and morbidity of which we are aware of is that published recently by Puffer and

Table 1. Information needed for assessment of nutritional status

Sources of Information	Nature of Information obtained	Nutritional implications
1. Agricultural data Food balance sheets	Gross estimates of agricultural production Agricultural methods Soil fertility Predominance of cash crops Overproduction of staples Food imports and exports	Approximate availability of food supplies to a population
2. Socio-economic data Information on marketing, distribution and storage	Purchasing power Distribution and storage of foodstuffs	Unequal distribution of available foods between the socio-economic groups in the community and within the family
3. Food consumption patterns Cultural–anthropological data	Lack of knowledge, erroneous beliefs and prejudices, indifference	
4. Dietary surveys	Food consumption	Low, excessive or unbalanced nutrient intake
5. Special studies on foods	Biological value of diets Presence of interfering factors (e.g. goitrogens) Effects of food processing	Special problems related to nutrient utilization
6. Vital and health statistics	Morbidity and mortality data	Extent of risk to community Identification of high risk groups
7. Anthropometric studies	Physical development	Effect of nutrition on physical development
8. Clinical nutritional surveys	Physical signs	Deviation from health due to malnutrition
9. Biochemical studies	Levels of nutrients, metabolites and other components of body tissues and fluids	Nutrient supplies in the body Impairment of biochemical function
10. Additional medical information	Prevalent disease patterns including infections and infestations	Interrelationships of state of nutrition and disease

From reference 2

Table 2. Mortality rates and ratios in comparison with Sweden in the same age in different countries

Country	Year	Post-Natal Mortality [a]		Infant Mortality [a]		1–2 yr Mortality [b]		1–4 yr Mortality [c]	
		rate 0/00 [a]	ratio	rate 0/00 [a]	ratio	rate 0/00 [b]	ratio	rate 0/00 [c]	ratio
Egypt	1970	96.8	42.1	116.3	10.5	107.0	118.9	39.3	98.3
Guatemala	1970	56.4	24.5	87.1	7.9	62.1	69.0	27.5	68.8
Chile	1970	53.1	23.1	86.5	7.8	24.3	27.0	3.2	8.0
Mexico	1971	39.9	17.4	63.3	5.7	30.9	34.3	10.9	27.3
India	1964	37.8	16.4	72.8	6.6	72.2	80.2	44.0	110.0
Philippines	1969	34.0	14.8	67.3	6.1	6.6	6.2	—	—
Thailand	1970	17.2	7.5	25.5	2.3	16.4	18.2	10.4	26.0
Italy	1970	9.2	4.0	29.6	2.7	3.2	3.6	1.1	2.8
Czechoslovakia	1970	6.5	2.8	22.1	2.0	2.0	2.2	1.0	2.5
Japan	1971	4.2	1.8	12.4	1.1	2.5	2.8	1.4	3.5
United Kingdom	1971	5.9	2.6	17.5	1.6	1.5	1.7	0.7	1.8
United States	1970	5.7	2.5	21.8	2.0	1.6	1.8	0.8	2.0
Sweden	1971	2.3	1.0	11.1	1.0	0.9	1.0	0.4	1.0

[a] Data from Ref. No. 2, p. 510
[b] Data from Ref. No. 3
[c] Data from Ref. No. 2, p. 564

Serrano[6], entitled 'The Inter America Investigation of Mortality in Childhood'. Data collected in 15 projects in American countries have shown that malnutrition was an underlying and associated cause in 11,913 cases of death in children under 5 years. Malnutrition was considered as an 'Underlying cause' when it was the direct cause of death and was evidenced by clinically severe malnutrition or a weight less than 60 per cent of normal for age. Malnutrition was an associated cause when it influenced the course of, but was not related to, the disease or condition directly causing death. The weight was 60–74 per cent for age (Figure 1). Mortality due to

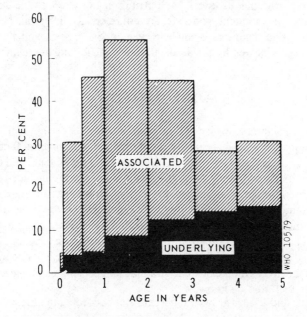

FIGURE 1. Percentage of deaths of children with nutrition as underlying or associated cause[6]

nutritional deficiencies was higher in the first year of life than in the age group 1–4 years. Mortality due to nutritional deficiencies was also higher in the rural areas than in cities. Kwashiorkor was the cause of death in 13.1 per cent of total nutritionally induced deaths, marasmus in 21.4 per cent and other non-identified forms in 65.4 per cent of the total cases. The mortality rate of kwashiorkor was highest in the second year of life and that of marasmus highest in the second and third month of life, after which it gradually declined. Therefore the mortality rate of the 2–5 month age group may not be a precise index of thiamine deficiency as indicated by Aykroyd and Krishnan[7] particularly in places where diarrhoea, pneumonia and marasmus are also prevalent. The second year[4] and the 1–4 years[8] mortality rates were also suggested as public health indices of protein–energy malnutrition. Corresponding rates in North America and European countries are much lower (Table 2).

Data on morbidity due either to nutritional disorders themselves or to other diseases that are known to affect man's nutriture such as malaria, intestinal parasitic and bacterial infections, tuberculosis, rubeola, pertussis, diabetes mellitus and degenerative heart diseases may provide approximate indices of the nutritional status of the community. These data should be available in health centres, private clinics or in hospitals, but if not may be obtained by rapid surveys or visits paid to some of these centres.

Limitations peculiar to the use of these records are the following. Doctors often tend to ignore nutritional disorders. Malnutrition is not a reportable disease. Most cases, especially the mild and moderate, are not referred to hospital. The classification of malnutrition disorders is unclear even to the experts and the presenting diagnosis is overshadowed by the associated or contributing acute infections.[9]

ANTHROPOMETRY

There is now considerable evidence that heredity may set certain limits on human growth, but nutrition may be regarded as the main environmental factor that will enable the body to achieve those limits. Infections and other acute and chronic diseases affect human growth only through nutrition. It may be concluded that growth standards chosen to represent optimal pre-school growth can be used in other less privileged communities regardless of racial differences.[10] Growth retardation may be the first response of the body towards nutritional deficiencies, while appearance of clinical signs may be the final stage. In overnutrition excess intake of some nutrients may appear, e.g. high energy intake will increase the body depot fat and its weight, while the excess intake of some vitamins and protein may have no obviously harmful effect, as far as we know.

Body organs and tissues grow at different rates according to age, sex and genetic potential, so that measurement of a body dimension at a certain age may be more revealing than at other ages. Anthropometric data are usually compared with standard norms of healthy, well-fed subjects either from the same locality (local standards) or internationally recognized standards such as those of Harvard.[11, 12] These reflect the growth of Caucasian children of predominantly middle-class origin. The Harvard growth charts were constructed by Reed and Stuart[11, 12] for children from birth to 18 years of age. Wetzel[13] devised a grid for height–weight–age data to represent the physical status of growing children. Seltzer and Mayer proposed tables for obesity standards from 5–50 years of age, giving minimum triceps skinfold thickness to measure obesity.[14] The Medico Actuarial mortality investigation tables[15] and The Metropolitan Life Insurance Company tables[16] contain data on adult men and women.

The anthropometric measurements of significance to nutrition workers are numerous and the most commonly used are listed in Table 3 together with their advantages and disadvantages and how they may be used for classification.

Somatic measurements, either alone or in combination, are the most frequently used method of assessing the nutritional status of young children, especially in

MCH and other centres for their long-term management (Chapter 15). The present trend under these circumstances is to use weight in relation to height allowing for age rather than relying on weight for age alone which is not standard for all children and fails to allow for growth retardation in the past.[17]

A certain degree of accuracy of the data is required; for length 0.5 cm; for weight 250 g and for skin-fold thickness it is 0.2 mm. Accurate age of subjects, especially children, may not be available. Use of a calendar of local events and a dental formula[18] may be helpful. The standards may be committed to percentile growth charts and cross-sectional data for many or longitudinal data for one child be plotted. Data may be classified according to the percentage deviation from norms, e.g. chest/head circumference and mid-arm circumference/head circumference as proposed by Kanawati and McLaren.[19] The mid-arm/head circumference ratio proved to be unrelated to the child's age and sex[19] and can be recommended in the age group 3–48 months, when the exact age of the child is not known. A simple steel or any unstretchable material tape measure can be used with minimum training and supervision. It is being increasingly appreciated that single measurements do not adequately denote nutritional status. It is reasonable that a subject of a given size (e.g. height) should have a certain mass (weight) which will vary to some extent with age. Standards and a classification of weight/height/age are available.[20]

The subject of Physical Anthropometry and Nutritional Status formed the topic for a recent symposium.[21] In this important review valuable contributions appear on such subjects as the degree of precision of measurements, the most useful measurements to make, statistical considerations and the merits of cross-sectional and longitudinal studies.

CLINICAL EXAMINATION

The clinical examination serves as a guide for recording the signs known to be related to inadequate nutrition and in detecting other diseases or conditioning factors which commonly influence the nutriture of an individual. It is usually simple to detect the clinical signs in the advanced stages of the deficiency conditions, but the less severe degrees may easily be overlooked. Sub-clinical stages remain unrecognized without the aid of a laboratory or other special techniques.

The interpretation of these signs requires careful judgment. They may be non-specific; produced by nutritional or even non-nutritional conditions. Some may be of multi-factorial aetiology; produced by more than one factor. Observer error is usually high and definition of signs and method of reporting have not been standardized. The diagnostic importance and the detailed description of the clinical signs have been discussed extensively.[2,3]

There are certain biophysical tests which have been found helpful in detecting functional changes in nutritional disorders: notably, dark adaptation ability, muscle exertion and deep tendon reflexes. Other tissue and morphological changes have been claimed to be useful in detecting early childhood malnutrition, e.g. changes in hair root and buccal mucous membrane.

Table 3. Some anthropometric measurements applied in nutritional assessment

Measurements	Age groups	Nutritional indication	Reproducibility	Advantages	Disadvantages	Observer error	Interpretation
1. Weight	All groups	Present nutr. status; under and over	Good	Common in use	Difficult in field; can't tell body composition; need accurate age; need proper scales	<100 g in children <250 g in adults	<60% severe 60–80% moderate 80–90% mild 90–110% normal 110–120% over 120% & over obese
2. Height	All groups; 7 yrs [a] child	Chronic nutr. status (under) Chronic under nutr. in early childhood	Good	Common in use Simple to do in field	Differs by daytime Other factors play a role	<0.5 cm child <3.0 cm in adults	<80% dwarf; 80–93% short 93–105% normal; >105% giant
3. Head circumference	0–4 yrs	Intrauterine & childhood nutr. (chronic undernutrition mental abilities	Good	Simple	Others factors play a role	<0.5 cm	
4. Mid-arm circumference	All groups	Present under- and overnutrition	Fair	Simple, age independent; child need not be denuded; suitable for rapid survey	No limits for over- nutrition; no standard for adult	<0.5 cm	<75% severe 75–80% moderate; 80–85% mild; >85% normal

	Age	Present	Rating	Characteristics	Requirements		Classification
5. Skin-fold thickness subscapula	All groups	Present under- and over nutrition	Fair	Measure body composition, detect obesity—adults	Needs expensive callipers difficult with child and in the field	1.0—1.5 mm	Similar to item(1)
6. Weight/height for age ratio	All ages	Present under and over nutrition	Good	Index of body build; age independent, 1—4 yrs and adults	Need proper scales; need trained personnel		<75% severe; 75—85% moderate; 85—90% mild; 90—110% normal; 110—120% over; >120% obese
7. Mid-arm/head ratio	3 mos-48 mos	Present undernutrition	Good	Simple; age independent; sex independent; any person can do it for field	No standard for adults		<0.25 severe; 0.25—0.28 mod; 0.28—0.31 mild; 0.31—0.35 normal; >0.35 obese
8. Chest/head circs. ratio	1—2 yrs	Present undernutrition	Fair or poor	Simple; age independent	For limited age; no classification method		<1 malnourished; >1 normal

[a] Reference 26.

Table 4. Signs known to be of value in nutrition surveys and their interpretation

	Signs	Associated disorder or nutrient
1. Hair	Lack of lustre Thinness and sparseness Straightness Dyspigmentation Flag sign Easy pluckability	Kwashiorkor, less commonly marasmus
2. Face	Naso-labial dyssebacea Moon-face	Riboflavin Kwashiorkor
3. Eyes	Pale conjunctiva Bitot's spots Conjunctival xerosis Corneal xerosis Keratomalacia Angular palpebritis	Anaemia (iron etc.) Vitamin A Riboflavin, pyridoxine
4. Lips	Angular stomatitis Angular scare Cheilosis	Riboflavin
5. Tongue	Scarlet and raw tongue Magenta tongue	Nicotinic acid Riboflavin
6. Teeth	Mottled enamel	Fluorosis
7. Gums	Spongy bleeding gums	Ascorbic acid
8. Glands	Thyroid enlargement Parotid enlargement	Iodine Starvation
9. Skin	Xerosis Perifollicular hyperkeratosis Petechiae Pellagrous dermatosis Flaky paint dermatosis Scrotal and vulval dermatosis	Vitamin A Ascorbic acid Nicotinic acid Kwashiorkor Riboflavin
10. Nails	Koilonychia	Iron
11. Subcutaneous tissue	Oedema Fat: decreased increased	Kwashiorkor Starvation, marasmus Obesity
12. Muscular and skeletal systems	Muscle wasting Frontal and parietal bossing Epiphyseal enlargement Beading of ribs Persistently open anterior frontanelle Knock-knees or bow legs Thoracic rosary Musculo-skeletal haemorrhages	Starvation, marasmus, kwashiorkor Vitamin D Vitamin D, ascorbic acid Ascorbic acid

13. Internal systems		
(a) gastro-intestinal	Hepatomegaly	Kwashiorkor
(b) nervous	Psychomotor changes	Kwashiorkor
	Mental confusion	Thiamine, nicotinic acid
	Sensory loss	
	Motor weakness	
	Loss of position sense	Thiamine
	Loss of vibration	
	Loss of ankle and knee jerks	
	Calf tenderness	
(c) cardiac	Cardiac enlargement	Thiamine
	Tachycardia	

BIOCHEMICAL ASSESSMENT

Biochemical changes of nutritional deficiencies occur in time after depletion of nutrient stores and depression of tissue levels, and before the appearance of anatomical lesions. Only occasionally can enzyme levels affected specifically by nutritional deficiency be measured in a convenient tissue, usually plasma or red cells; e.g. alkaline phosphatase for rickets* and red cell haemolysate transketolase in thiamine deficiency. Other tests that have been used in the field of nutritional status assessment fall into two groups. The first group reflects the dietary intake of individuals and the second represents metabolic changes that occur due to the deficiency state. Examples of the first group are the concentration of ascorbic acid in plasma or of vitamin A precursors that are in transit from one tissue to another. Examples of the second group are low plasma albumin due to decreased synthesis or high blood pyruvate accumulating as a result of metabolic pathway block. These latter are not nutrients but are synthesized in the body. The first group of tests may not be indicative unless great numbers of the population show exceptionally low levels. In individual cases some of these tests may be useful for confirming or ruling out the possibility of a specific deficiency, e.g. in a patient with spongy and bleeding gums, very low levels of vitamin C confirm scurvy and a high level will rule out such deficiency. Emphasis should be placed on tests related to the more common nutritional disturbances in the community. Use should also be made of simple tests that can be done in the field and are inexpensive.

Biochemical tests are often carried out in a sub-sample, e.g. 1 in 10 of the population studied. Other disadvantages peculiar to biochemical tests are the following: subjects may resent the drawing of blood or collecting of urine, especially young children; transportation of samples when acceptable conditions may not be possible; techniques may vary from one laboratory to another; normal ranges for most tests are wide; borderlines between categorizing 'poor' and 'low', 'fair' and

---

*Editor's note: doubt has recently been cast on the value of alkaline phosphate in detecting early rickets (Stephen, J. M. L. and P. Stephenson, *Arch. Dis. Childh.*, 46, 185 (1971).

'normal' and 'excess' have not been clarified. Interpretation of the data without the help of clinical or dietary and health history of the subjects is virtually impossible.

Table 5 shows various nutritional deficiencies and the related biochemical tests classified as 'first category' and 'second category' according to their practicality in the field. Suggestive criteria of interpretation of some biochemical tests are shown in Table 7.

Table 5. Laboratory tests for nutrients and metabolites

Nutrient	1st Category	2nd Category
1. Protein	Plasma amino acids, urinary hydroxyproline, serum albumin urinary urea/creatinine	Total serum protein
2. Lipids	Serum cholesterol, triglycerides, lipoproteins	
3. Vitamin A	Serum vitamin A and carotene	
4. Vitamin D	Serum 25OH cholecalciferol serum alkaline phosphatase	Serum calcium and phosphorus
5. Ascorbic acid	Whole blood ascorbic acid	
6. Thiamine	Urinary thiamine, erythrocyte transketolase activity	Blood pyruvate
7. Riboflavin	Urinary riboflavin, erythrocyte glutathione reductase	
8. Nicotinic acid		N_1-Methyl nicotinamide and its [6]pyridone in urine
9. Folic acid	Red cell folate	Serum folate, bone marrow film, thin blood film
10. Vitamin B_{12}	Serum vitamin B_{12}, serum thymidylate synthetase, urine methylmalonic acid	Bone marrow film Thin blood film Schilling test
11. Iron	Iron deposits in bone marrow, serum iron and % saturation of transferrin	Haemoglobin Haematocrit Thin blood film
12. Iodine		Urinary iodine Tests for thyroid function

ADDITIONAL MEDICAL INFORMATION

There is convincing evidence that all infectious diseases have some adverse metabolic effects and frequently influence the amount of food consumed, digested and absorbed by the diseased individual. Infection and malnutrition are interrelated and they interact usually in a synergistic way (Chapter 10).

An ecological approach is essential for a proper understanding of malnutrition. Field studies may need to be extended by laboratory experiments to study the disease as it occurs in nature rather than in individual persons. Number of episodes, severity and duration are of special importance. Diarrhoea and other intestinal diseases, rubeola, pertussis, tuberculosis, intestinal infestations, malaria, toxaemia of pregnancy, diabetes mellitus and hypertension are among the most common diseases known to affect nutrition in a community.

SAMPLING METHOD

The sample should be selected at random in order to represent the whole population. For nutritional surveys geographic distribution, dietary differences, ethnic background, age, sex, religion, socio-economic level and occupation have to be considered. Vulnerable groups of the population, e.g. pregnant and lactating women and young children, should be adequately represented. Recent census data have to be used in selecting the sites, the street, the houses or the families. The sizes of the clinical and the biochemical samples are chosen according to the desired level of representation and the available resources to provide sufficient number for a proper appraisal. Two simple techniques have been suggested, involving using either the standard error of the mean or the coefficient of variation of the mean:[22]

$$N = S^2/E^2 \tag{1}$$

N = Number of the sample
S = Standard deviation of the mean of previous studies
E = Standard error desired to deviate from the mean of the whole population

$$N = S^2/(\overline{X}.CV)^2 \tag{2}$$

CV = Coefficient of variation desired to deviate from the mean of the whole population
$\overline{X}$ = Mean of a previous study.

A full explanation and discussion of appropriate techniques is given by Kish[23] and Snedecor et al.[24]

INTERPRETATION OF DATA

In Tables 6, 7 and 8 several guides to interpretation of field and laboratory findings have been suggested. Table 6 shows the method of choice of tests that can be carried out in different degrees of malnutrition. In Table 7 some criteria are given for interpretation of various biochemical tests. Suggested criteria for community diagnosis of problems of public health magnitude are shown in Table 8 as quoted from McLaren.[25]

Table 6. Guide to methods of choice according to nutritional spectrum

Degree	Nutritional disorder	Method of assessment	Method of interpretation
	Dietary inadequacy	Dietary survey	As percentages of requirements
		Urine tests	Level of excretion
		Loading tests	As percentage of oral dosage
		Anthropometric measurements	As percentage of average standard
Mild	Depletion of stores	All above	Quantitative or in degree
		Liver biopsy	of concentration (grade I,
		Bone marrow biopsy	II, etc.)
	Tissue depletion	All above	Activity of the enzyme
		Enzyme assays	as compared with normal range
Moderate	Biochemical changes	All above	Quantitative grades as
		Blood nutrients level	compared with
		Urine tests	normal range
	Functional changes	All above	
		Tendon reflexes	Absent, weak, normal, hyperactive
		Night vision	normal, impaired
		Pulse rate	
		Electrocardiography	
		X-ray	Positive or negative
		Work performance	Weak, fair, normal
Severe	Anatomical changes	All above	
		Microscopic hair changes and mucous membrane changes	Degree of severity
		Clinical signs of undernutrition	Positive or negative
		Treatment trials	Positive or negative

Nutritional data are best interpreted jointly for clinical, biochemical, anthropometric and dietary data. The results are often presented as prevalence, e.g. a certain number or percentage of the population have low blood haemoglobin or xerosis of the eye etc. In some cases findings may support each other but sometimes they may not coincide. The best method of assessment should be based on a complete evaluation of all available findings. The background history, the anthropometric measurements, the biochemical results and quite often the therapeutic trials should be examined together.

Knowing the size, the kind and the distribution of nutritional problems in a community, the remaining questions will be: what are the curative and preventive measures that should be taken? and what is the sequence of priorities? The answers to these and other questions will depend entirely on the local and prevailing conditions in the studied community.

Table 7. Suggested guide to interpretation of some biochemical determinations in adults

	High	Acceptable	Low	Deficient
Blood				
Total Plasma protein, g/100 ml	7.0	6.5–6.9	6.0–6.4	<6.0
Serum albumin g/100 ml	4.25	3.52–4.24	2.80–3.51	<2.80
Haemoglobin, g/100 ml				
men	15.0	14.0–14.9	12.0–13.9	<12.0
women	14.5	11.0–14.4	10.0–10.9	<10.0
Haematocrit (PCV)%				
men	45	42–44	36–41	<36
women	43	38–42	30–37	<30
Plasma ascorbic acid (g/100 ml)	>50	20–49	10–19	<10
Urine				
Thiamine (μg/g creatinine)	⩾130	66–129	27–65	<27
Riboflavin μg/g creatinine	⩾270	80–269	27–79	<27

Table 8. Suggested criteria for recommending control measures against childhood malnutrition

Data collected	Guide for interpretation
1. Vital:	
Infant mortality	>50/1000 live births
1–4 years mortality	>10/1000 population of 1–4 years
2. Clinical signs:	
Frank marasmus, kwashiorkor, xerophthalmia	>1/100 of 0–5 years (hospital data)
Oedema, dermatosis of kwashiorkor	>5/1000 affected individuals 0–5 years field survey
3. Anthropometry:	
Weight or height	>20/100 below Boston standard 3rd percentile
4. Laboratory tests	>15/100 'low' ICNND standards or >5/100 'deficient' ICNND standards
5. Dietary evaluation	>20/100 below 75% of FAO/WHO recommended allowances

From reference 25.

REFERENCES

1. Liharzik, F. *Das Gesetz des menschlichen Wachstumes,* Vienna, Gerold, 1858.
2. Expert Committee, Medical Assessment of Nutritional Status, *WHO Technical Report Series No. 258,* Geneva, 1963.

3. Jelliffe, D. B. *The Assessment of Nutritional Status of the Community,* Geneva, WHO, 1966.
4. Gordon, J. E., J. B. Wyon and W. Ascoli. *Amer. J. Med. Sci.,* **254,** 121 (1967).
5. *U.N. Demographic Year Book,* 1972.
6. Puffer, R. R. and C. V. Serrano. *Patterns of Mortality in Childhood,* PAHO Sc. Pub. 262, 1973.
7. Aykroyd, W. R. and B. G. Krishnan. *Indian J. Med. Res.,* **29,** 703 (1941).
8. Bengoa, J. M., D. B. Jelliffe and C. Perez. *Amer. J. Clin. Nutr.,* **7,** 714 (1959).
9. McLaren, D. S. and A. A. Kanawati. *Trans. Roy. Soc. Trop. Med. Hyg.,* **64,** 754 (1970).
10. Habicht, J. P., R. Martorell, C. Yarbrough, R. M. Malina and R. E. Klein. *Lancet,* **1,** 611 (1974).
11. Stuart, H. C. and R. B. Reed, *Pediatrics,* **24,** 875 (1959).
12. Stuart, H. C. and R. B. Reed, *Pediatrics,* **24,** 904 (1959).
13. Wetzel, N. C. *J. Pediat.,* **22,** 329 (1943).
14. Seltzer, C. C. and J. Mayer, *Postgrad. Med.,* **38**(2), A101 (1965).
15. Association of Life Insurance Medical Directors and Actuarial Society of America. 1912 Medico-Actuarial Mortality Investigation, Vol. 1.
16. Metropolitan Life Insurance Company. 1942, Ideal weight of women. Metropolitan Life Insurance Co., *Statistic. Bull.,* **23,** No. 10, p. 6.
17. McLaren, D. S. and W. W. C. Read. *Lancet,* **2,** 146 (1972).
18. Jelliffe, E. F. P. and D. B. Jelliffe. Deciduous Dental Eruption, nutrition and age assessment. *J. Trop. Pediat. and Environ. Child Hlth.,* **19,** No. 2A Monograph 2, 193 (1973).
19. Kanawati, A. A. and D. S. McLaren. *Nature,* **228,** 573 (1970).
20. McLaren, D. S. and W. W. C. Read. *Lancet,* **2,** 219 (1975).
21. *ICNND Manual for Nutrition Surveys,* Washington, U.S. Government Printing Office, 1963.
22. Schllesselman, J. J. *J. Chron. Dis.,* **26,** 553 (1973).
23. Kish, L. *Survey Sampling,* New York, Wiley, 1965.
24. Snedecor, G. E. and W. G. Cochran. *Statistical Methods,* 6th edn., Ames, Iowa U.S.A., The Iowa State University Press, 1967.
25. McLaren, D. S. *Nutrition and its Disorders,* Edinburgh and London, Churchill Livingstone, 1972, p. 263.
26. Bengoa, J. M. In *Nutrition, National Development and Planning,* Massachusetts and London, The MIT Press, 1972, p. 110.

SECTION II

Malnutrition in the Community

CHAPTER 7

Multi-factorial Causation of Malnutrition

CARL E. TAYLOR AND ELIZABETH M. TAYLOR

Malnutrition is more than a medical problem. Its causes are dysfunctions in economic, demographic, cultural and ecological processes. The process of acquiring food permeates all aspects of human relationships with the environment and with society. The greater the poverty, the more ecological the causation of malnutrition and the larger the proportion of time and effort that individuals invest in getting and preparing food.

We have constructed a model (Figure 1) showing the interrelationships of factors that cause most of the malnutrition in the world. This required a selectivity that left out much more than was included. Causal factors are grouped under three headings: the production of food, its distribution and its utilization. The six groups of factors under production and distribution act to produce reduced, imbalanced or excessive consumption of nutrients. Alterations in the balance between these consumption factors and the three factors related to utilization then influence metabolic availability. Malnutrition results when deficiencies or imbalances are of specific nutrients or of energy generally. In affluent countries the major problem is obesity, caused by both excessive consumption of food and reduced levels of activity. There are several feedback loops of which two are shown in the model. Malnutrition lowers productivity of labour and thus contributes to poverty and decreased availability of food. Similarly, poor nutrition reduces resistance to infections which in turn aggravates malnutrition.

In the sections that follow, each of the nine groups of causal factors will be discussed in more detail.

LABOUR FORCE

Development planners now recognize the importance of agricultural labour. The growing world food crisis accentuates the importance of agricultural production which, in turn, seems to have a greater immediate potential for contributing to economic development than industry.[1] In most developing countries agriculture is the greatest source of employment, ranging between 50 and 70 per cent.[2]

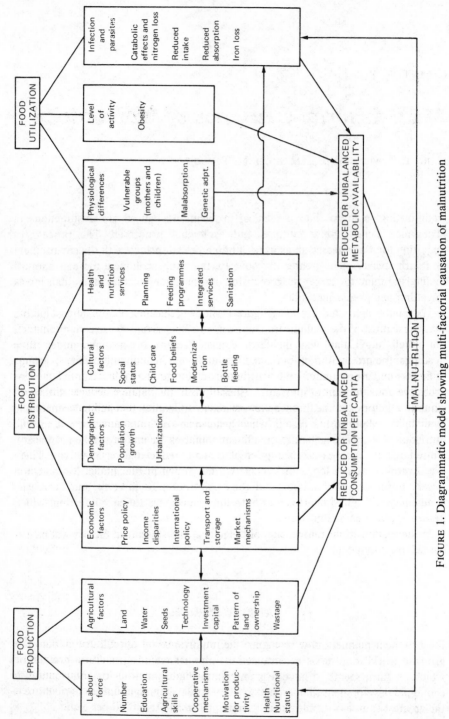

FIGURE 1. Diagrammatic model showing multi-factorial causation of malnutrition

Agricultural production is restricted by low productivity. High unemployment levels lead to a casual attitude towards work. Education may have either positive or negative effects on productivity. A common pattern is for workers to leave the farm to seek white-collar employment as soon as they become educated. Training in agricultural skills can, however, make food production as lucrative as most urban employment. New cooperative mechanisms are needed to adjust to new methods of agriculture and to ensure availability of fertilizer, irrigation, etc.

Health and nutritional status are important in improving labour productivity. Multiple studies on the controlled labour force of plantations demonstrated dramatic improvements when the prevalence of specific diseases such as malaria was reduced and when diets were improved.[3, 4]

One of the most important but least understood components of enhanced productivity is change in motivation.[5] Important cultural forces underlie these motivational variables. Better health and nutritional status may indirectly have their greatest effect on productivity through changes in motivation. As health and nutritional status improve, there is more energy to work harder. Where there is a greater survival of children and adults there is an intangible incentive to plan ahead and to work for improved levels of living.

AGRICULTURAL FACTORS

The low productivity of agriculture in most developing countries has limited any attempt to improve nutrition. Crop yields per unit of land remain low until there is general use of irrigation, new seeds, fertilizer, pesticides and precise timing of labour inputs. The promise of a rapid spread of these methods as part of the 'green revolution' has been sharply curtailed because of increasingly severe shortages of energy and fertilizer. Better technology, if it could be applied to the rich, alluvial Indus–Ganges–Brahmaputra plain of North India, is estimated to have the potential of producing up to ten tons of grain per acre per year—totalling more than ten times the present crop of all India.[6]

Inequities in the distribution of land are among the most obstinate barriers to agricultural development. High rents and sharecropping rates drain capital from farmers to non-productive land holders, often urban. In Asia and Latin America the problem is most obvious. In 1964, 24 per cent of the working agricultural population of Latin America owned 4 per cent of the agricultural land, but 2 per cent of the population owned 40 per cent of the land. The owners of *latifundios* (large estates) put nearly all their income into urban or foreign investment and luxury consumption.[7]

This is a prime example of the potent but indirect effect of politics on the nutrition of masses of people. Education, wealth and political power reside primarily in the landowning classes and this combination forms a formidable block to land reform.

Wastage of various kinds erodes the small agricultural yields. FAO has estimated world losses of food in field, storage, transportation or processing to be between $24 billion and $48 billion per year in low income countries. Estimates for crop losses are 40 per cent in Latin America and over 30 per cent in Africa. Rodents, insects and fungi probably consume two or three times the national food deficit in many countries.[8a] Inadequate transport allows localized or seasonal pockets of plenty in the midst of scarcity of certain foods. In Peru, the lack of refrigerated vans restricts the largest per capita fish catch in the world to the immediate coastal region.[8b] Wastage through soil erosion, overcropping, etc. can be assumed to be increasing.

Geographical variables determine some specific deficiencies. Endemic goitre and cretinism may be a severe if localized problem where iodine content of soil is low.[9]

ECONOMIC FACTORS

Poverty as a primary cause of malnutrition underlies most other causal factors. It tends to receive special attention because it is easily measured and directly influences food consumption.

The poor spend a larger proportion of available income on food than the rich. In many developing countries, two-thirds or more of income goes for food.[2] In South India, the poorest people spend 80 per cent of their income on food while the more affluent spend only 45 per cent. Nutritional problems are aggravated in urban situations because food has to be bought rather than grown and inappropriate foods are promoted by aggressive advertising.[8c]

Some development planners have maintained that with economic development people would improve their own nutrition. Current thinking recognizes, however, that better nutrition is both a means as well as a goal of development. As economic conditions improve, there is usually a lag in the rate at which benefits reach the poor. In Mexico, malnutrition is common but in Taiwan it is rare; the disparities in income distribution are much greater in Mexico, even though per capita income is twice as much: $530 versus $270.[8d] Direct measures to improve nutritional status among the poorest may equalize income distribution and also remove a major block to development.

National planning can stimulate increases in food production most readily by adjusting price policy. Such incentives to farmers, however, usually make food less available to the poor, so that in order to get better income distribution, appropriate mechanisms for food subsidization will have to be provided. Economic policies should also ensure distribution of food by providing good transportation and storage.

One of the largest components of foreign aid in the past 20 years has been shipment of surplus food. Any future surpluses will undoubtedly be needed to meet emergency situations arising from the increasing number of famines and droughts around the world as population growth leads to ecological devastation. In addition to population growth, the world food crisis is aggravated by growing affluence in developing countries. In poor countries the average person consumes about 400 pounds of grain per year. In North America, however, per capita grain utilization is approaching one ton per year, with only about 150 pounds being consumed directly as cereals and the remainder going into the inefficiencies of meat production.[10]

DEMOGRAPHIC FACTORS

An expected exponential rise in world population gives great urgency to efforts to solve the malnutrition problem. Population growth operates both directly, limiting the amount of food and arable land available per capita, and indirectly, exacerbating other social ills that foster malnutrition.

Increase in food production can bring no improvement in a people's nutritional state unless it exceeds the rate of population growth. In the developing nations, food production has approached a 3 per cent per annum increase over the last two decades but population growth has lagged behind only a fraction of a percentage point.

Population growth in much of Asia and Latin America is causing a land scarcity that has three nutritionally significant effects.[8, 11, 12] First, an increase in acreage cultivated that has accounted for most of the increase in food production is no longer possible in many areas. Second, in developing countries surplus rural labour leads to unprecedented migration to the city. The social dislocation attendant upon this demographic implosion accentuates most of the factors that cause malnutrition. Third, farming efficiency and the possible level of mechanization decline as land holdings become smaller. Significant capital investment then depends on a pooling of resources by a number of small-scale farmers.

Large family size lowers the quality of attention given to individual children.[13] In the clinic of the Indian National Institute of Nutrition, 61 per cent of all cases of protein–energy malnutrition were in children with three or more older siblings: a group that comprises 34 per cent of the child population.[14] The youthfulness of any rapidly growing population results in a high ratio of young dependents to economically active adults. One-half of the people in developing areas are below 19 years of age.

CULTURAL FACTORS

It would be ideal if a culture's food habits conspired to provide women and children, who are nutritionally most vulnerable, with an optimum diet within the limits of available food supplies. The opposite pattern, however, prevails in many areas; apparent causes are low socio-economic status and scientifically invalid belief systems about nutrition.

In scarcity situations, high-quality diet tends to accrue to high social status, which in turn depends on long-established cultural patterns, economic productivity or power. Unfortunately, those most vulnerable to undernutrition—young children, child-bearing women and the old—are usually economically dependent, and excluded from political power and high cultural status.

The nutritional status of females in many parts of the world is inferior to males, especially in times of shortages of food, and during child rearing and bearing. A greater demand for iron and other nutrients resulting from menstruation and pregnancy increases the prevalence of anaemia and other pregnancy-related conditions. Except for this, the generally poor nutritional status of women is clearly associated with dietary discrimination. That this discrimination may be evident early in life is indicated by many growth studies of children. At Narangwal Rural Health Research Center in the Punjab, girls in both high and low caste groups showed marked deficits at 3 years of age in mortality, weight, height and morbidity in comparison to males.[15] Mortality of females in South Asia is higher than of males at all ages.[11, 16]

Traditional patterns of child care lead to nutritive neglect of the young, often in the face of adequate adult diets. Surveys in Central and South America, Africa and South Asia found children's normal diets to be commonly 20 to 30 per cent inadequate, and sometimes as much as 55 per cent inadequate.[17] Malnutrition is the most important single cause of the extremely high child mortality in developing countries.[18]

Many of the most important rituals which identify cultures are built into acquiring food and eating it. Periods of unusual danger in the life cycle attract a number of ritual proscriptions of foods. It is common to withhold solids at the first signs of diarrhoea or other infections, precipitating protein–energy malnutrition. In the rural Punjab, the cause of infantile marasmus is believed to be a curse, transmitted involuntarily by the shadow of certain people. The cure is thought to be a restricted diet and isolation in a dark room.

The generally inadequate nutritive status of women is compounded during pregnancy and lactation in many areas by deleterious beliefs about specific foods. A study in North Carolina, U.S.A., among poor pregnant women found nearly one-third to have some nutritionally unsound food taboo (e.g. 'pork rots the uterus, . . . leafy vegetables mark the baby and cheese causes the baby's head to stick to the womb during delivery'.)[8e] Ignorance of dietary requirements and a nutritionally unsound cultural predisposition for certain foods causes deficits in some specific nutrients, particularly vitamins A, the B complex, C and D and iron.

Some of the cultural by-products of 'modernization' in the developing world are a threat to nutritional improvement. Paradoxically, an increase in income can result in lower quality nutrition as highly processed foods gain status. In Asia, increased income provokes a shift from home-pounded to commercially polished rice, which predisposes to beriberi.

Perhaps the most pernicious effect of 'modernization' is the sharp decline worldwide in the amount of breast-feeding (Chapter 8). The factors that we have discussed—demographic, economic, cultural and political—intertwine to form a severe epidemiological problem. This is primarily a problem of the city, generated by exposure to the urban élite and western influence. Advertisements for infant formulae and weaning foods, many inaccurate or misleading, spurred the transition, encouraging the image of bottle-feeding as prestigious, modern, 'scientific' and healthy. Women turned to bottle-feeding for convenience as they took up jobs outside the home. Low income results in insufficient purchase and variety of food stuffs. Lack of education, inconvenient means of preparation, and time demands from other children militate against proper, careful and sanitary preparation. Finally, the psychological stress of a rapid, tense city life-style seems to increase physical failure to lactate. The reactions of medical and political authorities have done little to change this trend. Medical textbooks give scant attention to the psycho-physical benefits of lactation. Governmental policy makers are not at present ready to deal with a subject so 'intimate'.

INADEQUATE HEALTH AND NUTRITION SERVICES

Inadequate services can be included among the major causes of malnutrition. There are more malnourished people in the world than ever before, even though a slight proportionate improvement in the overall levels of nutrition in the world may have occurred. In view of the tremendous investments in health and nutrition programmes, this slight increase cannot be considered a major achievement. Most efforts of organized services to improve nutrition have been inadequate and sometimes counterproductive. The most evident problem is the lack of planning. Nutrition programmes have been erratic in their coverage, inconsistent in their implementation and often misdirected in their policies. Implementation must begin with defined priorities (Chapter 13).

Inappropriate past policies are exemplified by the fact that 95 per cent of nutrition budgets in developed countries have gone into institutional child feeding. In child-feeding programmes in less developed countries, less than 10 per cent reached the vulnerable age groups of pre-school children.[8f] Give-away feeding programmes also tended to promote early weaning and discourage the local development of low-cost foods of good nutrient quality.

Much has been learned about ways in which services for nutrition, family planning and maternal and child health can be integrated. At the Narangwal Rural Health Research Center it was found that the key to an effective programme is to use auxiliaries to work in the community and the home.[19] The auxiliaries provide primary medical care and immunizations. Sanitation is also important. A new pattern of education of all members of the health team, including doctors, will be needed.

PHYSIOLOGICAL FACTORS

Physiological differences in nutritive requirements or ability to metabolize ingested food is included here as the first of the factors influencing utilization (Figure 1).

Pregnant and lactating women and young children are especially vulnerable to nutritional stress. Poor maternal diet is not only a health and humanitarian problem for the mother, it can traumatize children: perhaps irreversibly. The greater risk of maternal morbidity, mortality and apathy threaten the quality of child care. This maternal depletion is cumulative with repeated pregnancies. Maternal deficiencies of minerals and vitamins (especially iron and vitamins A and C) reduce foetal stores.

Sub-normal maternal height and weight, generally assumed to be indicative of childhood protein–energy undernutrition in low-income women, strongly increase the risk of complications during delivery and of producing nutritionally vulnerable underweight infants.[20] Information is rapidly accumulating on the specific effects on the foetus of maternal undernourishment and the mechanisms by which long-term defects in physical and mental development are produced.[21]

The period between the start of weaning and the fifth birthday is nutritionally the most vulnerable segment of the human life cycle. Rapid growth, loss of passive immunity and as yet undeveloped acquired immunity against infection produce dietary needs more specific and inflexible than at later periods.

Intestinal malabsorption is associated with wastage of nutrients, growth retardation and severe weanling diarrhoea. Non-specific intestinal abnormalities associated with acute malabsorption syndromes are common in any of the low-income countries studied so far.[22]

We know little about nutritional adaptation, both genetic and induced. There seems to be a genetic component to lactase deficiency in certain populations.[23] There is also some evidence that the human organism has considerable capacity for phenotypic adaptation to prolonged under- or overnutrition.[24]

LEVEL OF ACTIVITY

Energy intake must be balanced with levels of activity or malnutrition results. In undernutrition, physiological adjustments spontaneously lead to reduced activity. In overnutrition, however, there seems to be little spontaneous physiological adjustment. One of the commonest problems of affluent groups is obesity resulting from reduced physical activity and excessive intake of food (Chapters 9 and 20). There is increasing evidence that lack of exercise also has a specific effect in the causation of cardiovascular disease related to atherosclerosis (Chapters 9 and 19).

INFECTIONS

Interactions of malnutrition and infections are two-way and cyclic. Since synergism between malnutrition and infections was defined 15 years ago[25] there has been a rapid expansion of understanding and knowledge (Chapter 10).

Infections cause malnutrition through a variety of mechanisms. Perhaps most important is the direct effect of systemic infections on catabolism of tissues. Even minor infections produce nitrogen loss. Most acute infections also reduce appetite and tolerance of food. In many parts of the world, food is withheld in infections. Infections which involve the intestinal tract or treatments which include purgation can reduce the absorption of nutrients.

A number of clinical deficiency states are precipitated by infection. An epidemic of diarrhoeal disease or measles may be followed by kwashiorkor. Similarly, keratomalacia, scurvy and beriberi have been observed following infection.

Anaemia follows various parasitic infections including hook worm, *Schistosoma haematobium* and *Diphyllobothrium latum*. Weanling diarrhoea occurs because the child has to adjust to an adult diet while being exposed to a wide range of pathogens in an insanitary environment.

SYNTHESIS

Analysis of causal relationships is most useful if the findings are brought together in a synthesis that shows how they apply. Generalizations about the relative strength of causal factors and their interactions have to be adjusted to local situations. Similar patterns of malnutrition can result from different combinations of causes. Defining profiles of causal factors in particular situations should make it possible to move directly and rationally into control programmes.

Some simplified case studies will be presented to illustrate causal profiles that are likely to be found under various ecological and socio-environmental conditions.

Our first case study is from the Punjab, India (Taylor, 1974, unpublished data), a food surplus area where the green revolution has quadrupled agricultural production and led to rapid socio-economic development. At the start of our research, 25 per cent of children showed second and third degree malnutrition. Between 1968 and 1971 an intensive nutritional and infection control programme caused a 50 per cent reduction in child mortality and significant improvement in weight and height of study children as compared with control groups, but there was still 17 per cent second and third degree malnutrition in the village children after over two years of work. The causal factors which were most readily changed were mothercare and weaning practices. Infections were also reduced by providing early medical care and immunizations. The causal factor that seemed to be responsible for much of the residual malnutrition was large family size and short inter-pregnancy intervals.

The next case study is from Lebanon. Kanawati and McLaren[26] separated the relative strength of causal factors statistically. The variables associated with mothercare and home living conditions were shown to be most significant. Table 1 shows the relative importance of 20 variables, starting with weaning practices, income and mother's education.

The Newcastle upon Tyne Studies initiated by Spence are classic.[27] His detailed analysis of the causal factors influencing child health in a low-income industrial area showed that mothercare was the most important of a number of socio-economic variables.

In a field project in Bangladesh, however, we found drastically different causation (McCord 1974, unpublished data). Here the primary difficulty is lack of food due to overpopulation and inadequate agricultural production. The unusually good rice harvest in the autumn of 1973 was accompanied by a dramatic fall in the amount of third degree malnutrition from September to December. The food was used up in four to five months and by March 1974 the percentage of third degree malnutrition had again risen to earlier levels. The shortage of food was aggravated by other causal factors such as poor weaning practices and a high infection level, even

Table 1. Ranking of factors (X_2 test) causing malnutrition in a group of 3–48 month low-socio-economic Lebanese children and a control group

1. Introduction of supplementary solid food before 6 months of life	26.278	$p < 0.001$
2. Income more than 250 Lebanese pounds/month/family	20.541	$p < 0.001$
3. Mother's education (able to read and write)	18.990	$p < 0.001$
4. Refrigerator	17.910	$p < 0.001$
5. House size (more than 3 rooms)	16.190	$p < 0.001$
6. No vaccination	14.290	$p < 0.001$
7. Indoor bathroom	12.931	$p < 0.001$
8. Not hospitalized for a severe illness	12.350	$p < 0.001$
9. Indoor toilet	9.532	$0.01 > p > 0.001$
10. Weaned during 1st and 2nd months	9.347	$0.01 > p > 0.001$
11. Gastroenteritis for a period of more than 1 month	8.786	$0.01 > p > 0.001$
12. Water supply within the house	8.350	$0.01 > p > 0.001$
13. Family size (more than 4 children)	7.595	$0.01 > p > 0.001$
14. Bottle introduced during the first month	7.577	$0.01 > p > 0.001$
15. Father's education (able to read and write)	7.407	$0.01 > p > 0.001$
16. Energy intake (less than 85% requirement)	6.076	$0.02 > p > 0.01$
17. Indoor kitchen	5.770	$0.02 > p > 0.01$
18 Respiratory infection for more than 1 week	5.254	$0.05 > p > 0.02$
19. Protein intake (less than 85% of daily requirement) for the age period 4–6 months	5.082	$0.05 > p > 0.02$
20. Pertussis	4.960	$0.05 > p > 0.02$

From reference 26

though mothers have much time for child care because they are secluded with their children in purdah.

In Peruvian urban-fringe children, malnutrition was significantly associated with crowding, poverty and the education, marital status and height of the mother.[28]

We suggest that anyone planning a nutrition survey should go beyond the standardized descriptive data to include information which will permit the development of a local causal profile. From this profile, then, more rational programme development should be possible (Chapters 6 and 13).

REFERENCES

1. Lewis, J. *Quiet Crisis in India,* Washington, D. C., The Brookings Institute, 1962.
2. Myrdal, G. *The Challenge of World Poverty,* New York, Pantheon Books, N.Y., 1970.

3. Taylor, C. E. and F.-M. Hall. Health, population and economic development, *Science,* **157,** 651–657 (1967).
4. Williams, K. and T. D. Baker, *Health and Development, an Annotated Bibliography,* Baltimore, Dept. International Health, Johns Hopkins University, 1972.
5. Mallenbaum, W. Health and economic expansion in poor lands, *International Journal of Health Services,* **3,** 161–176 (1973).
6. Hopper, D. New directions in development, *The IDRC Reports,* Ottawa, International Development Research Center, Canada, 1974.
7. United Nations. *Economic Survey of Latin America, 1966, Part III,* New York, United Nations, 1968.
8. Berg, A. *The Nutrition Factor,* Washington, D.C., The Brookings Institute, 1973: (a) p. 70; (b) p. 201; (c) p. 40–48; (d) p. 48; (e) p. 47; (f) p. 160–161.
9. Stanbury, J. B., A. M. Ermans, B. S. Hetzel, E. A. Pretell and A. Querido. Endemic goitre and cretinism: public health significance and prevention, *World Health Organization Chronicle,* **28,** 220–228 (1974).
10. Brown, L. R. and E. P. Eckholm. Food: growing global insecurity, in *The U.S. and the Developing World,* J. W. Howe (Ed.), New York, Praeger, N.Y., 1974, pp. 66–84.
11. Myrdal, G. *Asian Drama,* Harmondsworth. Penguin Books, England, 1968.
12. Brown, L. R. *In the Human Interest,* New York, Norton, N.Y., 1974.
13. Williams, C. D. and D. B. Jelliffe. *Mother and Child Health—Delivering the Services,* London, Oxford University Press, 1972.
14. Rao, K. V. and C. Gopalan. Nutrition and family size, *Journal of Nutrition and Diet (India),* **6,** 258–266 (1969).
15. DeSweemer, C. *Growth and Morbidity,* Doctoral thesis, Johns Hopkins University, School of Hygiene and Public Health, 1974.
16. Wyon, J. B. and J. E. Gordon. *The Khanna Study: Population Problems in the Rural Punjab,* Cambridge, Harvard University Press, 1971.
17. Dema, I. S. *Nutrition in Relation to Agricultural Production,* Rome, Food and Agricultural Organization of the United Nations, 1965.
18. Puffer, R. and C. Serrano. *Patterns of Mortality in Childhood,* Publication No. 262, Washington, D.C., Pan American Health Organization, 1973.
19. Taylor, C. E. and C. DeSweemer. Nutrition and infection in *Food, Nutrition and Health, World Review of Nutrition, and Dietetics,* Vol. 16, Rechcigl, M. (Ed.), S. Karger, Basel, Switzerland, 1973.
20. Morley, D. *Paediatric Priorities in the Developing World,* London, Butterworth, 1973.
21. Metcoff, J. Intrauterine nutrition in *Textbook of Paediatric Nutrition,* D. S. McLaren and D. Burman (Eds.), London, Churchill Livingstone, 1976.
22. Rosenberg, I. H. and N. S. Scrimshaw. Malabsorption and nutrition, *American Journal of Clinical Nutrition,* **25,** 1047–1289 (1972).
23. Bayless, T. M. Lactose intolerance and milk drinking habits, *Gastroenterology,* **60,** 604–608 (1971).
24. Dubos, R. *Man Adapting,* New Haven, Yale University Press, 1965.
25. Scrimshaw, N. S., C. E. Taylor and J. E. Gordon. Interaction of nutrition and infection, *American Journal of Medical Sciences,* **237,** 367–403 (1959).
26. Kanawati, A. A. and D. S. McLaren. Failure to thrive, in Lebanon II, *Acta Paediat. Scand.,* **62,** 571–576 (1973).
27. Spence, J. S., W. S. Walton, F. J. W. Miller and S. D. M. Court. *A Thousand Families in Newcastle Upon Tyne,* London, 1954.
28. Graham, G. G. Environmental factors affecting the growth of children, *American Journal of Clinical Nutrition,* **25,** 1184–1188 (1972).

CHAPTER 8

Epidemiology of Undernutrition

DERRICK B. JELLIFFE

Nutritionists in pre-industrial, mainly tropical, resource-poor countries (RPC) are everywhere faced with undernutrition as their principal problem, both with such florid, easily diagnosable, advanced syndromes as kwashiorkor, marasmus and keratomalacia, and with the much commoner results of less severe malnutrition, all occurring in the context of an almost continuous barrage of bacterial, viral and parasitic infections.

Despite great variation in different ecologies, health profiles in the RPC show a common theme, with severe undernutrition mainly a problem in the physiologically vulnerable, especially young children and pregnant and lactating women. Similarly, undernutrition occurs in these groups to a limited and often unappreciated extent in disadvantaged communities all over the world.

Rational public-health plans to assist in dealing with undernutrition can only be based on epidemiological knowledge; that is, a continuing 'community diagnosis' of local forms of malnutrition, including their nature, dimensions and geographical location, the age groups involved, and the complex and interacting causes in the particular ecology. This is a similar process to that of clinical diagnosis in classical medicine, but needs to include an assessment of the resources actually or potentially available for mounting preventive programmes, including personnel, facilities, equipment and funds for relevant activities in health, agriculture, education, etc.

Information on the prevalence and aetiology of undernutrition is needed to convince planners and administrators of the magnitude of the problem in human and in economic terms (Chapter 13). It is needed to ensure the mobilization of limited resources for rational programmes geared to 'at-risk' areas (with, for example, low-protein tuber staple foods), to major problems (for example, rickets in Ethiopia and kwashiorkor in Southern Uganda), to vulnerable age groups (whether the first or second year of life), and to provide base-line information from which the effects of future developments, planned and accidental, may be measured ('nutritional surveillance').

Likewise, an assessment of the actual and potential resources for dealing with problems of community nutrition needs to be made, particularly including the type, location, function and coverage of existing health services, and the duties, interrelationships and training of available cadres of staff.

PREVALENCE OF UNDERNUTRITION

The nutritional status of a community and the prevalence of many forms of undernutrition often need to be measured by surveys, which can be of greatly varying degrees of complexity, and can be either longitudinal or, more usually, cross-sectional.[7] They often include the examination of statistically representative sections of the population for body measurements (anthropometry), for selected clinical signs, and using biochemical laboratory tests considered to be suggestive of various forms of malnutrition. Major difficulties here include problems of defining normal limits for such tests, as well as the selection of appropriate standards (Chapter 6).

Such cross-sectional surveys have the disadvantages of identifying more chronic forms of undernutrition, rather than those that are relatively acute: for example, marasmus rather than kwashiorkor. In addition, they give a picture of the situation in the community at one time of the year, and, ideally, need to be repeated at representative seasons.

Statistics concerning the occurrence of the more easily identified forms of malnutrition should also be sought from health service records, such as hospital admissions and health centre attendances. Plainly, these results are biased, but still helpful if interpreted with caution, as they can give some insight into year-round incidence and prevalence at different seasons. Analysis of cases admitted to the ward can be helpful in suggesting the causative factors responsible in the particular community.

In some circumstances, statistics on the mortality during certain age ranges known to be especially susceptible to malnutrition may be available, such as the second year of life for kwashiorkor, or 2–5 months for infantile beriberi. However, with the usual limited and inaccurate statistical data available, this is uncommon.

The community diagnosis should ideally include assessment of a wide range of non-medical factors, such as home food production, income and its expenditure, etc. Plainly, it can become a highly complex enterprise, taking considerable time, funds, trained staff and equipment. However, even with limited investigators, funds and all other resources, considerable data on prevalence, together with limited information on aetiology, can be acquired by means of rapid surveys (especially using anthropometry to assess protein–energy malnutrition of early childhood), combined with information from hospitals and health centres (and from their adjacent 'defined areas' when such exist). Such studies have, for example, been undertaken in Haiti[2, 3] and in a number of communities in East Africa.[1]

AETIOLOGICAL FACTORS

Human nutrition is the end-result of the interaction of all aspects of the ecology: that is, a whole range of different physical, biological and cultural factors in the human environment (Figure 1 and Chapter 7). Once this is appreciated, the practical question is to identify the main factors in the environment in the particular community, with special relation to the practical possibility of improving them at reasonable cost and in the near future as part of a realistic preventive programme.[4, 5]

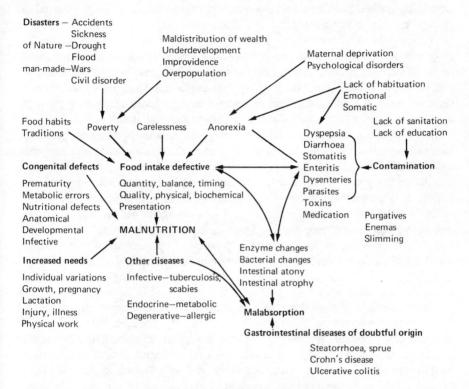

FIGURE 1. Some causes of undernutrition[12]

As an oversimplification and as a rough guide to thinking, the level of nutrition in a community, especially of its vulnerable young child population, may be considered as being due to the numerous complex, interacting ecological moulding forces, expressed in the following non-mathematical 'equation':

$$\text{Community level of nutrition} \propto \frac{\text{Education level} \times \text{Economic level} \times \text{Food Availability} \times \text{Aspects of health} \times \text{(Conditioning infections Preventive services)}}{\text{POPULATION SIZE}}$$

Each of the components of the equation affects the community nutrition level directly, and via the other factors indicated. Each is, of course, shorthand for a complex situation.

The *education level* includes not only the formal level of schooling and the limited technical personnel available in a country, including those in extension services, but also literacy in general. It operates through numerous channels, such as the number, quality and relevance of technical training establishments, and the existence of schools and their use for nutrition education. End-results include the supply of technically trained personnel and the numbers of literates likely to be exposed to modern knowledge concerning food, nutrition and related matters.

The *economic level* operates on a country basis, when an increased national income can, at least theoretically, make more governmental funds available for social services, such as schools and health services, as well as for specific nutrition programmes directed at major problems. At the family level, improved earning capacity means that there will be more money which can be used for the purchase of a greater range of foods, especially higher cost protein-rich items.

Food availability in the community nutrition-level equation is shorthand, both for the food present in the country as a whole (and its distribution and cost), and also for the food within the reach of a family, as well as its intra-familial distribution, especially to the young child, to pregnant and lactating women and to the elderly. Plainly, it is a composite of many activities: agricultural production, marketing, methods (and losses) during storage, and processing. It will be related to the emphasis given to cash crops versus foods in the nation's economic planning, the cultural significance of local foods in relation to physiologically vulnerable members of the family, and the dietary pattern in the community in general, but especially feeding during infancy, the transitional (or weaning) period, and in pregnancy and lactation.

Certain '*aspects of health*' particularly influence the community nutrition level, especially the ubiquity of nutritionally 'conditioning infections' (including, for example, diarrhoeal disease, measles, malaria and intestinal worms), and the health services concerned with the prevention or early rehabilitation of child malnutrition by nutrition education and growth supervision at Young Child Clinics, by the issue of food supplements, by measures designed to control relevant infectious diseases, as with immunization or the chemoprophylaxis of malaria, by child-spacing programmes, and by activities to improve environmental hygiene.

It is becoming increasingly apparent that the level of nutrition in a community is related to the number of mouths to be fed—that, in fact, *population size* (including family size and the closeness of child spacing) is the 'universal denominator' for all other components of the equation (Chapter 4). In fact, the present serious world food situation is due in large measure to the disproportionate, and currently geometrical, increase in population size, constantly outstripping not only economic, educational and social development, but also per capita availability of food. As is well-known, this trend particularly affects pre-industrial, largely tropical resource-poor countries (RPC) where food supplies are often already inadequate. The situation has recently become still further worsened in some such countries, especially those lacking petroleum, minerals and key foods, and dependent on imported foods and/or soil-products to continue modernizing their agriculture via the 'green revolution'.

In addition, a tremendous shift from the rural to the urban areas is now taking place in many developing countries; producing a different epidemiological situation, causing new problems altogether, which are nutritionally dangerous and of an obviously politically explosive nature. These are the new nutritional problems of comparatively recent years, related to rapid change from rural to urban community living, from a subsistence, food-growing economy, with the support of a closely knit pattern of relatives and kinship groups, to the often rather hostile world of the town, where all food has to be purchased, for which the 'new townsmen' have little preparation and in which the foods most available are often those which are cheapest and most easily transported and not necessarily the most nutritious. Particularly involved has been the pattern of infant feeding, as will be noted later.

Lastly, and impossible to include as a single item in the equation, is the *culture pattern* of the community. The system of values, attitudes, beliefs and customs is interwoven into every aspect of life and affects each component of the equation, ranging from the dietary pattern and methods of treating illness, to the sociopolitical priorities given to health and nutrition, particularly of mothers and young children, compared with other governmental activities, including defence.

CHANGING PATTERNS OF INFANT FEEDING

Patterns of infant feeding vary greatly in detail from culture to culture, and the precise use of terms in written accounts, such as 'weaning' and 'breast-feeding' differ markedly and are often not defined. It is, therefore, difficult to draw too specific conclusions from the reports available.[6]

Nevertheless, in general terms, four main patterns of infant feeding, modified from the classification of Raphael,[7] can be differentiated in the modern world in relation to lactation and weaning:[8]

(a) *traditional, pre-industrial* (total breast-feeder);
(b) *recently urbanized poor* (emerging bottle-feeder);
(c) *urban educated well-to-do* (élite bottle-feeder);
(d) *naturalist urban educated* (neo-élite breast-feeder).

(a) Traditional, pre-industrial (total breast-feeder)

Basically, in this type of community, breast-feeding is the norm and is prolonged for one to three years or more. Feedings are on demand, including the night, when the baby sleeps by the mother's side.

In some cultures, so-called pre-lacteal feeds are given in the early days of life, usually for a short period while colostrum is secreted prior to the coming in of 'mature milk'.

Apart from this, foods other than breast milk ('transitional' or weaning diet) are more usually introduced relatively late: that is, during the last months of the first year of life, or during the second year (so-called 'breast starvation', which can lead to 'late marasmus'). The first foods tend to be gruels, pastes or paps made of diluted or pounded, largely carbohydrate staples, such as cereals or tubers. In a few less sophisticated communities, these may be pre-chewed by the mother. Also, in some places, the first foods offered may often be ill-cooked items from the adult diet with little modification. The danger period is often mainly the 'transitional' second year of life, when undernutrition coincides with frequent infections. Kwashiorkor is the principal form of severe malnutrition, with mild–moderate protein–energy malnutrition usually common and avitaminosis frequently prevalent.

On the whole, semi-solids are introduced late from a nutritional point of view, especially more nutritious items, such as animal products, legumes and dark-green leafy vegetables. Large numbers of 'cultural blocks' exist in many communities which tend to delay or limit the introduction of these foods.

(b) Recently urbanized poor (emerging bottle-feeder)

By contrast, in recently urbanized poor communities, such as shanty towns and slums all over the world, there is usually a rapid decline in prevalence of breast-feeding. Breast-feeding is often only undertaken for a short period of time, frequently for only a few weeks or months (± 3). This is sometimes followed by a 'mixed milk feeding', in which breast-feeding and cow's-milk formula from a bottle are both employed.

For reasons of economics and home hygiene, dilute contaminated bottle-feeding result, with an increase in marasmus and diarrhoeal disease, especially in the first year of life.

In some areas of the world, processed infant-weaning foods in jars or cans have commenced to make an impact. While convenient and conferring status, they usually have a high cost/nutrient value and cannot be used effectively, as they are beyond the families' means.

(c) Urban educated well-to-do (élite bottle-feeder)

This has been the pattern in most of the western world for the past two decades or so, and among the usually very small westernized élite in developing countries. Breast-feeding is carried out by a small, but varying minority. Bottle-feeding with cow's-milk-based formula has become the norm, either from birth or from a few weeks after birth.

The trend, especially in the U.S.A., has been from the use of evaporated or powdered milks to convenient, but costly, 'ready-to-feed' liquid formulas. Likewise, the detailed composition of such formulas has been considerably modified in recent years, partly in attempts to emulate human milk, partly to add additional vitamins and minerals, and partly for economy. The final result may be surprisingly different from the 'parent' cow's milk.

Likewise, there has been a move from the preparation of home-made infant weaning foods towards commercial processed infant foods of high convenience. For various reasons, including pressure of advertising and lack of nutritional knowledge by health workers, these processed infant foods have become used earlier and earlier, so that it is common for them to be introduced in the first few weeks of life.

Because of the infant feeding pattern of cow's-milk formulas, with the volume and concentration under the mother's control, and the early introduction of semisolids, a form of 'double feeding' has developed, in which the most immediate nutritional risk is of developing infantile obesity (Chapters 9 and 20).

Overemphasis on cow's milk as an infant food has made iron-deficiency anaemia a considerable public health problem in some communities, and has drawn attention to the need to consider methods of increasing iron intake in bottle-fed infants (placental transfusion, iron-fortified cow's-milk-based formulas, iron-rich transitional foods).

The sugar and salt content of processed infant foods, geared to the mother's palate, have raised the possibility of their being related to the later development of such sugar-related diseases as dental caries and obesity, and of early habituation to a high level of dietary salt, with a possible link with hypertension in later life. Also, the excessive weight gain in infancy has been linked with possible persisting obesity into adult life, with the recognized associated risks of heart disease, diabetes, etc. (Chapters 9 and 19).

(d) **Naturalist urban educated** (neo-élite breast-feeder)

Partly in response to the overall striving for great degrees of 'naturalism', an increasing percentage of more educated women in western countries, including the U.S.A., Australia, Norway and the U.K., are becoming actively concerned with nursing their babies on the breast and with promoting breast-feeding as an important aspect of mothering.

The pattern usually advocated is breast-feeding *alone* for four to six months, with the introduction of semi-solids thereafter, especially in the form of home-prepared food mixtures ('multi-mixes'). Breast-feeding is advocated for one year or more.

It is of interest that the pattern of infant feeding advocated is protective against infantile obesity, neo-natal hypocalcaemia and cow's-milk allergy in RRC and, at the same time, helps to protect against the marasmus–diarrhoea syndrome and kwashiorkor in RPC.

USE OF EPIDEMIOLOGICAL APPROACH

The community nutrition-level equation approach is, in essence, an attempt to sort out the major causative factors in the local ecology on which a practical programme can be based. While this equation will be concerned with the whole community, it will inevitably relate in larger measure to the main vulnerable groups: young children, pregnant and lactating women, and the elderly.

A basic problem is always the question of the *range* of information to be sought. In the past, very large-scale surveys or studies have been undertaken, covering many different potentially causative factors. In fact, such are highly expensive and, anyway, often overwhelm the investigators with a mass of data which may never be analysed, or only after the situation has changed.

Selection is always necessary, depending on the expected nutritional situation and resources (funds, trained staff, laboratory facilities, etc.). A *limited* range of areas often needing to be considered is given in Table 1. At least qualitative data

Table 1. Miscellaneous factors in the aetiology of undernutrition

Geographico-climatic	Unproductive soil Climate (high temperature, extremes of rainfall)
Educational	Too few schools (illiteracy)
Social	Illegitimacy; family instability Absence of family planning (children too closely spaced; population pressure) Poor communications (food distribution) Alcoholism
Economic	National poverty (low gross national product) Family poverty (low per capita income) Low level of industrialization
Agronomic	Old-fashioned methods of agriculture Inadequate protein production (animal and vegetable) Concentration on inedible cash crops Poor food storage, preservation and marketing
Medical	High prevalence of conditioning infections (measles, diarrhoea, tuberculosis, whooping cough, malaria, intestinal parasites)
Sanitational	Unclean, inadequate water supply Defective disposal of excreta and rubbish
Cultural	Faulty feeding habits of young children Recent urbanization (changing habits) Limited culinary facilities Inequable intra-familial food distribution Overwork by women (limited time for food preparation for children) Sudden weaning (psychological trauma)

From reference 1

concerning the pattern of infant feeding can be obtained (Figure 2); while cost-nutrient calculations can be easily made for nutrients considered to be in most short supply (e.g. protein, vitamin A, riboflavin, etc.). These can be listed in relation to their cost per nutrient rather than for a given weight (Table 2).

Alternatively, the epidemiological investigation can be considered as an attempt to define community 'at-risk' factors, both biological and environmental (Table 3), and then to assess the practicability, feasibility and comparative cost-effectiveness of organizing appropriate preventive measures.

Table 2. Average cost[a] of foods in the West Indies as sources of protein and calories

Cost per 1000 calories		Cost per 20 grams of protein
0.25	Dry Skim Milk	0.05
0.22	Pulses	0.06
0.10	Cornmeal—Wheat Flour	0.08
1.20	Salt Fish	0.10
0.13	Rice	0.12
0.25	Macaroni—Rolled Oats	0.15
0.60	Sardines	0.18
0.55	Fresh Milk	0.20
0.60	Fresh Beef, Goat, Mutton, Cheddar Cheese	0.20
1.80	Fresh Fish	0.20
0.25	Bread	0.20
1.10	Chicken Necks and Backs	0.20
1.20	Corned Beef	0.20
0.47	Peanut Butter	0.22
0.55	Dry Whole Milk	0.23
0.25	Sweetened Condensed Milk	0.23
0.55	Evaporated Milk	0.25
0.90	Minced (Ground) Beef	0.25
0.25	Ground Provisions (Root crops)	0.28
0.40	Fresh Pork	0.35
2.20	Broiler Meat	0.35
0.60	Irish Potatoes	0.40
1.10	Frankfurters, Sausages	0.40
1.60	Fresh Eggs	0.40
0.80	Milk-Based, Cereal-Based, Infant Foods	0.51
0.80	'Health Promoting' Foods	0.56
0.29	Plantain, Green Bananas, Ripe Bananas	0.59
4.87	Infant Foods—Strained Meats	0.69
4.58	Infant Foods—Strained Vegetables and Meat	2.08
0.55	Arrowroot	13.00
0.09	Sugar	Infinity
0.15	Margarine, Cooking Oil	Infinity
0.80	Glucose	Infinity

[a]In Jamaican dollars, $1.00 = U.S. $1.10 (see also Chapter 26).
From reference 10

An ecological diagnosis of some major causative factors in kwashiorkor among the Baganda of East Africa is given in Table 4. This, it must be noted, is limited to epidemiological information gathered from health service data and as a result of cross-sectional surveys (including home visiting). The data are, then, by no means ideal for a full community diagnosis, but represent what can be collected with little extra resources and still give valuable guidance in programme planning.

Similarly, the diagnostic chain of events responsible for marasmus in Lebanon has been analysed by McLaren (Figure 3) and contrasted with that for

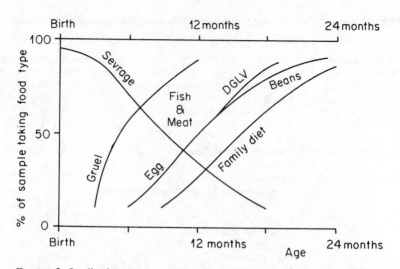

FIGURE 2. Qualitative pattern of infant feeding obtained by questionnaires in some West Indies Islands and graphed to show ages at which different foods are introduced into the diet[13]

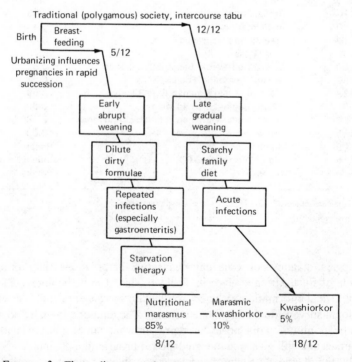

FIGURE 3. Flow diagram of pathogenesis of marasmus and kwashiorkor[9]

kwashiorkor. In this way indicators may be obtained concerning key aetiological factors possibly amenable to preventive measures.[9]

Undernutrition of all sorts is a result of a variety of different moulding forces, varying greatly from one country to another. Only by the understanding and insight obtained by epidemiological investigation can preventive programmes be launched which are logical and adapted to local needs and resources.

Table 3. Some at-risk factors in protein—energy malnutrition of children

	YOUNG CHILD
	Twins. Low birth weight. Some congenital abnormalities (e.g. cleft palate)
B	Close-spaced (<2 years). Large family size. Birth order
I	Transitional period (after second year)
O	Age range of maximal mortality
L	Growth failure (weight curve; other anthropometric indices)
O	Signs of malnutrition
G	Infections (measles; diarrhoea; whooping cough; 'non-immunized')
I	Family history (previous weanling deaths; previous malnutrition)
C	
A	**MOTHER**
L	Maternal illness and malnutrition (e.g. maternal height)
	M. presence. M. age (young or old). M. infections (malaria and low birth weight). M. death. M. intelligence/competence
	CULTURE
	Weaning practices (age; suddenness; separation; associated traumatic practices)
	Weaning food
	Child feeder
	Mother working
	Sex of child
E	Traditional practices with infections. Newly urbanized
N	
V	**SOCIO-ECONOMIC**
I	Economic level (relation to protein supply for young children in each economy,
R	especially urban)
O	Education considerations (literacy); language (for immigrants)
N	Incomplete family (absence or inadequate support by father, death or temporary
M	or permanent absence of mother)
E	Abandoned children
N	Alcoholism
T	
A	**GEOGRAPHIC-CLIMATIC**
L	Seasonal (especial relation to weaning)
	Geographically distant
	MISCELLANEOUS
	Non-attenders at health services

From reference 11

Table 4. Ecological diagnosis of causative factors of PCM among the Baganda of East Africa

	Present situation	Suggested preventive measures
Infant feeding	Breast feeding for 12–14 months, w:th a tendency to stop earlier	Encourage longest possible breast-feeding
	Starchy foods, especially 'matoke', beginning at 6 months	Attempt to widen diet from 6 months on (especially animal and vegetable protein, preferably as mixtures)
	Trend towards unnecessary bottle-feeding	Health education on dangers of bottle-feeding in local circumstances
Pattern of malnutrition	Nutritional marasmus (usually first year)	Breast-feed 12 months: Avoidance of bottle-feeding and associated diarrhoea
	Kwashiorkor (usually 1–3 years)	Breast-feed 12 months: Mixed diet with animal and vegetable protein from 6 months onward; prevention of conditioning diseases; avoidance of sudden separation at weaning
Pattern of relevant conditioning diseases	Tuberculosis	BCG campaign
	Hookworm	Health education, literacy
	Whooping cough	Immunization
	Measles	Vaccination
Available foods	*Village:* Plantain, sweet potatoes, cassava, groundnuts, beans, eggs	Encourage production of village protein foods (beans, eggs, fish ponds)
		Encourage parents to use protein food available for young children
	Shop: Fresh or dried skimmed milk, fish, meat	Raise standard of living and spending money available (diversified cash crops, industrialization)
Culture pattern	Prohibition of eggs, chicken, fish, mutton for women	Education
	Overemphasis on 'matoke' (steamed plantain)	Health education to use 'matoke' with other foods admixed
	Sudden separation of mother and child at weaning	Education
	Family instability	Education
Home economics	Foods usually steamed in plantain leaf packets	Preparation of infant food in traditional method (i.e. in plantain leaf packet)
Status of women	Subservient to men, with no say in household finances	Education of men, women and children: organization of parents' clubs and community development activities

From reference 1

REFERENCES

1. Jelliffe, D. B. *The Assessment of the Nutritional Status of the Community*, WHO Monograph No. 53 (1966).
2. Jelliffe, D. B. and E. F. P. Jelliffe. *Acta Tropica*, **18**, 1 (1961).
3. Jelliffe, D. B. and E. F. P. Jelliffe. *Amer. J. Publ. Hlth.*, **50**, 1355 (1960).
4. Antrobus, A. C. K. *J. Trop. Pediat.*, **17**, 187 (1971).
5. Morley, D., J. Bicknell and M. Woodland. *Trans. Roy. Soc. Trop. Med. Hyg.*, **62**, 164 (1968).
6. Jelliffe, D. B. *Infant Nutrition in the Sub-tropics and Tropics*, WHO Monograph No. 29 (second edn.) (1968).
7. Raphael, D. *Ecol. Food Nutr.*, **2**, 121 (1973).
8. Jelliffe, D. B., A. I. Ifekwunigwe and E. F. P. Jelliffe. *Breast Feeding and Weaning Foods*, in press. USAID.
9. McLaren, D. S. *Lancet*, **2**, 485 (1966).
10. McKigney, J. *J. Trop. Pediat.*, **14**, 55 (1968).
11. Jelliffe, D. B. and E. F. P. Jelliffe. *J. Trop. Pediat.*, **18**, 199 (1972).
12. Williams, C. D. *Lancet*, **2**, 342 (1962).
13. Gurney, J. M. *West Ind. Med. J.*, **20**, 227 (1971).

CHAPTER 9

Epidemiology of Overnutrition

J. I. MANN

An epidemiological approach to overnutrition must in the first instance attempt to examine the magnitude of the problem in different populations. Consideration of dietary practices and other environmental factors characteristic of communities in which disease frequency varies may help to identify aetiological factors and suggest means by which prevention may be practised at a community level. Epidemiological techniques may also be used to assess the value of programmes of prevention. Obesity and ischaemic heart disease are undoubtedly the two most common conditions associated with overnutrition and this chapter will deal principally with their epidemiology.

OBESITY

Definition and consequences to health

Obesity has been defined as adiposity in excess of that consistent with health. This would be a satisfactory definition if the point at which physiological adaptation ends and pathological disorder begins could be precisely defined. In practice the best that can be done is to define some arbitrary cut-off point beyond which morbidity and mortality show an unacceptable increase. Much of the evidence used for this purpose is derived from life insurance company statistics.

Statistics from the Build and Blood Pressure Study (based on pooled data from the largest life insurance companies in America) clearly demonstrate the excess mortality in heavier people.[1] Figure 1 shows an analysis of all policyholders aged 40–49 years. The death rate for the whole population in this age group was expressed as 100 per cent. The population was then divided into sub-groups according to deviation in weight from the mean and the relative death rates were compared. The minimum death rate occurred at 4–14 per cent below average weight and increased steadily with increasing body weight above this level.

Tables of 'desirable' body weight are derived from statistics such as these and suggest weight ranges (according to height) above which mortality tends to increase. Obesity has been varyingly defined as 10–20 per cent in excess of desirable body weight. Previously weight tables were based on 'average' rather than 'desirable' body weight. Clearly the former is not satisfactory since where many people are obese in a population such values are considerably higher than the ideal. Furthermore, in affluent societies, average weights show an increase with age,[3] a situation which mortality statistics suggest is not desirable. Tables of desirable body weight apply to people of all ages over 25 years.

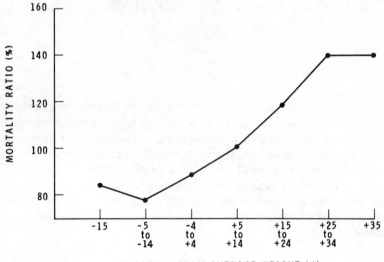

FIGURE 1. Effects of body weight on death rate in insured persons aged 40–49 years. (Taken from: Bray, G. A. Obesity: a serious symposium, Annals of Internal Medicine, **77**, 779 (1972))

All the statistics from which desirable body weight have been obtained have the disadvantage of being derived from a highly selected group of insured people and it cannot be stated with certainty that the findings apply to the general population. The tables commonly used are based upon persons examined during the years 1935 and 1953; this is more than a generation ago and the terms used to describe frame size have not been clearly defined. In addition, all information dates from the time the policy was taken out and no previous weight history is available. Finally, it is impossible to divide heavier individuals into those who weigh more because of muscular development and those who simply have too much adipose tissue. Despite all these disadvantages, however, these standards are probably the most useful that are currently available.

Methods are available for assessing the proportion of fat in the total body mass; the simplest of these entails the measurement of skin-fold thickness (subcutaneous fat) using one of the several varieties of callipers available. Results obtained from the skin-fold thickness measured at four sites (mid-triceps, sub-scapular, mid-biceps and supra-iliac) have been related to body density and formulae have been derived for estimation of total body fat. Standards for subcutaneous fat do exist[4] but because the patient needs to be partly undressed and experience is necessary to obtain accurate measurements of skin-fold thickness, this method has no great advantage over the use of desirable body weight for height in epidemiological studies. Various weight/height indices (e.g. weight/height^2) have also been used to describe obesity in epidemiological studies.[5]

Thus far, reference has been made to the excess in total mortality associated with obesity. Insurance company statistics also provide information as to the actual causes of death (Table 1) which may account for this excess, and other epidemiological studies have shown an association between obesity and morbidity from certain conditions. It has long been known that diabetes mellitus, presenting for the first time in middle age, occurs more frequently in the obese and the figures in Table 1 indicate that diabetes is a common cause of death in these people. Biliary

Table 1. Principal causes of death among men and women rated for overweight (standard insurance rate = 100 per cent death rate)

Cause of death	Per cent of standard death rate Men	Per cent of standard death rate Women
Diabetes mellitus	383	372
Cirrhosis of the liver	249	(147)
Appendicitis	223	195
Biliary calculi	206	284
Cardiovascular–renal diseases	149	177
Accidents	(111)	135
Pneumonia	(102)	(129)
Leukaemia and Hodgkins Disease	(100)	(110)
Cancer	(97)	(100)
Suicide	(78)	(73)
Peptic ulcers	67	—
Tuberculosis	21	35

Figures in parenthesis not statistically significant.

(Taken from Dublin, L. I. and Marks, H. H., Mortality among insured overweights in recent years. *Transactions of the Association of Life Insurance Medical Directors of America*, **35**, 235 (1951)).

calculi are also known to be more common in the obese, but part of the explanation for the excess number of deaths from this or from appendicitis may be due to the fact that such people are less satisfactory anaesthetic risks and more liable to postoperative complications. The excess number of deaths from cardiovascular and renal diseases is probably chiefly accounted for by the known association between obesity and hypertension,[6] diabetes and lipid abnormalities. However, some workers have claimed that an independent relationship exists between obesity and ischaemic heart disease.[7] The reason for the excess of deaths from cirrhosis of the liver is uncertain.

In this study no increase in total number of cancer deaths seems to have occurred in obese people but an association was found between obesity and cancers of the liver and gall bladder.[8] Retrospective case control studies have also suggested an association with cancer of the endometrium.[9] There are, in addition, several associated diseases which, although not usually fatal, cause a great deal of morbidity in the community, such as osteoarthritis, varicose veins, abdominal hernias and psychological stresses particularly during adolescence.

In infancy and childhood, obesity is associated with an increased tendency towards respiratory infections.[10] In one investigation 20 per cent of infants who had excessive weight gain in the first 6 months of life were found to be obese when re-examined between the ages of 6–8 years.[11] Furthermore, it would seem that between 50–75 per cent of children presenting with obesity remain overweight in adolescence and adult life when they are particularly resistant to treatment.[12, 13] Although before the onset of puberty the height of obese children tends to be above the standard, their ultimate height has been shown to be significantly below.[12] Several standards have been suggested for use in infancy and childhood, but it is important to realize that they all represent (in the words of Tanner) 'not what ought to be, but what is'. Standards based on average weights ought to be replaced, as they have been for adults, by desirable weights, but this can be done only when observations obtained from long-term prospective studies on children become available. Values for the mean and 'normal' range of height and weight of boys and girls up to the age of 18 are strikingly similar in Boston,[14] London[15] and Edinburgh.[16]

Effects of weight reduction

Weight reduction is well-known to result in improvement of both symptoms and glucose tolerance in maturity onset diabetics, to lower blood pressure in mild hypertension, and to provide at least some symptomatic improvement in osteoarthritis. Insurance statistics also suggest that weight reduction improves life expectancy.[17] Obese policyholders who were able to reduce their weight and maintain average body weight for a reasonable period of time achieved mortality rates approximately those of normal weight individuals. It should be stressed once again, however, that these data do not distinguish between different types of overweight, and overweight insurance policyholders may not necessarily be representative of the whole obese population.

Despite limited data and difficult interpretation the evidence still fits Shakespeare's warning:

Leave gourmandizing; know, the grave doth gape for thee thrice wider than for other men.

Shakespeare, *Henry IV,* Part II, Act V, Scene 5

Prevalence

It is extremely difficult to compare the prevalence of obesity in different countries.

Few random sample surveys have been carried out and different criteria have been used to define obesity.

In London, almost 50 per cent of men and women in all age groups were recently described as being overweight. The subjects were staff of the British Petroleum Company, and 'overweight' was defined as a weight greater than the mid-point of the weight range given in the tables for the largest frame, since no assessments of body build were available.[18]

In a careful analysis of heights and weights of British men, Khosla and Lowe have shown that since 1930 weight has increased at a much greater rate than height, so that the population is becoming progressively more obese and that a middle-aged man today probably weighs 15 lbs more than a man of the same age and height 30 years ago.[3]

Twenty per cent of over 1000 British businessmen attending the Medical Centre of BUPA (private practice medical insurance) have been found to weigh more than 20 per cent in excess of their desirable body weight.[19]

Amongst a random sample of urbanized Nigerians, using the same criteria, 5 per cent of men and 28 per cent of women were found to be obese.[20] Obesity tends to be more common amongst black South Africans than Nigerians, but it is still less common than in the American and British population. Amongst isolated Kalahari Bushmen in Botswana, who still lead their traditional hunter-gatherer way of life away from all westernizing influences, obesity, as measured by skin-fold thickness, has been found not to exist at all.[21]

In a recent survey carried out in Dudley (Worcestershire, England), 17 per cent of infants were defined as suffering from infantile obesity and a further 28 per cent as overweight. This very high prevalence of obesity was found to coincide with the early addition of solid foods to a full milk intake and a resultant daily energy intake well in excess of that recommended by the Department of Health and Social Security.[22]

Aetiology

Obesity can clearly only arise when energy intake is in excess of expenditure, but a number of factors seem able to influence the mechanism by which food intake is controlled to regulate body weight. Epidemiological studies have helped to clarify some of these.

The relationship of obesity to social class has been studied in some detail. In London, 329 adults were selected from two general practices so as to correspond to the social class distribution of the city as a whole.[23] Figure 2 shows the clear inverse relationship which emerged between social class and obesity in women, with a prevalence among the lower classes (IV and V) which was nearly twice that among the upper classes (I and II). The situation is more complex in men. Work habits of all subjects were studied, in an attempt to explain the unexpectedly low prevalence in the lower-class men as compared with lower-class women. This group turned out to be by far the most active, almost every man being engaged in vigorous manual labour.

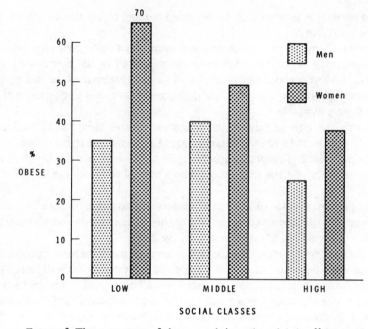

FIGURE 2. The percentage of obese people in each social class[23] (all ages)

There has long been a controversy over the role played by exercise in the regulation of body weight, but there does now seem to be an appreciable amount of evidence in favour of there being a relationship. Mayer has shown that above a threshold of physical activity, energy balance is well-regulated, but below this threshold regulation may fail and decreasing physical activity may actually be associated with increased energy intake.[24] A high level of physical activity may well account for the low incidence of obesity in this lower-class group of men by helping them to overcome the tendency to gain weight with increasing age. In affluent societies, the physical activity of many people falls below a threshold such as the one described by Mayer and the amount of physical activity is likely therefore to play little part in the regulation of their energy balance. A similar relationship between social class and obesity has been demonstrated in America and it appears also to be present in children.

In many developing countries, on the other hand, obesity is more often found in the upper classes and in some societies is regarded as a highly desirable state. In some countries the women are especially encouraged to consume as much food as possible.

The relationship between obesity and smoking habits raises an interesting point of conflict. A large survey in South Wales showed that men over 40 who had never smoked were on the whole nearly 6 kg heavier than smokers[25] (who were already 7 kg heavier than desirable). Men who had given up smoking for more than 8 years were approaching the body weights of men in the same age group who had never smoked. The health consequences of smoking are now well-established. It has therefore been suggested that, because of the inverse relationship of these two health hazards, more information is required concerning the relative importance of smoking and obesity.

There are undoubtedly many other aetiological factors in obesity. Obesity frequently runs in families. In one study, 80 per cent of obese children were found to have a family history of the condition. It is, however, difficult to distinguish between genetic and environmental factors here. In some cases psychological factors play a role and occasional cases are due to endocrine disturbances. Eating habits may also be important in individual cases. People who eat only three times a day are more likely to be overweight than those who eat on five or six occasions. Several surveys have suggested that obese adults and children may actually consume less than controls and here the physical activity factor may be very relevant. In one study, overweight children in a lower socio-economic class were found to eat a greater quantity of carbohydrate than their less obese peers in higher social classes.

Although genetic and biochemical determinants are still not fully understood, studies such as those outlined here do help to identify the sections of the population who are especially at risk and suggest some lines along which the problem might be approached at a community level.

ATHEROSCLEROSIS

Atherosclerosis is a disease process of complex aetiology but there can be little doubt that disordered nutrition plays a most important role. The process may affect any part of the arterial system and is associated with cerebrovascular and peripheral vascular disease, in addition to involvement of the coronary arteries resulting in ischaemic heart disease (IHD). Indications of the nutritional aetiology are based largely upon investigations concerning IHD, and for this reason the epidemiology will be considered chiefly from this point of view (Chapter 19).

Prevalence of ischaemic heart disease

Prevalence of IHD throughout the world may perhaps best be compared by examining mortality rates in different countries as is shown in Table 2.[26] Accuracy of diagnosis and death certification and care with which records are kept vary from country to country and may explain some of the observed differences, but there can be little doubt that mortality from this condition is high in affluent countries. In many prosperous countries IHD is the single commonest cause of death in middle-aged men, in some causing twice as many deaths as all malignant neoplasms, the second commonest cause of mortality in this age group in such countries. Furthermore, IHD is now being diagnosed with increasing frequency among the black peoples of East and Southern Africa amongst whom the disease was previously considered to be exceptionally uncommon, and it is the more affluent sections of these communities that are principally involved.[27] The incidence of IHD is considerably greater amongst Japanese living in California than those living in Japan.[28] There are, of course, certain anomalies in these international comparisons. Sweden can hardly be described as less prosperous than Finland, the United States of America and Scotland, and yet it has a much lower mortality rate.

Table 2. Deaths per 100,000 of the population from ischaemic heart disease in people aged 45–54 years in 1970

Country	Male	Female
Finland	403	55
U.S.A.	346	83
Scotland	343	81
Australia	297	77
New Zeland	273	18
Canada	270	48
England and Wales	259	42
Norway	213	23
Netherlands	201	25
Czechoslovakia	194	38
Israel	194	59
Federal German Republic	148	26
Hungary	146	38
Sweden	137	25
Italy	106	21
Bulgaria	72	26
France	66	12
Romania	61	20
Spain	50	10
Hong Kong	34	12
Japan	34	14

From reference 26

Many attempts have been made to relate death rates from IHD to certain environmental factors and in particular to dietary practices, in order to isolate which factors associated with prosperity might best explain a high mortality rate from IHD. Using data obtained from the 'balance sheets' of the FAO, Jolliffe and Archer found the intake of saturated fat to be the most important factor accounting for the differences in IHD death rates among countries. Animal protein also appeared to account for some of the variability in these rates.[29] Yudkin, however, using similar data, suggested a closer association between sucrose consumption and IHD mortality.[30] This apparent disparity may be explained by the very strong correlation which exists between consumption of sugar and saturated fat ($r = 0.92$) as compared with the relationship between heart disease mortality and sugar ($r = 0.80$) and saturated fat ($r = 0.82$).[31]

Population food consumption figures are notoriously unreliable as they are usually derived from local production figures, imports and exports of a particular commodity and no account is taken of quantities not utilized as food (Chapter 5). In addition, the accuracy with which data are recorded varies from country to country. Actual food consumption by people in defined samples and the diagnosis of IHD by standard criteria in these samples by international teams formed the rather more reliable basis for the correlations tested by Keys and coworkers in 7 countries.[32] The association between sucrose intake and IHD mortality ($r = 0.78$) was found to be greatly reduced when the partial correlation coefficient was computed holding saturated fat intake constant, whereas the association between saturated fat intake and IHD mortality ($r = 0.86$) was not markedly changed when the partial correlation coefficient was calculated controlling for sucrose.[33]

Temporal changes in ischaemic heart disease

It is also of interest to consider the way in which prevalence of IHD may have changed with time. Most older practising clinicians report a considerable increase in coronary arterial disease over the past few decades but it is extremely difficult to quantify this situation accurately. Electrocardiography and enzyme estimation have only been in routine use for a relatively short time and it is possible therefore that myocardial infarction (first described at the beginning of this century) is now simply being diagnosed more frequently. Furthermore, in most countries mortality statistics are classified according to the International Classification of Diseases (ICD) and before 1950 cardiovascular disease was grouped in such a way as to make isolation of deaths due to IHD extremely difficult. In 1950 the Classification was revised and the situation concerning heart disease clarified. Since this time, death rates from IHD would certainly appear to have increased in many prosperous countries and the increase seems to be particularly striking in younger men. Mortality rates from IHD in the United Kingdom since 1950 are shown in Figure 3.[34] It is interesting to note that the rate in young men seems not to have increased after 1965. A similar trend is apparent in the rates of other countries. It would seem then that death rates from IHD have greatly increased but it is difficult to be sure precisely when the increase first started, especially as the atherosclerotic lesion has been identified in corpses over 2000 years old.

Attempts have been made to relate these temporal changes within countries to changing dietary practices. Changes in the American diet over the past 70 years have been examined, with particular emphasis on fats and carbohydrates.[35] A decreasing consumption of total carbohydrate with a greater progressive decline in the intake of complex carbohydrate from flour, cereals and potatoes and a concurrent increase in simple sugars were found to be the principal changes. The increase in fat consumption was slight and due to increase of unsaturated fatty acids. The investigators felt that their data did not fit the hypothesis that low ratios of polyunsaturated:saturated fatty acids have contributed to the increasing incidence of IHD in the United States, but rather that changes in carbohydrate may be a factor. They do, however, overlook the possibility that the increased unsaturated fatty acids may have been hydrogenated. In Great Britain, the main increase in fat con-

110

sumption is said to have occurred during the 1930s, after the rise in IHD mortality is thought to have started, but sucrose consumption would hardly seem to offer an alternative explanation, as the major increase in consumption took place early in the last century.[36] These analyses, too, were based upon population consumption figures. In the United Kingdom, food surveys have been carried out since 1950 which provide rather more reliable figures and an attempt has been made to relate these to IHD mortality subsequent to 1950. Increasing consumption of coffee and a decreased intake of flour emerged as significant factors in addition to the less surprising association between IHD mortality and consumption of butter and eggs.

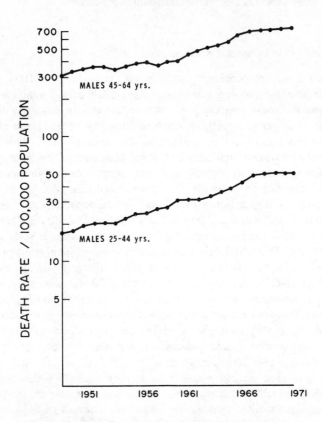

FIGURE 3. Mortality rates from ischaemic heart disease in the United Kingdom since 1950[34]

Many similar studies have been carried out and intake of saturated fat, measured at the population level, appears to be the dietary factor most consistently related to IHD prevalence. However, associations between IHD mortality and intake of different dietary components suggested by studies of this type need to be interpreted with great caution and the meaning of the associations tested by other techniques.

Diet and plasma lipids

It has already been stressed that IHD has multiple aetiology and it seems likely that the role of disordered nutrition may be largely via its influence on plasma lipids. Elevated serum cholesterol levels are associated with the development of IHD and recently it has been suggested that triglycerides may be equally important.[37] It is therefore necessary to consider the epidemiology of plasma lipids in relation to diet.

No other blood constituents vary so much between different people. From New Guinea to East Finland, the mean serum cholesterol ranges from 100–268 mg/100 ml when estimated by the same method in the same age and sex group. In East, West, Central and Southern Africa, levels are low amongst the black peoples who live nomadic or rural existences. Wealthy and more urbanized East and Southern African blacks have levels which do not differ significantly from the white Africans in these countries or communities in the United Kingdom or United States of America. The nomadic people of Somalia, Kenya and Tanzania, whose diets consist mainly of meat, milk and blood have always aroused particular interest since, despite this diet, they have usually maintained low blood cholesterols. It has, however, recently been pointed out that their diet is not in fact habitually high in saturated fat but that intake is subject to much irregularity in food supply on a seasonal basis. In Southern Africa, three different population groups resident were studied in parallel and an association demonstrated between income, saturated fat intake and serum cholesterol levels.

Some apparently conflicting results emerge from a study of serum cholesterol levels in the Pacific Islands. Maori men were found to have fairly high serum cholesterol levels but not quite as high as New Zealanders and Australians of European stock, despite a higher intake of saturated fat among the Maoris. Islanders from the more primitive Pukapuka eat more saturated fat (coconut oil) than those in the more urbanized Raratonga and yet have lower cholesterol levels. Similarly, in Guyana coconut oil is the major source of fat and yet cholesterol levels are low.

In South and Central America and the Caribbean, highly significant correlations have been found between atherosclerotic lesions and serum cholesterol levels and the percentage of total energy derived from saturated fat. The correlations with sucrose consumption and other variables were not significant.

In Israel, no appreciable correlation appears to exist between the current diet of Jewish men born in Africa, the Middle East or Europe and serum cholesterol levels. Mean age-adjusted serum cholesterol levels differed relatively little between the extremes (195 and 219) for North African and Central European Jews despite widely differing diets.

Epstein has pointed out that these seemingly inconsistent findings do not exclude type and amount of dietary fat as the major determinants of serum cholesterol levels, provided one concedes that these are not the only factors which determine the distribution of serum cholesterol levels within a population. It would seem that a diet which is also excessive in total energy, including that from carbohydrate, is an essential corequirement. Another factor which may be relevant is the fact that fat content and composition of animals varies widely. In Uganda, wild buffalo meat contains one-tenth as much lipid as beef from British cattle, and only 2 per cent of the British beef fatty acids are polyunsaturated as compared with 30 per cent of the meat fatty acids from woodland buffalo. Man's tissue lipids approximate the pattern of his dietary fat intake and carefully controlled dietary studies have confirmed the cholesterol-lowering effect of polyunsaturated fatty acids.[38] The amount of physical activity per se would not appear to be a major factor influencing plasma cholesterol levels.

Epidemiological factors influencing plasma triglyceride levels have been studied far less extensively because it is essential that measurements are carried out on fasting samples and because laboratory methods for their estimation are more difficult. In a recent study, exercise, either due to a direct effect or perhaps an indirect effect simply reflecting satisfactory energy balance, rather than diet, appeared to be the most important epidemiological factor influencing plasma triglyceride levels. Physically active, middle-aged men were found to have triglycerides significantly lower than men in the same age group with sedentary habits, despite a very similar diet, social environment and almost identical plasma cholesterol levels. The low levels of triglyceride found in these men did not differ significantly from the levels reported in nomadic and rural-living people consuming a non-westernized diet.[39] A diet habitually high in complex carbohydrate does not necessarily result in high fasting triglycerides and there would appear to be only one report in the literature concerning high levels of fasting triglycerides in rural people who are lean and physically active.[40]

Recently it has been recommended by WHO that elevations of serum lipids should be classified according to the lipoprotein abnormality since lipids (except for free fatty acids) do not occur in the blood in the free form.[41] Only three abnormalities are commonly present in populations. Type IIa is associated with an increase of β-lipoprotein (low-density lipoprotein), the lipoprotein principally responsible for carrying the cholesterol; Type IV with an increase of the pre-β lipoprotein (very low-density lipoprotein), which consists largely of triglyceride; and Type IIb in which both these lipoprotein fractions are increased. All three abnormalities are associated with an increased risk of IHD and the epidemiological factors influencing their prevalence in a community may be inferred from what has already been said about the epidemiology of the lipid fraction which characterizes each abnormality.

Several surveys have now been carried out in order to assess the prevalence of hyperlipidaemia and abnormal lipoprotein patterns. In one recent survey in London 17 per cent of healthy men aged 40–69 and 8 per cent of healthy women were found to have hyperlipidaemia of one of the above types.[42] Estimates of prevalence vary greatly and depend, of course, upon what upper limit of each lipid is regarded as the cut-off point. This is an extremely difficult decision since normal limits are perhaps best defined as below that level at which the risk of developing IHD starts to increase. The findings of the Framingham study (Figure 4) show that when cholesterol levels in men aged 40–49 have reached 260 mg/100 ml, the risk of developing IHD is twice as great as in men with a plasma cholesterol of 220 mg/100 ml.[43] In affluent communities, there are undoubtedly a great many men who have levels at and beyond this point, which would still be regarded by many as within the 'normal range'. The situation here is analogous to the problem of average and desirable body weight and perhaps in the not too distant future it may be possible to standardize laboratory methods for cholesterol and desirable ranges rather than average ranges will be widely introduced.

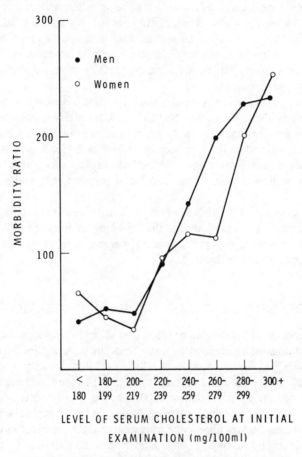

FIGURE 4. Risk of ischaemic heart disease (14 years) according to cholesterol levels: men and women ages 30–49 at entry[43]

Other predisposing factors

In addition to elevated plasma cholesterol (and perhaps also triglyceride) levels, no less than 26 other factors have been found to be associated with the premature development of ischaemic heart disease in the several prospective studies which have now been carried out. Elevated levels of systolic and diastolic blood pressure, hyperglycaemia and cigarette smoking have emerged most consistently. All the prospective studies have, however, been carried out in prosperous countries where mean cholesterol levels tend to be high. Hypertension and diabetes are relatively common in several population groups in Africa amongst whom IHD is rare and it has been suggested that the low plasma cholesterol levels, conditioned by diet, are, at least to some extent, responsible for the immunity from the disease.[44] People classified as obese were previously regarded as being at increased risk of developing IHD. It has now been established that obesity per se is not a strong risk factor, but diabetes, hypertension and elevated plasma lipid levels occur more frequently in obese people and this probably explains the apparent association. The role of heredity may be similarly explained (at least in part) by a familial predisposition to hyperlipidaemia and diabetes.

An inverse relationship has been found in some countries between water hardness (in particular, calcium content) and coronary artery disease, but in others no correlation was apparent. A rapid heart rate, increased blood coagulability, physical inactivity and certain personality types and blood groups are other suggested predisposing factors and may perhaps explain why a thin non-smoker with low plasma lipids, blood sugar and blood pressure may still have a heart attack.[38]

Epidemiological research, while not being able to define all the aetiological agents in IHD, has contributed a great deal to the knowledge of factors which predispose to or appear to protect against the disease and suggests lines along which efforts at primary prevention may be directed.

OTHER DISEASES OF MODERN CIVILIZATION

Cleave has recently elaborated his concept, first suggested in 1956, that many diseases common to western civilization result from the consumption of refined carbohydrate foods.[45] Overconsumption of refined carbohydrate in combination with the removal of dietary fibre and protein is suggested as the fundamental cause of such diverse conditions as diabetes, IHD, obesity, peptic ulcer, constipation, haemorrhoids, varicose veins, diverticular disease and *Escherichia coli* infections. The role of deficient dietary fibre in the causation of IHD and diabetes has been investigated further by Trowell[46] and Burkitt has considered its role in the epidemiology of large bowel disease.[47] As has already been indicated, it is extremely difficult to isolate one dietary factor in ever-changing dietary patterns in different countries, but the evidence in favour of fibre deficiency being an important aetiological factor in conditions such as diverticular disease is impressive[47] and we can expect epidemiological research (and other nutritional studies) to contribute further information in the future.

REFERENCES

1. Society of Actuaries: *Build & Blood Pressure Study,* Vols. I & II, Chicago, Society of Actuaries, 1959.

115

2. *Metropolitan Life Insurance Company Statistical Bulletin,* **41,** (Feb) 6, (Mar) 1, (1960).
3. Khosla, T. and C. R. Lowe, *Lancet,* **1,** 742 (1968).
4. Selzer, C. C. and J. Mayer, *Postgrad. Med.,* **38,** A101 (1965).
5. Goldbourt, U. and J. H. Medalie, *Brit. J. Prev. Soc. Med.,* **28,** 116 (1974).
6. Tibblin, G. *Acta Med. Scand.,* Suppl. 470 (1967).
7. Kannel, W. B., E. J. Le Bauer, T. R. Dawber and P. M. McNamara. *Circulation,* **35,** 734 (1967).
8. Dublin, L. I. and H. H. Marks. *Trans. Assoc. Life Insur. Med. Dirs Amer.,* **35,** 235 (1951).
9. Purcell, J. L. and P. B. Underwood. *Southern Med. J.,* **64,** 961 (1971).
10. Tracey, V. V., N. C. De and J. R. Harper. *Brit. Med. J.,* **1,** 16 (1971).
11. Eid, E. E. *Brit. Med. J.,* **2,** 74 (1970).
12. Lloyd, J. K., O. H. Wolff and M. S. Whelan. *Brit. Med. J.,* **2,** 145 (1961).
13. Asher, P. *Arch. Dis. Childh.,* **41,** 672 (1966).
14. Nelson, W. E. *Textbook of Paediatrics,* 9th Ed., Philadelphia, Saunders, 1971.
15. Tanner, J. M., R. H. Whitehouse and M. Tahaishi. *Arch. Dis. Childh.,* **41,** 454 (1966).
16. Thomson, J. *Hlth. Bull. Edinb.,* **13,** 16 (1955).
17. Marks, H. H. *Bull. New Jersey Acad. Med.,* **36,** 296 (1960).
18. Montegriffo, V. M. E. *Ann. Human Genetics,* **31,** 389 (1968).
19. Robinson, D. Personal communication (1974).
20. Johnson, T. O. *Brit. J. Prev. Soc. Med.,* **24,** 105 (1970).
21. Truswell, A. S., B. M. Kennelly, J. D. L. Hansen and R. B. Lee. *Amer. Heart J.,* **84,** 5 (1972).
22. Shukla, A., H. A. Forsyth, C. M. Anderson and S. M. Marwah. *Brit. Med. J.,* **2,** 507 (1972).
23. Silverstone, J. T. and R. P. Gordon. *Practitioner,* **202,** 682 (1969).
24. Mayer, J., P. Roy and K. P. Mitra. *Amer. J. Clin. Nutr.,* **4,** 169 (1956).
25. Khosla, T. and C. R. Lowe. *Brit. Med. J.,* **4,** 10 (1971).
26. *World Health Annual Statistics, 1970.* Geneva WHO Publications (1973).
27. Seftel, H. C., M. C. Kew and I. Bersohn. *S. Afr. Med. J.,* **44,** 8 (1970).
28. Keys, A. *Fedn. Proc. Fedn. Am. Socs. Exp. Biol.,* **16,** 204 (1957).
29. Jolliffe, N. and M. Archer. *J. Chron. Dis.,* **9,** 636 (1959).
30. Yudkin, J. *Lancet,* **2,** 4 (1964).
31. McGandy, R. B., D. M. Hegsted and F. J. Stare. *New Engl. J. Med.,* **277,** 417, 469 (1967).
32. Keys, A. *Acta Med. Scand.,* Suppl. 460 (1966).
33. Keys, A. *Atherosclerosis,* **18,** 352 (1973).
34. The Registrar General's Statistical Review of England and Wales 1950–1970, London, Her Majesty's Stationery Office.
35. Antar, M. A., M. A. Ohlson and R. E. Hodges. *Am. J. Clin. Nutr.,* **14,** 169 (1964).
36. Greaves, J. P. and D. F. Hollingsworth. *Wld. Rev. Nutr. Dietet.,* **6,** 34 (1966).
37. Carlson, L. A. and L. E. Böttiger. *Lancet,* **1,** 865 (1972).
38. Epstein, F. H. *Atherosclerosis,* **14,** 1 (1971).
39. Truswell, A. S. and J. I. Mann. *Atherosclerosis,* **16,** 15 (1972).
40. Sinnett, P. F. and H. M. Whyte. *J. Chron. Dis.,* **26,** 265 (1973).
41. World Health Organization Memorandum. Classification of Hyperlipidaemias and Hyperlipoproteinaemias. *Circulation,* **45,** 501 (1972).
42. Lewis, B., A. Chait, I. D. P. Worton, C. M. Oakley, D. M. Krikler, G. Sigurdsson, A. February, B. Maurer and J. Birkhead. *Lancet,* **1,** 141 (1974).
43. Kannel, W. B., W. P. Castelli, T. Gordon and P. M. McNamara. *Ann. Int. Med.,* **74,** 1 (1971).
44. Shaper, A. G. *Cardiovascular Disease in the Tropics,* A. G. Shaper, M. R. S. Hutt and Z. Fejfar (Eds.), London, British Medical Association, 1974, pp. 148–159.

45. Cleave, T. L. *The Saccharine Disease.* Bristol, Wright, 1974.
46. Trowell, H. *Proc. Nutr. Soc.,* **32,** 151 (1973).
47. Burkitt, D. P. *Proc. Nutr. Soc.,* **32,** 145 (1973).

CHAPTER 10

Nutrition, Infections and Immunity

Z. L. Awdeh

The overlap in the geographical distribution of malnutrition and infectious diseases
has long been observed by nutritionists and public health officers working in the
field. Because the two factors are mainly responsible for the high infant morbidity
and mortality rates in developing countries, the possibility of an association
between infection and malnutrition has received a good deal of attention.[1-3] Studies
made in several countries have suggested a cyclic relationship between malnutrition
and infections. Infections may precipitate malnutrition and malnutrition in turn
seems to increase the susceptibility of children to infections.

The factors that predispose to malnutrition are very complex and may vary from
one community to another. In general, environments where malnutrition is common
facilitate the spread of infectious diseases. These environmental conditions are
caused by overcrowding, improper sanitation, lack of vaccination programmes,
early weaning of infants and improper food storage facilities (Chapter 7).

Thus, even in the absence of any causal relationship between infections and
malnutrition, children who live in communities where malnutrition is common are
exposed more often to the risk of acquiring an infection as a result of environmental
factors. This chance association will amplify any causal relation there may be
between malnutrition and infections.

INFECTIONS AND NUTRITIONAL STATUS

The tendency of infections to precipitate malnutrition is not difficult to understand.
Most infections have an adverse effect on nitrogen metabolism. Even minor or sub-
clinical ones result in an increased loss of nitrogen and lead to a negative nitrogen
balance. In infections of the intestinal tract, although there is some decrease in
nitrogen absorption due to diarrhoea, the urinary nitrogen loss is the more important factor in the production of a negative nitrogen balance. Such infections have an
effect on the nutritional status of individuals of all age groups. However, this effect is
more evident among young children during the weaning period when infections
could lead to serious malnutrition. Infections also contribute to protein and other
nutrient deficiencies by decreasing appetite and diminishing food intake. Car-

bohydrate and fat metabolism is also affected by infections. Energy requirement in infections could be double the normal due to the increase in basal metabolism. All infections increase the demand on glucose and result in the depletion of muscle and liver glycogen.

An outstanding feature of protein–energy malnutrition (PEM) is the frequency with which it is precipitated by infections. In some cases outbreaks of diarrhoeal disease were followed three to four weeks later by outbreaks of kwashiorkor.[4] Measles also imposes a severe nutritional stress. A number of studies from Africa and South America suggested that measles in undernourished children precipitated kwashiorkor.[5] The association of chronic gastroenteritis and marasmus was also documented.[6] Infections are known to affect the levels of a number of vitamins. Keratomalacia might develop as a result of infections in persons with latent vitamin A deficiency.[7] Evidence also exists that scurvy and beriberi are precipitated as a result of infections in individuals living on diets that are low in ascorbic acid and thiamine.

Acute infections also affect iron metabolism. Chronic infections in general shorten the erythrocyte life span. Malaria and hookworm disease are known to produce iron deficiency as a result of iron loss. Infections may interfere with the metabolism of electrolytes such as calcium and phosphorus and diarrhoea causes potassium and chloride loss. Electrolyte imbalance associated with diarrhoea is of major clinical significance in many developing countries.

In general, infectious diseases result in reduced food intake, alter the metabolism of a number of nutrients, worsen the general nutritional status and may precipitate overt malnutrition in individuals whose nutritional status is sub-optimal.

MALNUTRITION AND INFECTIONS

(a) The Immune Response

The question of the nutrition of the host as a factor in resistance to infections is of great public health significance. If poor nutrition decreases resistance to infections, and infections precipitate malnutrition, then the prognosis of any child caught in this cycle is poor. Since the immune response in man accounts for most of the resistance to infections it is important to ask if malnutrition affects the immune response. This question is not easy to answer. Immunity is difficult to quantitate. The ability to resist disease is a very complex process which involves two main factors.

1. Humoral immunity is the production of specific antibodies following contact with foreign material such as a virus, a bacterium or a toxin. These antibodies, which in man are divided into five classes, G, A, M, D and E, are capable of binding specifically with the foreign material.

2. Cell-mediated immunity is the property of thymus-derived lymphocytes which respond to specific antigenic stimulation but do not secrete antibody. These lymphocytes participate in a number of immune processes such as: rejection of

grafts and tumours, delayed hypersensitivity reactions, activation of macrophages and cooperation with precursors of antibody-forming cells. Methods for the measurement of this form of immunity are complicated and the results are not easy to interpret.

The immune mechanisms also include other systems such as the complement proteins, a set of serum proteins which in the presence of specific antibodies are responsible for the lysis of foreign cells, the inflammatory response which increases the blood flow to infected areas, and the phagocytic cells.

Immunity depends on the cooperation of all these mechanisms and the exact measurement of immunity which involves all of these complex systems is not easy.

The other main difficulty is that malnutrition is a collection of diseases. Vitamin and mineral deficiencies together with PEM produce a mosaic of diseases each with its clinical and biochemical manifestations. PEM, the most common form of malnutrition, is a spectrum of disease with marasmus and kwashiorkor at the opposite ends of a spectrum and marasmic-kwashiorkor in between. The main features of marasmus are retarded growth with marked wasting of muscles and subcutaneous fat and no oedema, while in kwashiorkor the main features are oedema, dermatosis, fatty liver, misery, low weight and wasted muscles with some retention of subcutaneous fat. The immune response in severe marasmus might be quite different from that of mild or moderate marasmus. Also, what applies to kwashiorkor might not apply to marasmus. There are basic biochemical differences between marasmus and kwashiorkor and therefore it is not unlikely that the immune response in the different forms of PEM might be affected differently.

An added complication is the fact that most cases of malnutrition are accompanied by infections, and it is important to distinguish between the effects of pure malnutrition and those of infection on immunity. Furthermore, studies on experimental animals have shown that in some cases deficiencies of specific nutrients were antagonistic to viruses and intracellular parasites. Although such an effect has never been documented in humans, the possibility of an antagonism between some forms of malnutrition and certain infections should not be ruled out.

Studies of cell-mediated immunity in children suffering from kwashiorkor have indicated that this component of the immunological system is impaired. Skin testing for delayed hypersensitivity reactions for a number of antigens seems to be impaired. Lymphocyte transformation *in vitro*, another measure of cellular immunity, was also suppressed.[8,9]

Humoral immunity as measured by antibody response to specific antigens in children suffering from kwashiorkor was reported to be impaired[10] while the levels of the circulating immunoglobulin classes were found to be either low,[11] normal[12] or high.[13] The inconsistent immunoglobulin levels in this form of malnutrition could be attributed to the fact that some of the malnourished children studied were also suffering from infections. Some impairment of phagocytic activity of the circulating phagocytes was found. It would seem that in the kwashiorkor form of PEM the metabolic disturbance is such that some aspects of the immune system are adversely affected.

Marasmus, at the other end of the PEM spectrum, is the most common form of infant malnutrition in Asia and probably in the world. There is evidence to suggest that this form of malnutrition is becoming more prevalent even in areas where kwashiorkor is common.[14] In marasmus blood biochemistry is not remarkably affected. Humoral immunity in marasmus, as assessed by the levels of circulating immunoglobulins[15] and antibody response to specific antigens, seems to be normal.[16] Studies on cell-mediated immunity in marasmus are scarce but it would seem from these few studies that the cellular immunity is either normal or marginally depressed. Although a great deal of work remains to be done in this area, at this stage it would seem that neither the humoral nor the cellular aspects of immunity in marasmus are significantly affected.

The effects of specific vitamin deficiencies on immunity are important. These forms of malnutrition are less common than PEM. Consequently the effects of specific vitamin deficiencies on immunity have received little attention. From the few documented studies it seems that vitamin A deficiency has a serious effect on both the humoral and cellular immunity. It is thought that the high mortality rate of children suffering from xerophthalmia is due to their inability to respond to infections, usually of the respiratory tract. Deficiency of some of the B complex vitamins, particularly riboflavin, was found to result in a partial impairment of humoral immunity. Deficiency of ascorbic acid seems to reduce resistance to bacterial infections.

(b) Susceptibility

The pathological changes that result from malnutrition in general could possibly influence resistance to infections by mechanisms other than the effects on the immune system. Malnutrition may result in an increased susceptibility to infections, by its effects on the integrity of tissues which act as barriers against the penetration of infectious agents. Skin changes due to improper collagen formation are a usual feature of kwashiorkor. The skin manifestations in niacin deficiency are diagnostic in cases of pellagra. In vitamin A deficiency epithelial structures of the eye, the urinary tract, the lungs and the gastrointestinal tract undergo keratinizing metaplasia. Wound healing and collagen formation are adversely affected by deficiency of vitamin C. All of these nutritional deficiencies affect the function of epithelial tissues as an effective barrier against the penetration of infectious agents.

(c) Severity

Tissue mass, mainly protein and fat, is a reserve that provides the amino acids and energy during the course of an infection when the food intake is low, the energy expenditure is high and the nitrogen balance is negative. In children suffering from PEM the outcome of any infection tends to be more serious because of the low protein and fat reserves. This may partly explain why the common childhood infections, such as measles, that leave no permanent damage in the well-nourished child may be fatal to a child suffering from marasmus or kwashiorkor.

PRACTICAL CONSIDERATIONS

Nutrition programmes in developing countries have been very effective in eliminating specific vitamin and mineral deficiencies on a national scale. Unfortunately the impact of such programmes on childhood PEM has not been significant. It would seem that this form of malnutrition will remain as the main problem for a significant fraction of children living in developing countries. In such a situation it is important to know if immunization programmes in these countries are effective. At present it seems that immunization against DPT, poliomyelitis and measles is effective in malnourished children and should be implemented. Immunization programmes in areas where malnutrition is common may also result in some improvement of the nutritional status of the community.

REFERENCES

1. Scrimshaw, N. S., C. E. Taylor and J. E. Gordon. *Wld. Hlth. Org. Mongr. Ser. No. 57,* 1968.
2. A survey of nutritional-immunological interactions. *Wld. Hlth. Org.* **46,** 537 (1972). (1972).
3. Faulk, W. P., E. M. Demaeyer and A. J. S. Davies. *Am. J. Clin. Nutr.,* **27,** 638 (1974).
4. Jelliffe, D. B., B. E. R. Symonds and E. F. P. Jelliffe. *J. Pediat.,* **57,** 922 (1960).
5. Morley, D. C. and K. M. MacWilliam. *W. Afr. Med. J.,* **10,** 246 (1961).
6. McLaren, D. S. *Lancet,* **ii,** 485 (1966).
7. Oomen, H. A. P. C. Proceedings of a conference on beriberi, endemic goiter and hypovitaminosis A, Kinney T. D. and R. H. Follis, Jr. (Eds.), *Fed. Proc.,* **17** Suppl. 2 part. II, 111 (1958).
8. Smythe, P. M., M. Schonland, G. G. Brertor-Stiles, H. M. Coovadia, H. J. Grace, W. E. K. Loening, A. Mafoyane, M. A. Parent and G. H. Vos. *Lancet,* **2,** 939 (1971).
9. Sellimeyer, E., E. Bhettay, A. S. Truswell, O. L. Meyers and J. D. L. Hansen. *Arch. Dis. Childh.,* **47,** 429 (1972).
10. Reddy, V. and S. G. Srikantia. *Indian J. Med. Res.,* **52,** 1145 (1964).
11. Aref, G. H., M. K. Badr El Din, A. I. Hassan and I. I. Araby. *J. Trop. Med. Hyg.,* **73,** 186 (1970).
12. McFarlane, H., S. Reddy, K. Adcock, H. Adeshina, A. R. Cooke and J. Akene. *Brit. Med. J.,* **4,** 262 (1970).
13. Keet, M. P. and H. Tom. *Arch. Dis. Childh.,* **44,** 660 (1969).
14. McLaren, D. S. *J. Trop. Pediat.,* **12,** 84 (1966).
15. Najjar, S. S., M. Stephan and R. Y. Asfour. *Arch. Dis. Childh.,* **44,** 120 (1969).
16. Awdeh, Z. L. and S. Alami, in preparation.

CHAPTER 11

Nutrition and Mental Development

U. S. YATKIN

It has been suggested that undernutrition is the most common disease in the world to affect the physical and psychological development of the child. Pre-school children appear to be the major risk group all over the world. Approximately 300 million pre-school children (60 per cent of the total pre-school population of the world) suffer from some degree of moderate-to-severe protein–energy malnutrition.[1] One can immediately understand the importance and urgency of the problem. The literature on human, as well as animal subjects, shows that undernutrition affects behavioural development. Dobbing[2] and Winick et al.[3] have demonstrated that when undernutrition occurs either pre-natally or during the first two years of life, when brain growth is at its maximum, the damage to the brain cells will be permanent, thus leading to mental impairment.

Other researchers have been concerned with the causation of undernutrition. They have suggested that many causes lead to a syndrome of deprivation. In fact, undernutrition has been mostly associated with the low-income groups, and is more prominent in the developing countries. Cobos and Guevara[4] proposed an interaction between the nutritional status of the individual and his food intake, physical health, psychological make up, family function and social group factors. All these elements are related to one another and to the total system in a manner not yet well understood. The various factors interact and are interdependent. Cobos and Guevara argue, for example, that food intake is dependent upon food availability, size of family, economic status, food habits and other factors. They propose that the psychological damage associated with undernutrition may, therefore, be secondary to a total syndrome of deprivation. Whether or not undernutrition is only a minor member in a total syndrome of deprivation does not alter the fact that is demonstrated in many studies of mental abilities, that undernourished children score lower than their healthy siblings. Furthermore, their scores are directly related to their nutritional status.

Although this chapter deals in general with the area of undernutrition and mental development, some methodological issues of the use of mental tests will be presented. Of particular concern is the use of mental tests in a culture different from the one on which they were standardized. This is critical to the quantification of the data.

MENTAL DEVELOPMENT AND ITS MEASUREMENT

For more than a century, psychologists have been trying to identify and measure cognitive functions in children. Definitions of intelligence were offered implying various degrees of contributions from the environment or from inheritance. Today, however, there is a tendency to consider many causal elements for intelligent behaviour. Those factors currently considered are culture, level of education of parents, family-social condition, the child's opportunities for experience, his needs, motivations, aspirations and biological conditions. Undoubtedly, all these variables are pertinent to the interpretation of the test's findings. However, our problem in the practical sense is to find reliable ways of assessing an index of cognitive functions, and then to try to identify the reasons for the functioning.

It has been argued that it is inappropriate to use a child's obtained score and compare it to a culturally different reference population. This argument is totally valid when one considers IQ scores as a theoretical abstraction. For the purpose of comparison within cultural groups, the obtained numbers serve as reliable indicators relative to the groups, but should in no way be construed as IQ scores. For example, it is nonsense to compare a child from Mexico with an American child on an American test. One might, on the other hand, consider that after appropriate changes are made in the test, it retains some correlative value within the same population. One can further argue that the transformed tests are capable of assessing and comparing the behaviour of children who have suffered nutritional deprivation with children who have not experienced such nutritional stress.

UNDERNUTRITION AND ANIMAL BEHAVIOUR

For many reasons, Dobbing[2] strongly advocates the use of animal experiments to elucidate the human problem of undernutrition and brain development. The most important one is that it is not ethically acceptable to perform certain experiments on healthy human brains. In a series of experiments, he demonstrated that undernutrition leads to growth retardation. More specifically, if this growth retardation occurs during certain vulnerable periods of brain development, it will lead to permanent distortion in the functioning of the adult brain. Zamenhof[5] reported that maternal undernutrition significantly affects brain weight in the newborn rat. In humans, the most rapid increments of brain weight occur in the last trimester of pregnancy,[6] and by the age of one year, two-thirds of the final weight is achieved. It is believed that if undernutrition occurs during that period, the growth of the brain will be retarded and damaged, thus the age of onset of undernutrition seems to be an important factor.

There are many factors affecting learning; among them are the level of motivation, the emotional state, and the value of the reinforcement. If food is used as reinforcement for animals which have been undernourished, it is doubtful whether the reinforcement has the same incentive value as in the control group. Griffiths and Senter[7] reported that protein–energy-deficient rats made fewer errors when running the maze to a goal consisting of a balanced diet than when the reinforcement was a low-protein diet. When compared to a healthy control group, the protein-deficient animal performed better when the reinforcement was the balanced diet. The value of the food reinforcement being greater for the undernourished animals explains the findings of several studies where no detrimental effect on learning was observed.

One possible solution to the problem of incentive is simply to avoid food as a reinforcement. Several studies have utilized a water maze where the reinforcement was escape from cold water.[8,9] Others have used the avoidance of an electric shock as the source of motivation.[10,11] Such an approach seems quite appropriate, except that the effect of early undernutrition and stress tolerance must first be examined. In fact, Levitsky and Barnes[12] reported that rats which have been undernourished during their early life exhibited stronger behavioural responses to a loud noise and to avoidance of an electric shock. Thus, it seems that animals which experience protein–energy undernutrition early in life exhibit greater emotionality when confronted with aversive stimulation. Thus, it is not possible to draw any definite conclusions concerning the relationships between undernutrition and animal performance.

MODERATE UNDERNUTRITION AND MENTAL DEVELOPMENT

Sulzer et al.[13] conducted a study on Head Start children in the United States. They found that children suffering from anaemia, as defined by low haemoglobin or low haematocrit, performed less well on a vocabulary test than non-anaemic Head Start children. These results suggest that anaemic children have a slower reaction time and a poorer level of motivation and, therefore, poorer learning ability. These data do not, however, allow us to conclude whether this effect is chronic or acute.

McKay, McKay and Sinisterra[14] reported that young children who suffer from chronic nutritional and other health deficits in their first few years of life have retarded developmental characteristics which, however, are found to be remediable through treatment beginning in the pre-school years. One might conclude that mild nutritional deficiency during early childhood retards behavioural development but, at least for some forms of undernutrition if treated properly, the damage may not be permanent.

In Beirut we tested a group of 15 children who showed *failure to thrive*.[15] This group was identified according to a low *Index of Thriving* composed of weight, length, head circumference and mid-arm circumference. The children in this group who were suffering from mild chronic undernutrition scored lower on general intelligence tests than their siblings and a healthy control group matched for age, sex, and socio-economic class. Moreover, they obtained lower scores on memory, visual motor, reasoning and social intelligence tasks. On the other hand, they received slightly higher scores on the learning tasks. This difference was not statistically significant. Table 1 lists the means of the three groups and their scores on the various dependent measures. Inspection of the data indicates the overall inferiority of the *failure to thrive* group. The exception of the learning task can be seen to be small in comparison to the other differences.

Table 1

Means and standard deviations for the 6 measures

	IQ	Learning	Memory	Visual motor	Reasoning	Social and intelligence
Failure to thrive	87.7 ± 7.8	8.8 ± 1.5	9.5 ± 1.4	8.6 ± 1.3	10.0 ± 1.6	7.8 ± 2.2
Siblings	94.9 ± 7.1	8.2 ± 2.1	10.0 ± 5.3	11.6 ± 6.9	12.4 ± 6.4	9.8 ± 6.2
Control healthy	98.7 ± 7.1	7.6 ± 1.6	9.0 ± 4.2	11.6 ± 4.6	19.9 ± 12.1	11.3 ± 3.1

From reference 15

In a study of 500 pre-school children in the city of Santiago, Mönckeberg[16] found a strong relationship between nutrition and intellectual development. He studied 3 different groups: Group A consisted of middle-class children who were not under-nourished, and both of whose parents had an average secondary education. Groups B and C were of lower-class children, with parents having an average of two years of schooling. Group B had participated for a period of 10 years in a programme of nutritional supplementation with milk and free medical care. Group C did not receive special medical care. These children had poor physical health with the average height at one year being below the third percentile of the Iowa norms. They reported that in Groups A and B the subnormality rate was 3 per cent and 5 per cent respectively, while in group C it reached 40 per cent. Although these results demonstrate a strong relationship between nutrition and intellectual level, the experimenters did not conclude that the differences in intellectual performance were due only to nutrition. They feel that the extra feeding and medical care programme of group B may have had an effect on the environment and cultural and maternal motivations. These results, as well as the results of other studies, demonstrate the difficulties of isolating the exact effect of undernutrition on mental capacity.

SEVERE PROTEIN–ENERGY MALNUTRITION AND MENTAL DEVELOPMENT

The majority of studies in the area of undernutrition have examined the effects of severe protein–energy malnutrition on cognitive development. There are several factors involved which are believed to have significant effects on the long-term consequences of severe undernutrition: (i) age of onset; (ii) severity; (iii) duration; (iv) health and environmental rehabilitation.

Human studies relating to the effect of undernutrition on mental development present major problems which are not easily overcome. Warren[17] presents a critical review of some of the pioneering studies and examines the methodological problems involved. He cites the studies of Cabak and Najdanvic,[18] Stoch and Smythe[19,20] and several others, where age of onset of undernutrition, severity, duration and rehabilitation were unknown. Furthermore, most of these studies employed a crude matching control group, and when siblings were used only a few were tested. Another weakness of these studies is that undernourished children were selected on the basis of their height, weight and head circumference and very little was known about their previous health background.

For an ideal assessment of behavioural and psychological development in undernourished infants, certain methodological considerations should be kept in mind. It is essential to distinguish between immediate short-term and long-term effects of undernutrition and to trace the patterns of behavioural recovery. Thus it is important to assess the undernourished infant's behaviour during nutritional treatment and recovery, and to assess the longitudinal effects through early puberty. In addition, it is essential to establish well-defined control groups. A matched control reference group should be drawn from well-nourished infants from other families of the same socio-economic class. Healthy siblings in fact may constitute a better control group, whose genetic and environmental backgrounds are more similar. However, it should be noted that such controls come from the same home that led to undernutrition in one child.

Other possible factors contributing to the effects of undernutrition could be the age of onset and duration of undernutrition. Cravioto and Robles[21] suggested that the younger the child at the time of hospitalization for severe undernutrition the less complete his behavioural recovery. This is in line with the views of Dobbing[2] and Winick[3] who stress that the greatest risk to the structure of the nervous system is in the young undernourished organism. Chase and Martin[22] reported that children who became severely undernourished before the age of 4 months showed less mental impairment when tested about $2\frac{1}{2}$ years later, than those who suffered undernutrition after 4 months. Hertzig et al.[23] found no association with age of onset, nor did Evans et al.[24] Yaktin et al.[25] reported an inverse relationship between age on admission and IQ on discharge from the Rehabilitation Unit. The differences between their 3 age groups (birth–6 months; 6–12 months; 12–18 months) were significant at the 0.01 level. In the follow up study 3 years later,[15] we reported no association with age of admission and subsequent IQ. We suggested that this lack of relationship may stem from two major factors. Firstly, older children would tend to have been undernourished for a longer period of time, with a more adverse effect on later intellectual level. Secondly, the effects of undernutrition on mental performance are likely to be more severe during an earlier rather than a later period of post-natal life. These two main factors operate with mutually antagonistic effects. Therefore, the duration of, as well as the age of onset of, undernutrition is a contributing and interacting factor affecting mental growth.

Several further points arise from our longitudinal study in Beirut.[26] The subjects were 55 infants suffering from acute and severe protein–energy malnutrition of the marasmic type. They came from a low socio-economic class, with a family income of about 150 Lebanese pounds per month (about $50). This amount represents a mere subsistence-level income. The majority of the fathers and almost all of the mothers were illiterate. The children were between $2\frac{1}{2}$ and 19 months at admission to the Rehabilitation Unit. During their stay of 4 months, they were tested for mental development every 2 weeks.

Many researchers have observed that the general stimulus milieu of the institution during medical rehabilitation contributes to the overall progress of the subjects. In order to study and control for the stimulation factor, half of the infants, or the unstimulated group (US), were roomed in the usual clinical environment. The other half, the stimulated group (S), received extra perceptual and emotional stimulation consisting of a colourful room decorated with pictures, red curtains and bright-coloured linoleum on the floor. A variety of toys, baby chairs, a pram, a play pen and music were provided for the children. The most important source of stimulation was the warm nurse–child relationship given to these children. Nurses spent a good part of their time with the children, playing with and singing to them. From the point of view of standard nursing and medical care, the two groups were treated similarly. Both groups were matched for sex and age at admission. A control group consisted of 30 healthy children selected according to an *Index of Thriving*[27] from the same community and matched in age and sex with the experimental groups.

During their stay in hospital the children were assessed every 2 weeks for 8 testing sessions on the 1955 revision of the Griffiths Mental Development Scale. This Scale gives a general development quotient (DQ) and measures of 5 mental functions: locomotor, personal-social, learning and speech, eye and hand coordination, and performance. The control group was tested in a similar fashion: 8 times, every 2 weeks.

During hospitalization, both experimental groups (S and US) improved consistently and significantly regardless of the environmental stimulus conditions. The differences between all 8 test sessions were significant at the $p < 0.01$ level. The greatest improvement occurred during the first 3 test sessions, i.e. during the first month that the children spent in hospital. Moreover, the stimulated group improved significantly more than the unstimulated group. The difference became significant ($p < 0.05$) at the fourth session. From the fifth session onward, or 8 weeks after admission, the difference was highly significant ($p < 0.001$). However, despite the fact that both groups kept on improving steadily throughout the 4 months, they never attained the level of the normal control group. The results are presented in Figure 1. The control group kept more or less to the same rate of mental development during the 8 testing sessions. It is of interest to note that, in the experimental groups, of the 5 mental functions studies, the greatest improvement occurred in the personal-social function. The scores for hearing and speech seemed the most retarded over the entire period of recovery.

A follow-up study of 30 of the severely malnourished children and 15 of their controls was carried out 3 years later.[15] The results were compared to their 3 respective control groups: data were collected on 3 additional groups for purposes of comparison with the follow-up data. Measurements were taken with 30 young siblings of the original marasmic group. An additional 15 children with 'failure to thrive' who had never received nutritional treatment, and 15 of their healthy siblings were examined. Of the 30 previously marasmic children, 15 were of the stimulated group and 15 were of the unstimulated. All children were assessed on the adapted Lebanese version of the Stanford–Binet Intelligence Scale. The results presented in

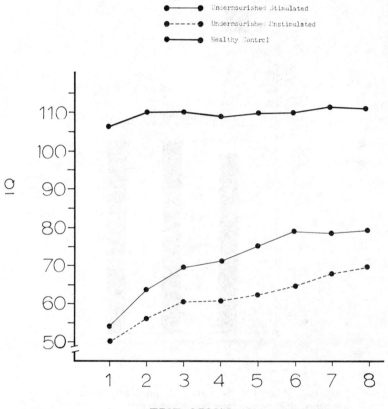

FIGURE 1. Mental development in recovering malnourished children and healthy controls[26]

Figure 2 show that all the previously marasmic children obtained poorer scores than the other groups on general intelligence, memory, visual motor, reasoning and social-intelligence tasks. The best scores were obtained by the healthy children. These results are remarkably similar to two recent follow-up studies of severely undernourished children who were fully rehabilitated.[23,28] Another interesting finding in our study was a significant correlation between the present IQ of previously marasmic infants and their present physical growth ($r = 0.56$, $p < 0.01$).

130

Mental abilities of parents of all children were measured. Fathers had consistent-ly higher scores than mothers, regardless to which group they belonged. Both mothers and fathers of the healthy control group had higher scores than the other groups. This is a significant finding in that recent work related to the effect of home environment and intelligence of children has suggested that the intelligence of the mother affects the language system she employs in her interaction with her child.

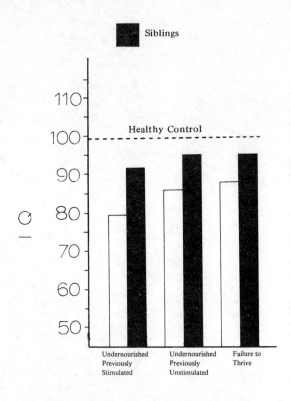

FIGURE 2. Mental performance in previously under-nourished children and their healthy siblings[15]

This is believed to be a critical factor in the development of language and cognitive skills in the child. Thus, the higher IQ of the healthy control group may be the result of the better home environment which the more intelligent mother is providing for her children. This, in turn, may be related to the nutritional state of the family. This demonstrates again that the cause of undernutrition is probably multi-factorial, but it does not change the fact that undernutrition during early childhood has an adverse on subsequent mental growth.

There are large numbers of children in the world who, because of undernutrition and of other social and economic conditions, will not reach their full intellectual potential. Some believe that investments in education are to a certain degree being wasted and suggest that these funds be spent on improving nutritional and preventive measures. Others, however, feel that improvement in education will bring permanent improvement in all social and economic conditions.

REFERENCES

1. Kaplan, B. J. Malnutrition and mental deficiency, *Psychol. Bull.,* **78,** 321 (1972).
2. Dobbing, J. Undernutrition and brain development: The use of animals to elucidate the human problem, *Proc. XIII Intern. Congr. Pediat.,* **2,** 39 (1971).
3. Winick, M., J. A. Bresel, P. Rosco and M. Nelson. The effect of undernutrition on certain control mechanisms of cell division, *Proc. XIII Intern. Congr. Pediat.,* **2,** 53 (1971).
4. Cobos, F. and L. Guevara. Assessment of cognitive development in deprivation and malnutrition, in *Nutrition, Development, and Social Behavior.* Proceedings of the Conference on the Assessment of Tests of Behavior from Studies of Nutrition in the Western Hemisphere (NIH) 73–242, 1970, p. 173.
5. Zamenhof, S., E. Van Marthews and F. L. Margolis. DNA-cell number and protein in neonatal brain: alteration by maternal dietary protein restriction, *Science,* **160,** 322 (1968).
6. Davison, A. N. and J. Dobbing. Myelination as a vulnerable period in brain development. *Brit. Med. Bull.,* **22,** 40 (1966).
7. Griffiths, W. J. and R. J. Senter. The effect of protein deficiency on maze performance of domestic Norway rats, *J. Comp. Physiol. Psychol.,* **47,** 41 (1954).
8. Cowley, J. J. and R. D. Griesel. The development of second generation low protein rats, *J. Genet. Psychol.,* **103,** 233 (1963).
9. Barnes, R. H., S. R. Cunnold, R. R. Zimmermann, H. Simmons, R. B. MacLeod and L. Krook. Influence of nutritional deprivations in early life on learning behavior of rats as measured by performance in a water maze, *J. Nutr.,* **89,** 399 (1966).
10. Frankova, S. and R. H. Barnes. Effect of malnutrition in early life on avoidance conditioning and behavior of adult rats, *J. Nutr.,* **96,** 485 (1968).
11. Barnes, R. H., A. U. Moore and W. G. Pond. Behavioral abnormalities in young adult pigs caused by malnutrition in early life, *J. Nutr.,* **100,** 149 (1970).
12. Levitsky, D. A. and R. H. Barnes. Malnutrition and animal behaviour, in *Nutrition, Development and Social Behavior.* Proceedings of the Conference on the Assessment of Tests of Behavior from Studies of Nutrition in the Western Hemisphere. (NIH) 73–242, 1970, p. 3.
13. Sulzer, J. L., W. J. Hansche and F. Koeing. Nutrition and behaviour in Head Start Children: results from The Tulane study, in *Nutrition, Development and Social Behavior.* Proceedings of the Conference on the Assessment of Tests of Behavior from studies of Nutrition in the Western Hemisphere (NIH) 73–242, 1970, p. 77.
14. McKay, H. E., A. McKay and L. Sinisterra. Behavioral intervention studies with malnourished children: A review of experiences, in *Nutrition, Development and Social Behavior.* Proceedings of the Conference on the Assessment of Tests of Behavior from studies of Nutrition in the Western Hemisphere (NIH) 73–242, 1970, p. 121.
15. McLaren, D. S., U. S. Yaktin, A. A. Kanawati, S. Sabbagh and Z. Kadi. The subsequent mental and physical development of rehabilitated marasmic infants, *J. Ment. Def. Res.,* **17,** 273 (1973).
16. Monckeberg, F. E. Nutrition and behaviour in practical problems in field studies in an urban community, in *Nutrition, Development and Social Behavior.* Proceedings of the Conference on the Assessment of Tests of Behavior from studies of Nutrition in the Western Hemisphere (NIH) 73–242, 1970, p. 107.
17. Warren, N. Malnutrition and mental development, *Psychol. Bull.,* **80,** 324 (1973).

18. Cabak, V. and R. Najdanvic. Effect of undernutrition in early life, *Arch. Dis. Childh.*, **40**, 532 (1965).
19. Stoch, M. B. and P. M. Smythe. The effect of undernutrition during infancy on subsequent brain growth and intellectual development, *S. Afr. Med. J.*, **41**, 1027 (1967).
20. Stoch, M. B. and P. M. Smythe. Does undernutrition during infancy inhibit brain growth and subsequent intellectual development? *Arch. Dis. Childh.*, **38**, 546 (1963).
21. Cravioto, J. and B. Robels. Evolution of adaptive and motor behavior during rehabilitation from kwashiorkor, *Amer. J. Orthop.*, **35**, 449 (1965).
22. Chase, H. P. and H. P. Martin. Undernutrition and child development, *New Eng. J. Med.*, **282**, 933 (1970).
23. Hertzig, M. E., H. G. Birch, S. A. Richardson and J. Tizard. Intellectual levels of school children severely malnourished during the first two years of life, *Pediatrics,* **49**, 814 (1972).
24. Evans, D. E., A. D. Moodie and J. D. L. Hansen. Kwashiorkor and intellectual development, *S. Af. Med. J.*, **45**, 1413 (1971).
25. Yaktin, U. S., D. S. McLaren, A. A. Kanawati and S. Sabbagh. Effect of undernutrition in early life on subsequent behavioural development, *Proc. XIII Intern. Congr. Pedia.*, **2**, 71 (1971).
26. Yaktin, U. S. and D. S. McLaren. The behavioural development of infants recovering from severe malnutrition, *J. Ment. Def. Res.*, **14**, 25 (1970).
27. Kanawati, A. A., N. Haddad and D. S. McLaren. The arm circumference as a public health index of protein–calorie malnutrition of early childhood, *XIV J. Trop. Pediat.*, **15**, 233 (1970).
28. Birch, H. G., C. Pineiro, E. Alcade, T. Toca and J. Cravioto. Relation of kwashiorkor in early childhood and intelligence at school age, *Ped. Res.*, **5**, 579 (1971).

CHAPTER 12

Dietary Toxins

A. H. Hallab and R. I. Tannous

INTRODUCTION

Dietary toxins are usually described as substances naturally found in foods, which interfere in the processes of living cells and tissues. However, one would soon discover the inadequacy of such a definition. Hypervitaminosis A caused by the ingestion of polar-bear liver or seal liver and resulting in acute disturbances to arctic explorers has been documented.[1] Many other substances that normally promote growth also act as toxic substances when found in excess amounts. For example, when the soil is rich in absorbable selenium wheat grown in that soil will contain large amounts of selenium, thereby rendering it poisonous.[2] To add to the confusion, selenium in trace amounts, was recently found to be essential for biological reactions.[3]

The problem of dealing with toxic substances in food is made difficult by the fact that the amount of these factors consumed daily may be extremely small, and therefore no apparent adverse effect may result from single doses. The present review will be restricted to an outline of the major toxic substances that are hazardous to man's health.

ENDOGENOUS TOXINS IN FOODS

These dietary toxins include: enzyme inhibitors; haemagglutinins, the toxin(s) of favism, lathyrogens, cycads and cyanogenetic glycosides.

Enzyme Inhibitors

Foods consumed by man such as cereal grains, legume seeds, oil seeds, egg white and some vegetables have been shown to contain such inhibitors.[4]
˗ The best known and most extensively studied of these toxic factors are trypsin inhibitors which interfere with tryptic digestion in the gastrointestinal tract, and thus alter the nutritive value of dietary proteins. It has been amply demonstrated that antitryptic factors from unheated soybeans exhibit growth-depressing effects in rats

and mice that could not be associated with decreased food intake. Pancreatic hypertrophy has been observed in rats and chicks fed raw soybean meal. Trypsin inhibitors have also been found in a large number of other legumes.

Ovomucoid, one of the constituents of egg-white proteins, has been identified as an inhibitor of trypsin.[5] Commercial egg-white powder may contain the antitryptic factor because it is not readily destroyed by ordinary cooking. However, it has been reported that feeding egg white with known ovomucoid activity has no effect on nitrogen retention in human subjects.[6]

The destruction or elimination of enzyme inhibitors is generally attained by proper processing or adequate heating. The nutritional value of several legume proteins derived from soybean, horse bean, lentils and peas increased upon the destruction of trypsin inhibitor by heat treatment or autoclaving.[7] However, autoclaving other legumes such as peanut, guar bean and common vetch did not improve their nutritive value, suggesting that other heat-stable toxic factors may be present in some legume seeds.

Other enzyme inhibitors have been isolated in foods. A chymotryptic inhibitor, isolated from white potatoes and unusually resistant to heat, acid and alkali, has been reported.[8] The substance inhibits chymotrypsin which mediates proteolysis and milk clotting.

Haemagglutinins

Haemagglutinins, sometimes referred to as phytoagglutinins, are proteins which when ingested agglutinate red blood cells from various animal species. They are widely distributed among legumes such as peanuts, horse bean, soybean, lentils, sweet pea, lima bean, navy bean, kidney bean, fava bean and common vetch. The most familiar of the haemagglutinins is ricin, which is derived from castor bean. Ricin is extremely toxic and must be detoxified by heat before castor bean meal can be fed to animals.

Several investigators have demonstrated the toxic effect of haemagglutinins, isolated from different legumes, on the growth of rats and chickens.[9] A possible explanation for this depression in growth is that haemagglutinins combine with cells lining the intestinal wall, in a similar manner to their combination with red blood cells, causing general interference with the intestinal absorption of nutrients.

Haemagglutinins, like trypsin inhibitors, are heat-labile and are destroyed by adequate cooking of the legumes.

Favism

Favism is a condition that results from the ingestion of fresh or uncooked broad beans (*Vicia faba*) and occurs commonly in some Mediterranean countries.[10] A characteristic feature of favism is haemolytic anaemia, which may be precipitated in certain cases simply by exposure to the blossoms of this legume. It is believed that susceptibility of individuals to this disease is transmitted by a sex-linked gene of intermediate dominance.

Changes in the erythrocytes of susceptible individuals include reduced glutathione content, reduced glucose-6-phosphate dehydrogenase activity, and increased activities of blood transketolase and transaldolase.[11] The identity of the causative agent remains unknown, because of the difficulty of reproducing the disease in experimental animals. It has been claimed, however, that the nucleoside vicine is the active principle of *vicia faba* responsible for favism. When vicine was fed to animals, it retarded the growth of rats (at 0.6 per cent of the diet), induced mild haemoglobinuria in the dog when stomach fed at the level of 0.2 g/kg body weight, and inhibited *in vitro* activity of glucose-6-phosphate dehydrogenase.[12]

Lathyrogens

Lathyrism is a disease in man that is characterized by paralysis and muscular weakness of the legs, and has been commonly encountered in India and countries of the Mediterranean. The disease is generally associated with the consumption of certain peas of the genus *Lathyrus* such as *L. sativus* (chicken vetch) and *L. cicera* (flat-podded vetch).

Two clinical manifestations are associated with the disease, namely neurolathyrism and osteolathyrism. The main active principle that causes osteolathyrism is believed to be aminopropionitrile, BAPN, $(NH_2-CH_2-CH_2-CN)$.[13]

However, other toxic substances have been isolated from vetch that can cause neurolathyrism in rats, mice and chicks. It remains to be investigated as to which of these compounds is the causative agent of human neurolathyrism.

Cycads

Cycads are palm-like tropical and sub-tropical trees. The kernels and the stems of the trees are eaten in south-west Pacific islands in climatic emergencies such as drought and typhoons. The toxicity of cyads has been suspected of precipitating amyotrophic lateral sclerosis, which is characterized by progressive paralysis of limbs and death within five years from onset of the disease. Soaking the kernels in water for several days, with frequent changes of water, may lead to the elimination of the active toxic substance.[14] Pregnant and nursing mothers can transmit the toxic factor, if raw cycads are eaten, to the foetus or through milk to infants, who are most vulnerable to the toxicosis of cycads.[15]

Cyanogenetic Glycosides

Glycosides that yield hydrocyanic acid (HCN) upon hydrolysis are widely distributed in plants.[16] The toxicity of these cyanogenetic glycosides is attributed to the liberation of HCN by hydrolytic enzymes present in the plants.

Amygdalin is a well-known glycoside which is found in almonds and stone fruit kernels. Upon hydrolysis amygdalin yields gentiobiose, hydrocyanic acid and benzaldehyde.

Another example is phaseolunatin, found in lima beans, chick peas and common vetch. Upon hydrolysis, phaseolunatin yields glucose, hydrocyanic acid and acetone.

Lima beans contain the hydrolytic enzymes that liberate HCN from the glycosides if the bean is crushed prior to cooking.

Another important example is the presence of the glycoside linamarin in cassava. Cassava provides a major source of energy to many millions of people of the developing regions of the world. The greater part of HCN is normally liberated from cassava glycosides during processing and cooking; nevertheless, there are often sufficient residual quantities to produce chronic toxic symptoms, and occasionally even acute poisoning.[17]

Since the liberation of HCN from the glycoside is an enzymatic reaction, heat treatment would be expected to render the food non-toxic. However, outbreaks of poisoning from cooked lima beans have been reported in many countries.[17] It is believed, therefore, that this toxicity in humans may arise from the absorption of HCN liberated in the colon through the action of bacterial enzymes.

EXOGENOUS TOXINS ASSOCIATED WITH FOODS

Toxic substances which find their way into our food include pesticide residues, mycotoxins and bacterial toxins.

Pesticide Residues

The extensive use of systemic poisons and potentially hazardous substances in fields to protect crops from pests has justifiably attracted the attention of public health workers as well as governmental regulatory agencies. Attention was further increased by Rachel Carson's book *Silent Spring* in 1962. As a result, a report was prepared in 1963 by John F. Kennedy's Science Advisory Committee.[18] This report pointed out the advantages of pesticides, while at the same time suggesting that there are some risks involved in their application. Pesticides can be divided into two major groups.

(1) *Chlorinated pesticides.* This class includes DDT, Aldrin, Dieldrin, Endrin, Heptachlor, Lindane and Toxaphene. As a group, chlorinated pesticides are the most noxious and dangerous from a public health standpoint. They possess long residual activity, are very stable compounds, are virtually insoluble in water and are fat-soluble, thus find their way into the adipose tissue to exert their cumulative hazardous effect.

(2) *Non-chlorinated pesticides.* This class includes the organophosphate insecticides such as Malathion, Parathion, Methyldematon, Dimethoate and Dichlorvos. Herbicides and carbamate chemicals such as 2,4-D, carbaryl dithiocarbamate, inorganic bromides and arsenic compounds also belong to this category.

Recent studies monitoring the intake and levels of pesticide residues point to the low detectable intake of the organophosphates due to their fast degradation to non-toxic compounds after their application. In direct contrast to this, several studies have shown the persistence and continuous increase in dietary intake of chlorinated hydrocarbons in foods.[19]

Because most of the research work on pesticides is carried out on experimental animals, it is difficult to evaluate the safety of pesticides and extrapolate animal data to humans. Careful application and supervision of these pesticides and their levels should always be maintained, especially in developing countries where ignorance, coupled with indifference and haphazard usage, could lead to disasters of large magnitude.

Mycotoxins

The secretion by some air and soil moulds of certain chemicals as metabolic by-products which become associated in feed and foods characterizes the subject of mycotoxins. Environmental conditions that are favourable for the activity of these moulds include temperature above 20°C, humidity exceeding 80 per cent R.H. and moisture content of substrate not below 8 per cent.

Direct involvement of man by mycotoxicosis includes poisoning by:

   (i) mushrooms, especially by Amanita species;
  (ii) infected cereals with Claviceps species causing ergotism;
 (iii) infected yellow rice with several toxigenic fungi such as *Penicillium islandicum, P. toxicarium, P. citreoviride, P. citrinum* and *P. rugulosum*;
 (iv) infected overwintered grain with a mould belonging to the genus *Fusaria* and precipitating a condition known as alimentary toxic aleukia (ATA).

Mycotoxicosis is characterized by profound blood disorders, hepatoma, degeneration of kidney, heart and central nervous system, and gangrene of the limbs.[20]

Many recent investigations have been undertaken to isolate, identify and characterize new mycotoxins. Aflatoxins derived from the mould *Aspergillus flavus* have been extensively studied. They have been amply demonstrated to cause death in turkeys, chickens and ducklings when the feed was found to contain only a few parts per million of this toxin. Four aflatoxins are recognized at present; Aflatoxin B_1, G_1, B_2 and G_2, the letters being derived from the colour of the fluorescence, blue and greenish-blue when the compounds are chromatographed on thin-layer and examined under ultraviolet light. Other fungal metabolites worth mentioning are the ochratoxins which have been isolated from maize cultures of *Aspergillus ochraeus*. The ochratoxins are toxins as highly potent as the aflatoxins. The liver cells of animals ingesting the toxins show gross fatty infiltration but not the necrosis or bile duct proliferation which characterizes aflatoxins.[20,21]

Animal toxicosis does not necessarily exclude their association with human disorders. A possible aetiological relation between mycotoxins and the high incidence of liver cancer in some African and Far Eastern countries is under investigation.*

   * Editor's note: Aspergillus contamination of glutinous rice is thought to be responsible for the high incidence of Reye's syndrome in Northern Thailand, characterized by liver necrosis and frequently fatal.

BACTERIAL TOXINS

This group of toxic substances can be divided into the following.

(1) *Enterotoxins*. Substances which are formed intra-cellularly by viable bacteria after invading the host. Enterotoxicosis occurs upon the invasion of foods by micro-organisms such as Salmonella and Shigella.

(2) *Exotoxins*. Substances that are usually polypeptides in nature, secreted by the micro-organism outside the host. They cause disease without the presence of the bacteria which secrete them. *Clostridium botulinum, C. perfringens, Staphylococcus aureus* and *Bacillus aureus*, are examples.

Bacterial toxins vary in their effect from enteritis caused by a staphylococcus infection to the more drastic and severe condition typified by gastric distension, failure of the pupil to respond to stimuli, and respiratory paralysis caused by *C. botulinum*. The heat-labile status of both enterotoxins and exotoxins means that cooking proteinaceous foods and refrigerating unused portions suppress the bacteria and inactivate the toxins produced. Proper care and attention should be given to canning foods that have relatively high pH such as meats, fish, peas, beans and corn.

REFERENCES

1. Rodahl, K. Hypervitaminosis A, Norsk Polar-Institutt Skrifter Nr. 95, Oslo, 1950.
2. Rosenfeld, I. and O. Beath. *Selenium: geobotany, biochemistry, toxicity and nutrition*, New York, Academic Press, 1964.
3. Schwarz, K. and C. M. Foltz. Selenium as an integral part of Factor 3 against dietary necrotic liver degeneration, *Am. Chem. Soc., J.*, **79**, 3293 (1957).
4. Sohonie, K. and A. P. Bhandarkar. Trypsin inhibitors in Indian foodstuffs. I. Inhibitors in vegetables, *J. Sc. Ind. Res.*, **13**, 500 (1954). From *Chem. Abs.*, **49**, 534a (1955).
5. Lineweaver, H., and C. A. Murray. Identification of the trypsin inhibitor of egg white with ovomucoid, *J. Biol. Chem.*, **171**, 565 (1947).
6. Scudamore, H. H., G. R. Morey, C. F. Consolazio, G. H. Berryman, L. E. Gordon, H. D. Lightbody and H. L. Fevold. Nitrogen balance in men consuming raw or heated egg white as a supplemental source of dietary protein, *J. Nutr.*, **39**, 555 (1949).
7. Tannous, R. and M. Ullah. Effect of autoclaving on nutritional factors in legume seeds, *Trop. Agr.*, **46**, 123 (1969).
8. Ryan, C. A. and A. K. Balls. An inhibitor of chymotrypsin from Solanum Tuberosum and its behavior towards trypsin, *Proc. Nat. Acad. Sci.*, **48**, 1839 (1962).
9. Liener, I. Toxic factors in edible legumes and their elimination, *Am. J. Clin. Nutr.*, **11**, 281 (1962).
10. Hedayat, H. Natural toxins in foods, beans and favism, *Cahiers Nutr. Dietet.*, **5**, 23 (1970).
11. Bowman, J. E. and D. Walker. Action of *Vicia faba* on erythrocytes: possible relationship to favism, *Nature*, **189**, 555 (1961).
12. Lin, J. Y. and K. H. Ling. Studies on favism, *J. Formosa Med. Assoc.*, **61**, 484 (1962).
13. Rao, S. L., K. Malathi, and P. S. Sarma. Lathyrism, *World Rev. Nutr. Diet.*, **10**, 214 (1969).
14. Yang, M. G., O. Mickelsen, M. E. Campbell, G. L. Laquer and J. C. Keresztesy. Cycad flour used by Guamanians: effects produced in rats by long-term feeding, *J. Nutr.*, **90**, 153 (1966).

15. Michelsen, O., E. Campbell, M. Yang, G. Mugera, and C. K. Whitehair. Studies with cycads, *Fed. Proc.*, **23**, 1363 (1964).

16. Palma, V. R. Hydrocyanic acid content of different varieties of beans, *Nutr. Abs. Revs.*, **43**, 4426 (1973).

17. Nestel, B. and R. MacIntyre (Eds.). *Chronic Cassava Toxicity.* Proceedings of an interdisciplinary workshop, London 29–30 January, 1973. International Development Research Center, Ottowa, Canada.

18. Kennedy, J. F. Use of pesticide, reprint, President's Science Advisory Committee, *Chem. and Eng. News.*, **41**(21), 102 (1963).

19. Duggan, R. E. and J. R. Weatherwax. Dietary intake of pesticide chemicals, *Science,* **157**, 1006 (1967).

20. McLean, A. E. M. and E. McLean. Diet and toxicity, *Brit. Med. Bull.*, **25**, 278 (1969). (1969).

21. Purchase, I. F. M. Fungal metabolites as potential carcinogens with particular reference to their role in the etiology of hepatoma, *S. Afr. Med. J.*, **4**, 406 (1967).

SECTION III

Measures to Combat Malnutrition

CHAPTER 13

Nutrition Policy and Programme Planning

H. GHASSEMI

INTRODUCTION

The science of nutrition was born when the pioneering students of this subject began to recognize the relation between food and health. In the relatively short history of nutrition a number of major developments have been recorded.

The untiring search by leading scientists during the last two centuries has resulted in the discovery of the chemical nature and metabolic role of various nutrients in the body and the daily needs of human beings for these nutrients. This work is still incomplete and a great deal remains to be learned on human nutritional requirements.

Parallel to the advances in basic nutrition, substantial progress was made in the study of clinical aspects. Pioneering work done by outstanding clinicians has provided much knowledge on the clinical profile, aetiology and methods of treatment of diseases due to nutritional deficiencies or excesses.

By means of helpful techniques in analytical chemistry, it has become possible to learn about the composition of foods and rich sources of various nutrients. Advances in this area have served as a basis for some important developments such as dietary intake studies, food supply planning and development of foods.

In recent decades, with the use of nutritional tools and particularly through the application of epidemiological techniques, community nutrition has made its beginning.

Although scientific knowledge is expanding in a remarkable way, its application in assessing the nature and magnitude of food and nutritional problems and genuine attempts for their solution have proved to be painfully slow. This seems to be partly due to the fact that a general 'awareness' in this respect took a long time to develop. Worldwide appreciation of nutritional problems is a recent phenomenon. However, the initial phase of the community nutrition era was limited to an expanding awareness and consciousness of the problems and this was followed by fact-finding efforts. In this phase, assessment of the nature and scope of food and nutrition problems and their epidemiology, ecology and sociology has been the main concern among many developing countries and will remain so for a long time to come. Some countries have made less significant progress than others along this line, but there is no doubt that, on the whole, the vast amount of information which has accumulated within the last two or three decades is of immense value. A great deal has been learnt about human food consumption, nutritional problems of various vulnerable groups, and the causal relationships in precipitation of nutritional problems. The methodology of investigation has improved and there is now a much better grasp of the multi-dimensional nature of nutrition problems while much more is known about food, population, urbanization and health.

Naturally, out of all this increasing information has grown the urge for problem-solving. In the history of the evolution of nutrition this may be described as the Intervention Era.

INTERVENTION ERA

During this era, which dates back to the mid-20th century, various efforts were made to control malnutrition in many developing countries. Nutrition in this era was approached primarily as a Public Health Problem. In the intervention approach the solution was sought through two main channels: increase in food production, particularly protein-rich food, and feeding and education programmes. It was implicit in this approach that increase in food supply plus direct distribution and education to the malnourished would provide an effective solution to the problem.

After two or three decades of experience there is now doubt as to whether intervention of this type will by itself be effective in controlling nutritional problems. Although there is no systematic analysis at hand to explain the failure a number of explanations come to mind.

Nutrition has suffered from a low priority status and a wide gap exists between the nutrition worker and the office of the decision-maker. Therefore, nutrition programmes have remained as a welfare service of very small size with a poor management.[1] Furthermore, overall understanding of the causal relationships in precipitation of nutritional problems has been far from adequate. The causes of malnutrition have been dealt with in a narrow context. Programme formulation has been strikingly non-systematic and nutrition intervention programmes very often lacked clear nutritional objectives. It is interesting to note that, in common practice, a programme often becomes an end rather than a means for achievement of certain objectives.

Even within the philosophy and approach of intervention, there is often a lack of comprehensiveness and entirety in the programmes. For instance, feeding without education, feeding in absence of infection control, focus on one age group and neglect of others, are among such examples. Nutrition assistance is usually offered in isolation from other social assistance and development efforts. Therefore it provides, primarily, for symptomatic, rather than causal, treatment of the problems.

Finally, beneficiaries of nutrition programmes were, in reality, not the vulnerable groups of top priority. A good example is limited nutrition service provided for infants and pre-school children when access is a major constraint. Very often school children become the accessible substitute.

Although intervention did not produce the expected impact in terms of control of malnutrition, there certainly were a number of major accomplishments in this brief era. In spite of its shortcomings, nutrition intervention has been instrumental in providing assistance to millions of needy people under most difficult conditions. Furthermore, significant progress was made on various fronts. As mentioned before, worldwide awareness of malnutrition was created, vast amounts of information on food and nutrition accumulated and analysis of the problem causation improved. Furthermore, numerous institutions for research and training were established and an increasing number of skilled people joined the small core of nutrition workers in developing countries. Further major progress in this era has been the development of capacity and building of machinery for delivery of nutrition care in both urban and rural areas. On the whole, the expansion and improvement in survey, research, training, service and promotion which have taken place since the Second World War will undoubtedly serve as a most valuable basis for future progress in the field of nutrition.

CHANGING CONCEPTS

Among major developments in the field of nutrition in recent times, two are most significant.[2] The first is the recent appreciation of the multi-factorial nature of nutrition, that is that nutrition is determined by the interaction of a number of factors. Inter-disciplinary thinking in the field of nutrition developed as a result of continuous search for a better causal analysis of malnutrition. This has set into motion radical changes in concepts and approaches to the solution of nutrition problems. In the inter-disciplinary context, nutrition has experienced a sudden rise in status and there is no doubt that cross-fertilization among various disciplines has been most instrumental in such developments.

As a consequence, malnutrition began to be seen as a social problem and not purely as a public health problem. Nutrition has acquired a great deal of significance as an instrument and outcome of national development.[3] This is a dramatic improvement over the recent past, when nutrition was looked at as only a relief item within the frame of social welfare activities. Therefore, as a parameter in development, nutrition now has to be integrated into the national development planning process. This calls for application of planning techniques to the problems of nutrition. Even more important, in this context, is the equal emphasis to be given to the treatment of the causes as well as of the symptoms of malnutrition—as a social problem—at the same time. Such an approach represents a drastic departure from the intervention approach in which symptomatic treatment of the problem is focused upon. This brings us to the present era of planning which is the outcome of drastic changes in concepts and approach to the solution of nutritional problems over the last few years.

It is in these recent times, that planning for food and nutrition policies and programmes has been strongly advocated. In fact, food and nutrition policies and programmes are given as comprehensive and effective multi-disciplinary instruments in integrating nutrition into national development.

At present, matters are in a transition state. The trend is towards a full-fledged planning situation, where a unified approach for improvement of the food and nutrition situation in developing countries is expected to become effective. Current changes in concepts and approach naturally open new doors and introduce new difficulties. The prospects are undoubtedly impressive. New trends will help the status of nutrition to rise further. It is also expected to be instrumental in closing the gap between the nutrition worker and the office of the decision-maker. Furthermore, in the new direction in which we are moving, there will be much more room for systematic thinking and practice. As a result of integration into the planning process, there will be a sharp focus on objectives, priorities, selection of alternatives and strategy of implementation. Food and nutrition activities are expected to change from a catalogue of scanty, small and uncoordinated programmes into a single integrated movement of national proportion. Consequently, increasing support for nutrition should be generated. This will result in rapid advances in research, training, organizational development, capacity building and leadership.

On the other hand, we know progress means change and change imposes its own problems. Among the major problems peculiar to our present transition in the field of nutrition, a few merit special consideration. The approach to an inter-disciplinary subject requires clear and constructive communication among the disciplines involved. At the moment, there is a communication problem mainly due to the absence of a language that could facilitate communication at a technically satisfactory level within and among the disciplines concerned. Continuous effort from all sides for development of a medium of satisfactory communication is a fundamental requisite for progress in an inter-disciplinary field. Also, very much related to the communication snags, is a lack of clear understanding of the specific role of each discipline in the new approach. There will definitely be some difficulties in arriving at an equilibrium where balanced emphasis is given to different dimensions of a multi-dimensional situation such as nutrition. In other words, the pendulum should hopefully swing to balance the emphasis with respect to the roles of different disciplines.

The planning and administrative difficulties peculiar to any inter-disciplinary work hardly need to be emphasized. Among such difficulties, particular mention should be made of problems of leadership, organization, simultaneous commitment and financing arrangements among a number of agencies involved. There is another problem in transition which presents itself with a great deal of complexity. That is the desirable pace of transition in various situations. Our ultimate purpose is to have full-fledged and operational food and nutrition policies as an integrated part and parcel of national development plans.

For all practical purposes, we are not dealing with a homogenous situation and the definition of an approach which is both effective and adaptable to various situations characterized by substantial diversity is a great challenge before us.

DEFINITION

Over the past few years a number of definitions have been offered. Changes in definition over time reflect substantial progress in our understanding of the complexity and multiplicity of factors involved in the genesis of nutritional problems.

Johnston and Greaves[4] gave the following definition in 1969:

'Food and nutrition policy concerns the complex of measures which promote changes in food consumption that lead to adequate levels of nutrition'.

In 1973 Ganzin et al.[5] offered the following definition:

a complex of educational, economic, technical and legislative measures designed to reconcile, at a level judged feasible by the planner, projected food demand, forecast supply and nutritional requirements.

Also in early 1973 the Food and Agriculture Organization of the United Nations (FAO), The World Health Organization (WHO), The Pan American Health Organization (PAHO), The United Nations' Children's Fund (UNICEF) and other United Nations agencies concerned in an inter-Agency Meeting in Santiago, Chile, adopted the following definition:[6]

The coherent ensemble of principles, priorities and decisions adopted by the State and applied by its institutions as part of the national development plan in order to supply, in a given time, the population with the food and economic, social and cultural conditions necessary for adequate nutrition and nutritional welfare.

There is substantial difference in approach and substance between the definitions given above. From a nutritional point of view, the ultimate objective of policies and programmes is to arrive at a situation where the nutritional condition of nearly all people in the state is adequate. In this context, it is quite obvious that the definitions given by Johnstone and Greaves and by Ganzin et al. are inadequate. This is because reconciliation of supply and demand of food in the aggregate without prior consideration for distribution aspects does not necessarily solve the nutritional problems. They are also inadequate in an inter-disciplinary context, with their emphasis on agriculture and total neglect of the socio-economic aspects which are equally important in order to ensure sufficient food for the undernourished and malnourished population. As a matter of fact these definitions are geared to nutrition *in* food policy rather than nutrition *and* food policy.

The definition adopted in Santiago is more directed to the inter-disciplinary requirements of adequate community nutrition. Within the frame of this definition balanced emphasis is given to the agricultural, social, economic and cultural aspects. There is one observation to be made that seems relevant to both definitions. It is implicit in the definition given by Ganzin *et el.* that once food supply and food demand are reconciled, in relation to nutritional requirements, adequate nutrition for all would result. However, the definition adopted in Santiago implies that with adequate food supply, sufficient income and proper food habits the problem will be solved. In other words, when the problem of ignorance and poverty is overcome, malnutrition should disappear. This is largely but not entirely true. The best historical evidence is the case of the United States. This is a country where food supply and demand have been reconciled for a long time and desirable social, economic and cultural affluence have been achieved. In such a situation, it was nevertheless concluded after a national survey that considerable nutritional problems prevail in the country[7] (see also Chapter 31). It is further interesting to note that affluence has produced a different pattern of malnutrition in the country. Therefore, it is not unreasonable to argue that malnutrition is not a problem of poverty alone, and the need for promotion of a healthy environment and a healthy life-style should be equally emphasized in a definition.

WORKING MODELS

Three working models have been proposed so far. First, a model proposed by Joy[8] which has been applied in a nutrition planning exercise in Iran by Joy and Ghassemi (1971). In this model estimates of the nutrition gap are derived through quantification of nutritional problems and shortages of specific nutrients among the undernourished and malnourished. This is followed by the determination of the specific kind and quantity of extra food supply—both natural and synthetic, selected by criteria of least cost and acceptability—needed in order to satisfy the nutritional needs of the undernourished and malnourished. As another related part of this model, consideration is given to generating effective demand on the part of the consumers: the malnourished and undernourished. In order to ensure adequate dietary intake, a number of policy instruments such as income, food prices and employment are of special consideration in this context. Simultaneously, intervention programmes to be directed to the vulnerable groups are systematically considered in this model. Furthermore, continuous planning, administration, research, training and evaluation are given proper consideration.

Second, in the working model proposed by the United Nations Inter-Agency Meeting in Santiago,[6] three correlated elements are considered. These are supply, demand and biological utilization of food. Food supply policies refer to governmental measures directed to ensure an adequate food availability in the country, both in quality and quantity, according to the nutritional needs of the population. Major policy considerations on the supply side are to be given to food production, marketing, industrialization and international food trade. Policies related to food demand include the various aspects pertaining to the acquisition and consumption of food. Major policy instruments in this regard are income distribution, employment, food prices, supplementary feeding, consumer education and population policy. Finally, policies related to biological utilization of foods mainly refer to programmes for control of parasitic and infectious diseases which are the causes of nutrient losses. It includes strengthening and expansion of health services, prevention and control of communicable diseases, nutrition and health education and environmental sanitation.

Third, in a model by Berg,[9] a systematic approach to nutrition planning is proposed. This model calls for definition of nutritional problems, analysis of causes, clear nutritional objectives and a systematic approach to identifying problem causes and solutions. Practical application of systematic planning techniques, in the context of national development, is recommended in this model. Also, strong emphasis is given to sharpening of nutritional objectives, rational selection of alternative measures, forceful administration and promotion of applied research.

The three working models given above present different approaches and emphases from a nutritional point of view. The comparison given below is an attempt to focus on the similarities, differences and nutritional significance that they present. In the beginning it should be pointed out that any given population at a given time consists, in terms of nutritional status, of three categories (Figure 1).

(O) The overnourished.

(A) The adequately nourished.

(U & M) The undernourished and malnourished.

The size and characteristics of the population in each category vary according to the circumstances. Nutritionally speaking, the ultimate purpose of nutrition policy is to arrive at a situation where almost all the population is brought to and maintained in a satisfactory state. This is the same as bringing categories (O) and (U & M) of the population to join category (A). In the dynamic situation of real life, there is most probably a constant movement of the population from one category to another. The process of nutritional improvement should continuously enlarge the relative size of category (A).

In comparing the above three working models, it becomes evident that the Santiago model takes the entire spectrum of population as its terms of reference in planning. In this model, a comprehensive food policy designed for feeding the entire population and concomitant, nutritional improvement is the focus of attention. Therefore, the approach here centres on food policy, of which nutrition is only one dimension. Attention to the problems of the overnourished may be implicit but certainly not explicit, in this model.

In contrast, the models proposed by Joy and Berg both concentrate on the malnourished and undernourished. In other words, the reference population in these models is limited to category (U & M) of Figure 1. They are both nutrition-policy oriented and do not explicitly include a food-policy dimension for the entire population spectrum. Also, they both consider nutrition in the context of poverty. It is important to note that these models both focus on nutrition intervention in a modern sense. That is to say that both causal and symptomatic treatment of malnutrition are taken into account. Furthermore, these models provide for integration of nutrition into national development planning. It should be noted that Joy's model goes one step further; and that is identification and quantification of food supply and demand to be generated for nutritional improvement purposes. Actually this model includes a food-policy component specifically geared to the fulfilment of nutritional objectives.

As mentioned before, lack of proper consideration for the problems of overeaters is one shortcoming of all these working models. This is due to the fact that these

150

models focus so much on poverty, and therefore on socio-economic aspects, while the problems of the affluent are obviously of a different nature. It is true that the relative size of the affluent population in developing countries is small. Still, in a comprehensive model and in the long run this matter should not be overlooked.

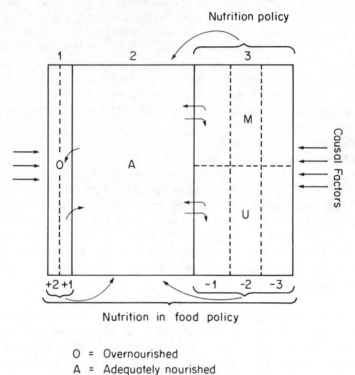

FIGURE 1. Static classification of population in terms of nutrition status for definition purposes[10]

It is fairly clear by now that each of these models has certain weak and strong points. The most important factor is the possibility of application under the difficult conditions of the many developed countries. For instance, the Santiago model is the most difficult in terms of immediate practical application. That is because, first, it requires complete and comprehensive data on food, agriculture, nutrition and health, and other social and economic aspects. Second, a fairly advanced planning and administrative machinery is necessary for application of this model. Third, it moulds nutrition deeply into the total development process. Therefore, in the absence of strong political commitment to a poverty-focused planning it may even become counterproductive so far as nutrition is concerned.

There has already been some warning on the practical aspects of various approaches proposed. Pines,[11] in referring to the political, technical, administrative and coordination barriers involved in the formulation and implementation of a national nutritional plan, proposes a review and advocacy approach. This approach calls for short-term improvement of nutrition through systematic review of government policies and programmes by well-placed nutrition advocates which would ensure necessary adjustments for nutrition purposes.

THE NUTRITION PLANNING SEQUENCE

The planning sequence would be somewhat different depending on which of the three working models is to be applied. Making plans for national nutrition improvement is not a very difficult task. It is the successful implementation of plans and programmes that presents the real challenges. The whole process of planning and action can become a success only if it begins with a genuine commitment on the part of the government and the public at various levels. In the following lines Berg[12] has ably described the nature and depth of commitment required before the formulation of nutrition plans is attempted.

Nutrition programme planning begins with the assumption that the decision maker recognizes the problem, is aware of its relationship with broad national objectives, accepts the notion that good nutrition can be an investment in human capital, analogous to education, and has decided to give increased attention to the nutrition sector. However, it is based on the premises that malnutrition will not be alleviated widely or quickly under current development policies and trends, that important shifts in policies and practices may be required to effect changes, and that the scope of such shifts may involve many people, activities and entities, not now regarded as part of the nutrition universe.

The following sequence is essentially an adaptation of established planning techniques and is quite in line with Berg and Joy's working models.

DEFINITION OF THE PROBLEM

The aim is to assess the nature, size and distribution of the nutritional problems. In determining the distribution aspects, it is most important to classify explicitly the population at risk in terms of ecologic, demographic, geographic and socioeconomic characteristics. In practical terms, such problem definition amounts to a set of answers to the following questions: What are the specific nutritional deficiencies? How severe are they? Who is affected and where are they? What are the trends? Information on dietary intake, clinical, biochemical and anthropometric measurements, consumer expenditure survey, agriculture and vital statistics and food balance sheets are to be used for this purpose (Chapters 5 and 6).

Although the technique is fairly straightforward, invariably data are scarce and incomplete. Whatever is available is not always comparable and it is based on poor samples and inadequately presented. This is party due to poor survey planning and partly because of inadequacies in survey methodology. In this situation difficulties should be expected particularly in problem quantification and assessement of trends. Needless to say, improvements in data collection and problem assessment are to be considered as a part of the national nutrition plan.

CAUSAL ANALYSIS

For intervention purposes, it is essential to know the determinants of the problems and the causal relationships involved. In a causal analysis three strata of causes of malnutrition have been described.[12] The most immediate causes, from the health point of view, are insufficient nutrient intake, poor utilization of nutrients and increased nutritional needs due to infection. At the other extreme are such factors as general inadequacy of national resources, rapid population growth, and the entire causes of underdevelopment. In between these two strata, which is the area in which a nutrition planning analysis should concentrate, lie those socio-economic factors directly influencing diet and utilization that can possibly be manipulated to improve nutritional status.

Determining factors are classified by Call and Levinson[13] into direct and indirect. For instance, food deficiency is a direct factor, while low purchasing power, commodity prices and poor selection may be amongst the indirect factors in precipitation of a nutrition deficiency.

On many occasions, causal analysis is found to be of a general type. For instance, poverty, ignorance, shortage of food, etc. are given as the causes. For practical planning purposes, systematic and quantitative analysis in depth is required. There are always a number of determinants and their relative weight and relationships should be known. Causal analysis should focus strongly on major determinants of nutritional status, in particular the malnourished and undernourished population, and be subject to policy levers. This approach would be valuable in pinpointing the links in the chain of causation, where intervention might effect changes for better nutrition.

As a part of the causal analysis, Joy and Berg[8,12] have both proposed nutritional profile studies, as a useful tool in designing intervention measures. The nutritional profile is an analytical description of important variables which characterize a population group and determine its nutritional status. For example, low-income small farmers, urban poor and landless agricultural labourers have their own typical profiles in which certain determinants of nutritional status, peculiar to that particular system, are to be described.

PRELIMINARY STATEMENT OF BROAD OBJECTIVES

Once the scope and nature of the problem are defined and both immediate and distant causes become relatively clear, the possible nutritional objectives should be identified. Objectives should be specific, numerical and ambitious at first sight. The sources required in order to achieve objectives are to be defined as sub-objectives. In defining the objectives, selection of targets is an important element. Should the programmes be directed to the infant, pre-school child, school child, the pregnant woman or, more realistically, which combination of these groups?

There are three important considerations in defining a meaningful objective; (i) giving a specific and numerical target, (ii) it must have a time frame, and (iii) an estimation of resources is required, provision of which will become sub-objectives. For instance, production of special foods, control of infection or necessary leglisation become sub-objectives in the control of child malnutrition. In short, increasing precision in the definition of objectives ensures a systematic approach to the analysis and formulation of action programmes. In this context, the following is an example of a clearly described objective:

Reducing from thirty per cent to twenty per cent the number of children below three years of age suffering from all degrees of malnutrition within three years beginning on a specified date when the plan operation commences.

In this case, components of the programme such as training or the development of special foods become sub-objectives. While a statement of objectives is explicit in Berg's model, it is only implicit in the model proposed by Joy.

IDENTIFICATION AND COMPARISON OF ALTERNATIVE MEASURES

When the problem is defined, its anatomy is known, and its broad objectives are stated, alternative possible measures to be taken in controlling the problem should be identified and compared in terms of their cost and relative effectiveness. Alternative measures are obviously influenced by the frame of analysis and the working model to be chosen. For instance, Call and Levinson[13] refer to variability in intervention measures with regard to cost, nutritional effectiveness, acceptability and administrative viability. Intervention measures also differ with respect to the time frame, selection of target and presence or absence of economic and social multipliers.

Interventions of a long-term nature, such as education and fortification, are more commonly applied in developed countries. Short-term measures such as child-feeding are more peculiar to developing countries. Intervention may attempt to reach only a selected group. This is called a 'target approach' like child-feeding. By contrast, there is a 'blanket approach' in which the selected group may be reached by covering the entire population. Food fortification is an example of blanket approach in intervention. Table 1 shows the long-run and short-run intervention approaches.

In Joy's working model (Figure 2) there is a specific component spelled out in intervention that may be called 'Food-Policy Component' of a nutrition plan. That is

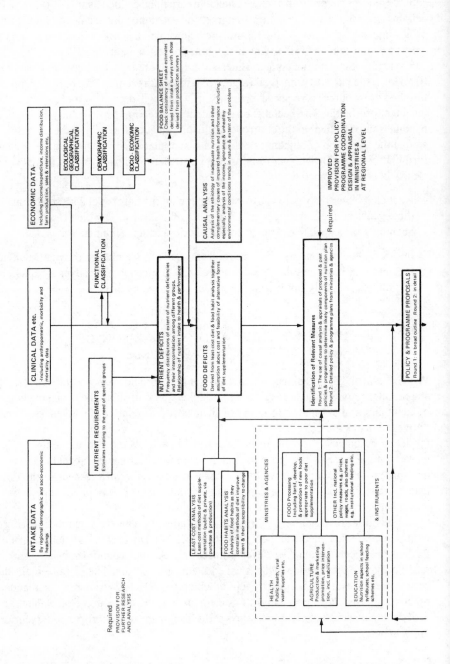

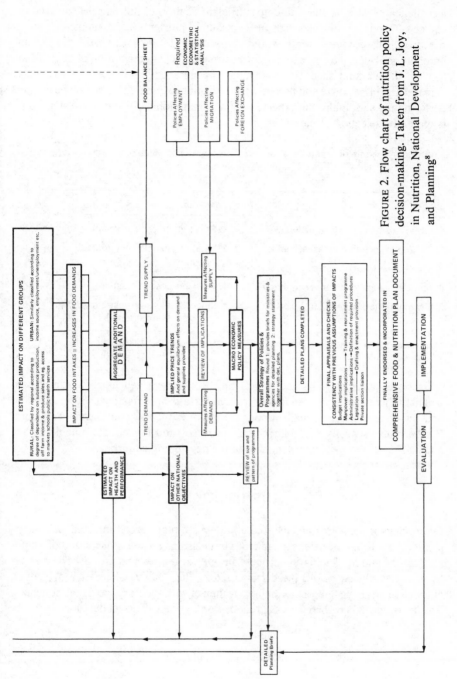

FIGURE 2. Flow chart of nutrition policy decision-making. Taken from J. L. Joy, in Nutrition, National Development and Planning[8]

a sequence of various steps aiming at (i) identification of nutrient deficiencies; (ii) choice of foods or other sources of the required nutrient intake supplementation, based on least-cost diet analysis and study of food habits; (iii) estimation of additional food supply for nutritional improvement; (iv) augmentation of demand for food by the malnourished; (v) assessment of general equilibrium effects on supply, demand and prices. Size and pattern of intervention, estimated impact on health and performance and finally the expected impact on national objectives are steps to be taken in the selection of measures.

Table 1. Long-run versus short-run interventions: 'blanket' versus 'targeted' approaches[a]

Long-run	Short-run
1. Increasing per capita income (blanket)	1. Government price intervention (blanket)
2. Commodity supply increases (blanket)	2. Rationing (blanket or targeted)
3. Plant breeding for nutritive quality (blanket)	3. Child-feeding (targeted)
4. Nutrition education (blanket or targeted)	4. Food fortification (blanket)
5. Environmental sanitation (blanket)	5. Innoculations and mass anti-parasitic programmes (targeted)

[a] Taken from Call and Levinson in *Nutrition, National Development and Planning*, Berg *et al.* (Eds.) 1973. Page 172 (Ref. No. 13).

Proposed alternative measures will have to be reviewed against several constraints inherent in a particular country and certain circumstances. Budgetary and political constraints are usually among the major elements to be taken into account. Furthermore, scarcity of management resources and inadequate machinery are among major limiting factors in most of the developing countries.

THE DECISIONS

Once relevant measures are selected and detailed plans are completed, a final appraisal is made and decisions are taken. The decisions are made as a result of a complex debate and an eliminating process among various interest groups. The planner by now has placed before the decision-maker the options, alternative objectives, alternative strategies and potential programmes with their expected consequences. The decision-maker, therefore, is in a position to make rational decisions.

IMPLEMENTATION

A nutrition plan is only as good as its implementation. Success in implementation depends on strong leadership, sound organization and administration, extensive training and research, and continuous planning. At present, experience in nutrition administration is quite limited, and, in fact, development of effective implementation machinery within the administrative hierarchy needs at least as much attention as is being given to planning. In a broad sense, the complete national nutrition machinery should have three wings: political endorsement, planning and implementation. The wing for political endorsement is envisaged in the form of a high-level inter-ministerial body. Inter-ministerial Councils for food and nutrition have been established in many countries. These Councils are often meant to produce coordinated food and nutrition policies and plans but frequently little or no technical support is given to them. It is totally unrealistic to expect a council or committee made up of high-level political figures, without adequate technical staff support and in isolation from national planning machinery, to succeed in producing plans and programmes. It is for these reasons that Councils of this nature have rarely been functional.[8,10] Bodies of this type could become more effective if they were primarily concerned with political endorsement of the proposed plans and programmes. In this case, technical aspects of nutrition planning should become the responsibility of a planning body to be established as a part of the national planning machinery. Planning is to be considered a continuous process. In the same context, national nutrition research strategy is to focus on finding those facts that are most needed for plan and programme formulation, effective operation and evaluation. The planning body should include a variety of expertise in subjects such as nutrition, economics, health, agronomy, sociology and statistics.

The executive side consists of nutrition units in the various ministeries most concerned with nutrition, such as health, agriculture, education. A somewhat similar network would be required at a provincial level for programming, implementation and evaluation. Within the national network, room should be made for advocates of nutrition to be placed at the highest possible level in order to build strong leadership within the system.

Development of leadership and large-scale administrative capacity largely depends on innovation and expansion of training activities. Actually, there is need for a radical change in approach to training in nutrition. Training of this kind should aim at producing nutrition practitioners, prepared to accept totally new responsibilities. So far, training programmes offer a great deal in nutrition science and very little in nutrition practice.

Finally, there are other aspects of implementation such as financial management, procedures and legislation, to which proper attention should be given.

EVALUATION

Evaluation is the measurement of the degree to which the original objectives have been accomplished. It measures the actual performance, it informs the planner of weaknesses, need for adjustments and further research and how costs and benefits compare under operating conditions. In other words, evaluation provides for improvements from one planning cycle to the next. It is very important that evaluation

158

should be built into the design and operation of a programme and that the data required for this purpose are automatically generated. Evaluation is the element which no one opposes but generally it receives very little attention.[14]

REFERENCES

1. The Food and Agriculture Organization of the United Nations. Food and nutrition: A new view of an old problem, *Nut. Newsletter*, **11**, 4 (1973).
2. Ghassemi, H. Changing concepts in nutrition, *Proceedings International Conference on Social Sciences, and Problems of Development*, Persepolis, Iran, May 1974 (in press).
3. Barg, B. Nutrition and national development, in Berg, A. Scrimshaw, N. and D. Call (Eds.), *Nutrition, National Development and Planning*, Cambridge, Mass., MIT Press, 1973, p. 49.
4. Johnston, B. F. and J. P. Greaves. Food and nutrition policy, FAO, Rome, 1969, *Nutrition Studies*, No. 22.
5. Ganzin, M. In Rechcigl, M. *Man, Food and Nutrition*, London, CRC Press, 1973.
6. FAO/WHO/PAHO/UNESCO/UBICEF/ECLA Inter-Agency Consultant Meeting on Food and Nutrition Policy, Santiago, Chile, 1973.
7. Center for Disease Control, Ten-State Nutrition Survey 1968–1970, U.S. Department of Health, Education and Welfare, Atlanta, Georgia.
8. Joy, L. Nutrition intervention programs: Identification and selection, in Berg, A. Scrimshaw, N. and D. Call (Eds.), *Nutrition, National Development and Planning*, Cambridge, Mass., MIT Press, 1973, p. 198.
9. Berg, A. and R. Muscat. Nutrition program planning: An approach, in Berg, A. Scrimshaw, N. and D. Call (Eds.), *Nutrition, National Development and Planning*, Cambridge, Mass., MIT Press, 1973, p. 247.
10. Ghassemi, H. Nutrition policy and program planning, in *WHO/FAO/UNESCO/UNICEF/ Second Regional Seminar on Food and Nutrition*, Beirut, September 1973, p. 113.
11. Pines, J. *Review and Advocacy, First Steps in Nutrition Planning*, PAG Doc. No. 1. 17/13, May 1974.
12. Berg, A. *The Nutrition Factor: its Role in National Development*, Washington D.C., The Brookings Institution, 1973, p. 233.
13. Call, D. and F. J. Levinson. A systematic approach to nutrition intervention programs, in Berg, A. Scrimshaw, N. and D. Call (Eds.), *Nutrition, National Development and Planning*, Cambridge, Mass., MIT Press, 1973, p. 165.
14. Wray, J. D. Evaluation: Everybody talks about it, in Gyorgy, P. and O. Kline (Eds.), *Malnutrition is a Problem of Ecology*, S. Karger, Basle, Switzerland, 1970, p. 144.

CHAPTER 14

New Sources of Food

N. W. PIRIE

New sources of food are of three fairly sharply distinguishable types: foods that are familiar in some communities but would be regarded as new elsewhere, foods that are often eaten in small amounts but that would be regarded as new if eaten in quantity, and foods that are not now eaten anywhere. The first type raises fewest problems. These foods are clearly neither intrinsically unacceptable nor a serious health hazard. They may, however, be minor health hazards and deserve close scrutiny before their more widespread use is advocated. We are not concerned here with plants such as some species of *Lathyrus* or *Argemone* that are eaten only in emergency or through inadvertence, but with those such as the djenkol bean which is esteemed, and *Cycas* flour which is a staple, though each is hazardous. Fortunately, plants in this group do not seem to have any particular merits that make their more widespread use probable. Individuals are sensitive to certain foods, e.g. the sensitivity to wheat and rye in sufferers from coeliac disease. In regions where such sensitivity is widespread, e.g. in the Eastern Mediterranean where favism (sensitivity to broad beans) is common, the introduction of a food that is safe elsewhere may be unwise. This is an argument for diversifying rather than restricting the diet. Some commonly used methods of preservation are in a different category. There is good reason to suspect that some methods of fermentation used with cassava and fish, and some methods of preservation by smoking, are not without risk. The argument that because a certain type of food is traditional it is therefore safe should be examined in the light of the local health statistics.

The production of food, from both traditional and new sources, depends on various inputs. The four most important are energy, water, carbon and nitrogen. Foods must also contain elements such as phosphorus, sulphur and several metals, but the amounts needed are between a tenth and a millionth of the amount of carbon and nitrogen needed therefore, except perhaps for phosphorus, few problems are likely to arise over the world supply though there are well-known regional deficiencies. Sunlight is the main source of energy and will continue to be so for the foreseeable future. It is abundant, but is used inefficiently in conventional agriculture. An important reason for envisaging new sources of food is that their use may open the way for more efficient systems of agricultural photosynthesis. Modern agriculture also depends on large injections of energy other than sunlight. It is salutary to remember that a farmer in New Guinea gets 11 times as much energy from the sweet potatoes he grows as he expended in clearing and cultivating the land,[1] whereas there is as much energy in the oil fuel used by an up-to-date farmer as in the edible part of the crop grown. New sources of food are particularly important if they enable sunlight to be used more efficiently, if they use up smaller amounts of increasingly expensive fossil fuels, and if they make more complete use of all the products of photosynthesis.

SOURCES THAT ARE EDIBLE AFTER MINIMAL PROCESSING

Vegetables

Leaves are used throughout the world, from the far North where the rumen contents of reindeer are eaten, to tropical deserts where the most abundant vegetation may be buds from bushes. But the amount eaten is rarely as great as is nutritionally desirable. Two groups of countries are contrasted in Table 1 and it is clear that

Table 1. Grams of protein, per head per day, supplied by commercially grown vegetables

Chile	3.3	Brazil	0.5
France	5.0	Ceylon	2.0
Israel	3.7	Denmark	1.7
Italy	5.1	Guatemala	1.0
Japan	5.1	India	0.1
Portugal	7.8	Mexico	0.4
U.K.	2.6	Nigeria	1.1
U.S.A.	3.8	Venezuela	0.2

From FAO Production Yearbook 1971, Table 137.

vegetables tend to be eaten less in those countries most in need of improved food supplies. Dark green leafy vegetables (DGLV) are not distinguished from the others in published figures, but a few show that some communities get 5–10 g of protein per head per day from DGLV. In other communities their use is declining. This is partly a consequence of urbanization; it is mainly a consequence of the declining prestige of vegetables. An increased consumption of DGLV in those countries where they are eaten rarely would be, in effect, the introduction of a new source of food. The first reaction of agricultural advisers to the suggestion that there should be an increase in market gardening in a tropical region is to import seeds of species and varieties cultivated in Europe and North America. This is unlikely to be the best policy. Species such as *Basella,* or *Amaranthus,* even in their present semi-wild state, probably do better than imported varieties and they will do better still after some skilled selection. One reason for expecting this is that many indigenous tropical vegetables have a photosynthetic mechanism which enables them to use strong light better than temperate zone plants.

DGLV have been strongly advocated as sources of carotene (pro-vitamin A). This role is undoubtedly important but should not overshadow their role as protein sources (they contain 20–30 per cent of true protein in the dry matter) nor as the most productive way of using land. Comprehensive results are seldom published from which yields can be calculated. In Britain the annual protein yield can be more than 1 ton per ha;[2] in Nigeria it can be 3–6 tons per ha.[3] These yields greatly exceed the yields of protein concentrate from any conventional form of agriculture.

For more than 30 years, and in several countries, there has been active research on *Chlorella* and other green algae in the hope that they would produce food by photosynthesis more cheaply and abundantly than the higher plants. Algal products are available commercially as pharmaceutical and flavouring agents, and a mixture of algae and bacteria grown in sewage is produced as animal feed. The blue-green alga *Spirulina* is produced commercially in Mexico and elsewhere. It shows promise as a human food because it grows in saline and alkaline water that would not otherwise be used, and because it is a traditional food in Mexico and parts of Africa.

Seeds

Cereal seeds are now the main source of food and they are likely to remain so. Many of the new varieties contain 15–20 per cent protein whereas the older varieties contained only 7–12 per cent. This increase in protein is usually the result of changes in the ratios in which the component proteins occur in the grains;[4] that change may affect cooking quality. Thus, strains of maize (*Zea mays*) with increased lysine are said not to make tortillas with the familiar texture. In spite of these changes in quality, the new varieties will probably soon become acceptable, as will species such as *Sorghum,* that are unfamiliar in most regions, and the new wheat/rye hybrid (*Triticale*).

The recent dramatic increase in the yields attainable with well-manured cereals, the 'green revolution', has led in several countries to an unfortunate diminution in the area devoted to seed legumes. There is now a welcome increase in interest in them[5,6] and recognition that the existing varieties were primarily selected by farmers because they would give a moderate yield in adverse conditions.[7] This resistance to adversity explains the otherwise surprising cultivation of *Lathyrus* in India in spite of the toxicity of some varieties. Most of the other species of seed legumes are slightly toxic, perhaps because the toxic substances help to protect the seeds from insect and fungal attack. With improved conditions of cultivation and storage, this protection will be less advantageous, so that plant breeders can try to produce varieties that do not need fermentation or prolonged cooking to render them safe when eaten in quantity. In climates where there is a period of drought or cold weather the seeds must be allowed to ripen and produce a dry storable product. The yield is, however, often as great, but reached more quickly, if the seeds are harvested green[8] and the yield may be even greater if the perishable green pod is eaten and not the seed only.

There is scope for research on the improvement of seeds from plants other than the cereals and legumes. In parts of France and Italy chestnuts (*Castanea*) are a useful source of starch; in Bolivia, the seeds of *Quinoa* are eaten and those of another chenopodium, *C. nutalliae*, in Mexico. Chenopodium seeds were at one time eaten in western Europe; they may be worthy of reinvestigation because they tend to be richer in protein than cereal seeds and it may be possible to select varieties that would yield both seeds and edible leaves. Remembering what has been achieved in turning wild grasses into cereal crops, there is no reason to assume that similar potential is not latent in many other groups of plants. Any such uncovering will be slow; in the meantime, the non-cereal and non-legume seeds that contribute significantly to human feeding do so after some form of processing, e.g. cotton seed and rape.

SOURCES FROM WHICH EDIBLE PRODUCTS CAN BE MADE BY MECHANICAL FRACTIONATION

There is no novelty about extracting sugar and oils mechanically from inedible material, and the amount of novelty involved when dried starchy products are produced from sources such as cassava and potato is small. Attention in this section is therefore concentrated on protein sources.

Leaves

Human food is not at present made on a commercial scale by fractionating leafy crops. They are discussed first, partly because the leaf is the main site of photosynthesis, and partly because leafy crops are potentially the most abundant source of food protein. Protein is extracted by pulping the fresh forage and pressing, the extract is then coagulated, and the protein is filtered off and washed if necessary. Such simple equipment is used that leaf protein could be made in a village or a large farm. Material made in laboratories is used in demonstrations and human feeding experiments in Britain, India and Nigeria. The techniques of extraction and the quality of the product have been fully described.[9] Less refined leaf protein, cheap enough to be used for pig and poultry feeding, is produced commercially in Hungary and the U.S.A. The fibre residue is used as fodder for ruminants.

Oil-seed residues

When made in the traditional way, oil-seed residues are so contaminated that they cannot be used as human food. During the last 30 years, soya (*Glycine max*) bean residue has been prepared more hygienically and it, or protein separated from it by standard methods, is now so extensively used in the food industry that it can no longer be considered a new source of food. Similarly, there is nothing new about using the smooh paste of whole groundnuts (*Archis hypogaea*) as peanut butter; the residue, containing 40–50 per cent protein, after expressing oil from groundnuts, is used extensively in India as a component of 'balahar'. Where protein deficiency is the paramount problem, and where there is a market for the extracted oil, this separation is advantageous. In other regions it seems more sensible to encourage greater use of unfractionated groundnuts as 'butter' or in soups. There is some prejudice against groundnuts through fear of aflatoxin poisoning. But mycotoxins can be formed in most other foodstuffs when fungal damage results from storage in unsuitable conditions and, in domestic cooking at any rate, damaged seeds are easily recognized.

Cotton (*Gossypium hirsutum*) seed is an abundant by-product; it usually contains the phenolic aldehyde, gossypol. Some new varieties are free from gossypol, and there are mechanical techniques for separating the gossypol-containing glands from the meal. This restraint on the use of cotton-seed meal has therefore been removed and interest in it is increasing. Opinions differ about the success of projects in Central America, especially Guatemala. Cotton-seed meal does not dominate the nutritional scene there; on the other hand, advertising has been very restrained and the amount spent on promoting this new form of food is less than a commercial concern would have spent on promoting a new brand or even a new packaging style of a familiar food.

Unlike cotton seed, rape (*Brassica napus*) seed is not a by-product. It is being grown on an increasing scale because it is a temperate zone oil-producing crop. Use of the residue was restricted by the presence of toxic sulphur compounds; these can be eliminated by breeding and by washing the meal carefully. Rape-seed meal is already used as food for non-ruminant animals, it will probably soon appear as human food in aid programmes, but rape has no obvious merits as a tropical crop to be grown and used in protein-deficient regions. Although coconut (*Cocos nucifera*) is eaten by many people, the amount eaten is small because use is restricted by the amount of fibre in the meat. As with cereal seeds, and unlike legume seeds, use is not restricted by the presence of toxic substances. There is therefore increasing interest in processes for separating the protein and fibre. Initial attempts were unsuccessful because dried or autoclaved coconut was used; now that protein, oil and fibre are separated from fresh material by methods similar to those used traditionally in the South Pacific it is reasonable to expect more of the coconut crop to be used as human food rather than being turned into copra which, after oil expression, leaves a residue suitable only for animals.

FOODS MADE BY BIOLOGICAL CONVERSION

The foods considered so far come from plants that produce organic matter when supplied with light and a few simple substances. Animals and micro-organisms have to be supplied with organic matter which, with varying degrees of inefficiency, they convert into more useful or attractive forms. At one time, domestic animals were esteemed as sources of fat, now people tend to think of animals primarily as sources of protein. There is little carbohydrate in animals. The composition of micro-organisms can be controlled by varying the conditions in which they are grown; they too were initially cultivated as sources of fat but are now usually valued as protein sources.

Mammals

It is difficult to assess the nutritional importance of the smaller wild animals because the amount of meat supplied by them is seldom accurately measured. Den Hartog and de Vos[10] point out that they are usually caught and eaten by women and children and that there is a risk that any attempt to organize hunting would lead to increased consumption by adult men. The larger herbivores, caught by hunting, already supply about half the meat eaten in some African countries. It can be argued therefore that the cull of 10,000 tons of elephant and hippopotamus meat from the parks in Uganda[11] introduces no great novelty. If wild animals are to be used more extensively, more people will have to accept meat with a slightly different flavour from that of domestic animals and, if the animals come from their natural environment, with much less depot fat. There is at present no evidence that the absence of fat is a species characteristic and that the meat from wild and domestic animals, if they were fed on the same forage, would not be similar.

Kay[12] assembled, with references, the arguments for using more species of herbivore. Until there has been intensive selection, domestic animals are likely to out-yield any others on well-tended sward, but animals that are already adapted to rough country are likely to do better on it. It is logical to expect a mixture of animals, grazing and browsing at different levels, to make fuller use of mixed vegetation than would be made by a single species. There is much inconclusive evidence for these propositions. Thus, with improved management,[13] red deer are thriving in Scotland and it thought that Labrador could carry 0.5 million reindeer. The animals most often considered for use and eventual domestication are African buffalo, capybara, eland, elephant, elk, hippopotamus, impala, kangaroo and manatee. Less originality has been shown in thinking of new domesticated birds.

Fish

In spite of much research and publicity, products made from fish by industrialized processes have not fulfilled early expectations. The Swedish (Astra) project seems to be the only one that is still operating on a large scale, though methods for small-scale drying and smoking are being continually improved. In simple large-scale processes, bones and guts are included in the product; this may make it hazardous because of fluorine, and aesthetically unacceptable. Material made by more elaborate processes, such as that used by Astra, can be incorporated in bread and baby food[14] and it should be a valuable component of aid programmes.

Because it is at present being made in a country with a high standard of living, it is not likely to contribute much to the permanent food supply of those regions now most in need. That must await the development of processes of an intermediate degree of sophistication which could be used locally. In the meantime, improvements in the distribution of fresh and lightly preserved fish seem preferable to the conversion of fish into flavourless powders with a long shelf-life.[15]

Invertebrates

A few years ago, a reasonable estimate for the live-weight of unexploited cephalopods was 9 million tons. A more recent estimate,[16] based on the quantity eaten by sperm whales, is about 100 times larger; much of this population lives at depths where catching would be difficult. Various species of cephalopod are already eaten in many countries in spite of their rubbery texture; popularization should therefore not be difficult. Antarctic krill is nearly as abundant. Human food has not yet been made from it, and problems will arise because the individuals weigh only 5–20 g and have an indigestible chitinous covering. Mussels and other shellfish are being cultivated and protected from predation on an increasing scale; they are already eaten by so many communities that they should be acceptable wherever there is not a religious prohibition. Although large land snails are relished in Southeast Asia and West Africa, it is unlikely that they will be deliberately cultivated because there is no evidence that they convert vegetable matter into human food more efficiently than mammals. Insects and their larvae are often eaten as delicacies but they are probably not worth cultivating. Insect eggs are so abundant on the surface of some lakes that they are collected and eaten. If they are nutritionally valuable, this form of production may be worth exploiting: Yount[17] records standing crops of 7.5 tons (fresh weight) per ha and annual yields of 18 tons.

Micro-organisms

Yeasts have been eaten in small amounts in bread and turbid 'native' beers for millennia. They are now being cultivated industrially, mainly for use as animal feed. Their use as human food has been investigated for 30 or more years and there seems little doubt[18] that 5–10 per cent (dry weight) can be added to bread without serious effects on quality. Yeast contains 10–20 per cent of nucleic acid, the amount that can be eaten is therefore restricted by individual tolerance of the uric acid that is formed.[19] *Candida* grown on molasses is most often used, it has little flavour; a *Rhodotorula* grown on coconut water has a pleasant strawberry flavour.[20] Cultivation on substances such as these is suited to local production and use. The recent intense interest in industrialized countries in yeasts grown on the n-alkane fraction of oil will probably have little impact on nutrition in the less developed countries because of the complexity of the technology with this substrate. But the interest is welcome because it will increase the prestige of yeast grown on other substrates and it will produce a protein concentrate for feeding animals in industralized countries and thus safeguard such protein sources as fish and legume seeds which the less developed countries now export.

Bacteria are being grown as animal fodder; there are disturbing reports[21] of human sensitivity to them and there seem to be no proposals to use them as food. Funguses are more likely to be used and they, unlike yeasts and bacteria, have a mycelial structure which makes it easy to separate the product as a fibrous or felted mass that can be handled almost as if it were meat or fish. Funguses contain a more diverse range of hydrolytic enzymes than yeasts and can therefore grow on more types of agricultural by-product. Although fungus mycelium is a substantial component of many traditional fermented foods, especially in Southeast Asia, no product consisting predominantly of mycelium appears to be on sale as a human food. *Fusarium* is being grown commercially in Britain, *Aspergillus* in Britain and Switzerland, and *Paecilomyces* in Finland. All these are intended ultimately for use as human food when their safety and value have beem demonstrated.[22] Mushrooms, the large spore-bearing caps that grow from the mycelium of some funguses, are already familiar foods in many countries and their more extensive cultivation raises no novel problems.

PARTIAL AND TOTAL SYNTHESIS

There is no reason to think that the synthesis of protein, fat and carbohydrate will be cheaper than their production biologically. However, some chemical manipulation of indigestible material will probably be advantageous. The most obvious example is the hydrolysis of wood with acid or enzymes. This may not be relevant in the present context because the resulting glucose does not differ from glucose made in more familiar ways. Similarly, semi-synthetic vitamin A does not differ from vitamin A in foods such as milk; furthermore, the carotene in a modest helping of green vegetables is a substitute for it. The most probable products of the chemical industry are amino acids such as methionine and tryptophan, made either by fermentation or partial synthesis. These would probably be used to fortify foods containing a protein that is deficient in one or two amino acids, and this fortification, if it is considered beneficial, would be done centrally so that the consumer would not be aware of it. The early prejudice against the use of amino acids was largely based on the unpleasant taste of inadequately purified material. Protein analogues (plasteins) can be reconstituted enzymically from hydrolysates but they are not yet on the market.

CONCLUSION

Those new foods that can be produced locally by simple techniques will have the greatest effect on world nutrition. When large-scale industrial production is advantageous or essential, attention must be paid to the amount of power that will be used both in running the equipment and in making any chemicals needed. Attention must also be paid to the manner in which effluents would be disposed of or, preferably, used. With increasing fuel costs and increasing ecological awareness, these are points that will get more attention than hitherto. The development of practical processes for making new foods calls for much skilled research. This is wasted if the foods are not eaten. A comparable amount of research is needed on methods for winning acceptance for novel foods of proven merit.[23] Too little work is now being done on that subject.

REFERENCES

1. Oomen, H. A. P. C. Evaluation of subsistence patterns in New Guinea, *Overdruk uit Voeding*, **34**, 563 (1973).
2. Shepherd, F. W. Vegetables, in *Food Protein Sources*, N. W. Pirie (Ed.), London, Cambridge University Press, 1975.
3. Schmidt, D. R. Comparative yields and composition of eight tropical leafy vegetables grown at two soil fertility levels, *Argon J.* **63**, 546 (1971).
4. Kaul, A. K. Protein-rich cereal seeds, in *Food Protein Sources*, N. W. Pirie (Ed.), London, Cambridge University Press, 1975.
5. Protein Advisory Group. A note on required legume research, *Protein Advisory Group Bulletin*, **3**, (4), 11 (1973).
6. Milner, M. (ed.) Nutritional improvement of food legumes by breeding, New York, Protein Advisory Group, United Nations, 1973.
7. Swaminathan, M. S. and H. K. Jain, Food legumes in Indian agriculture, in *Nutritional improvement of food legumes by breeding, M. Milner (Ed.) New York, Protein Advisory Group, United Nations, 1973*.
8. Bradfield, R. Soybeans intercropped with maize and eaten young, *Cajanus*, **6**, 218 (1973).
9. Pirie, N. W. (ed.) *Leaf protein: Its agronomy, preparation, quality and use*, International Biological Program Handbook 20, Oxford, Blackwell, 1971.
10. Den Hartog, A. P. and A. De Vos, The use of rodents as food in tropical Africa, *Nutr. Newsletter*, **11**, (2), 1 (1973).
11. Myers, N. National parks in savannah Africa, *Science*, **178**, 1255 (1972).
12. Kay, R. N. B. Meat production from wild herbivores, *Proc. Nutr. Soc.*, **29**, 271 (1970).
13. Blaxter, K. L. Deer farming, *Scott. Agric.*, **51**, 225 (1972).
14. Hallgren, B., L-B. Sjoberg, and J. Stelleman. New uses for fish proteins, in *Proteins in Human Nutrition*, J. W. G. Porter and B. A. Rolls (Eds.), Academic Press, 1973.
15. Burgess, G. H. O. Increasing the direct consumption of fish, in *Food Protein Sources*, N. W. Pirie (Ed.), London, Cambridge University Press, 1975.
16. Denton, E. J. On buoyancy and the lives of modern and fossil cephalopods, *Proc. R. Soc.* (B), **185**, 273 (1974).
17. Yount, J. L. A method for rearing large numbers of pond midge larvae, with estimates of productivity and standing crop, *Am. Mid. Nat.*, **76**, 230 (1966).
18. Yanez, E., H. Wulf, D. Ballester, N. Fernandez, V. Gattas and F. Monckeberg. Nutritive value and baking properties of bread supplemented with *Candida utilis*, *J. Sci. Fd. Agric.*, **24**, 519 (1973).
19. Walsen, C. I., D. H. Calloway and S. Margen. Uric acid production of men fed graded amounts of egg protein and yeast nucleic acid, *Am. J. Clin. Nutr.*, **21**, 892 (1968).
20. Baena-Arcega, L. Philippine contribution to the utilisation of micro-organisms for the production of foods, *Biotech. Bioengng Symp.*, **1**, 53 (1969).

168

21. Waslien, C. I., D. H. Calloway and S. Margen. Human intolerance to bacteria as food, *Nature, Lond.,* **221,** 184 (1969).
22. Protein Advisory Group. New information from the MIT conference on single cell protein, *Protein Advisory Group Bulletin,* **3,** (3), 27 (1973).
23. Pirie, N. W. The direction of beneficial nutritional change, *Ecol. Fd. Nutr.,* **1,** 279 (1972).

CHAPTER 15

Centres for Combating Childhood Malnutrition

I. D. BEGHIN

INTRODUCTION

Undernutrition is a disease: it affects the health of the child, its well-being, and its chances of survival. But the causes of undernutrition are mainly economic, social and cultural. A solution, therefore, cannot be expected from health measures alone (Chapter 7). Health measures are palliative, and affect only in a limited way the underlying causes of undernutrition.

Full integration of nutrition activities with other health activities is not only a necessity which results from the epidemiology of undernutrition; it is also justified by the fact that health is seen in a unitarian way in most cultures, and that artificial separation of health and nutrition may limit the involvement of the community. More than anything else, however, integration is made mandatory by the need to use scarce resources in the most efficient manner, and to save on facilities, personnel and time.

Another lesson from epidemiology is the observation, made on all continents, that as a rule the siblings of the undernourished child are also affected, since the causes of malnutrition lie in environmental characteristics which affect the whole family. Various terms have been used to express this concept: the 'risk family', the 'affected family', the 'risk mother', etc. A few years ago we suggested calling the siblings; contacts.[1] The extension of the concept of risk to the whole family, and its practical consequence that programmes must reach the whole family and not just the child, in turn imply the need to reach all those families: i.e. to identify them, and provide them with either treatment or protection. The problem therefore is to define clearly what minimal health and nutrition care should be delivered to every affected family or risk family in the country, including the most neglected or most remote community, and how to train and supervise the auxiliaries and volunteers who will deliver such care. To do so, obviously, the active participation of the community is essential.

Paternalistic 'vertical' programmes have as a rule failed, and the need for the people concerned to participate in health programmes is now generally accepted. But community participation in the diagnosis of their own health or nutrition status, or in the selection of priorities and type of services to be organized, still meets with reluctance, or even opposition, from some health workers. The word 'community' is understood here in its broadest sense, meaning 'the people'. The élite, the natural leaders, mass organization, unions, church groups, etc. are *part* of the community, but should not be confused with the community (Chapter 2).

In some cases the service 'package' (an example of which is given in Table 1) would be delivered by a formal health structure, in others by paramedical personnel or even by volunteers linked to the health system. But in all instances there should be a strong input from the people of the community.

Table 1. Components of a 'package' of minimal mother-and-child health nutritional attention at the community level

---

1. Immunizations: (i) measles; (ii) BCG and whooping cough; (iii) others

2. Elementary medical care: (i) treatment of diarrhoea and respiratory infections in children; (ii) treatment of major illnesses such as TB and malaria; (iii) first aid

3. Surveillance of growth and development of young children, and minimal pre-natal care centred on the nutritional status of the pregnant woman

4. Supervised supplementary feeding in selected families

5. Referral of severe and/or complicated cases to a more sophisticated health facility

6. Family planning, with emphasis on the spacing of children and on breast-feeding (or just promotion of family planning and referral)

7. Minimal health education, including nutrition education and family planning

8. Collecting and reporting a minimum of statistical information

9. Motivation and mobilization of people to participate in each of the eight previous components

---

SURVEILLANCE OF GROWTH AND DEVELOPMENT OF THE YOUNG CHILD

Surveillance of growth and development of the young child has traditionally been, and still is, the major single health activity related to nutrition. It is important both for the individual and for the community. It allows early detection of undernutrition in the individual child, and identification of risk families and contacts. In addition it serves the purpose of monitoring the nutritional status of the community as a whole, while at the same time keeping alive the interest of the community in its own health. Surveillance of growth and development, however, has meaning only to the extent that it generates prompt action. Weighing of so-called 'well babies' is too often seen more as a ritual than as the essential public health measure it is. The information not only needs to be collected: it must be interpreted and utilized (Table 2). (See Chapter 6 for full discussion of the use of anthropometry.)

The periodicity of weight and height controls should be realistic. The norm, too often, is beyond the capacity of the clinic. One should be practical, not require mothers to bring their children too often, have the courage to drop less important groups such as older or better nourished children and increase the frequency of controls among higher risk groups. Surveillance of growth and development, furthermore, should be comprehensive and include surveillance of the general health status of the child, of its diet, and of its motor and behavioural development, and it should also be used as an opportunity for immunizing the child and educating its mother. As much as possible, it should be *delegated to properly trained and supervised personnel* such as auxiliaries, 'health promotors', or volunteers from the community.

Table 2. Cases of protein–energy undernutrition in children under 5 years, per country and per degree, in Central America and Panama, 1965–1967, in percentages

| | Undernutrition | | | |
Country	Normal	1st Degree	2nd Degree	3rd Degree
Guatemala	18.6	49.0	26.5	5.9
El Salvador	25.5	48.5	22.9	3.1
Honduras	27.5	43.0	27.2	2.3
Nicaragua	43.2	41.8	13.2	1.8
Costa Rica	42.6	43.7	12.2	1.5
Panama	39.3	48.8	10.8	1.1

Source: INCAP

Lastly, there should always be a place, even if distant, where problem cases can be referred and will be taken care of.

What was said above for post-natal growth and development also applies to the ante-natal period. When the incidence of low birth weight in a population group is high, it indicates a poor nutritional status of the mothers in that population. It also indicates a higher risk of malnutrition and of death in young children.[2] Low birth weight is therefore a good indicator of the nutritional situation of the community. At the individual level, although height and weight are commonly used to monitor the growth and development of pregnant women, adequate risk criteria are still not available. In any case, pregant women must be put under control. Surveillance, both post-natal and pre-natal, serves the same purpose, and this should never be lost from sight: to save lives; to protect the health of those who are more at risk; and to promote better health and nutrition for the greatest possible number.

EARLY DETECTION AND DIAGNOSIS OF NUTRITION

Early detection of undernutrition

Three factors must be met before attempting to improve the nutrition of young children in a community: recognition of the existence of undernutrition, quantification of it, and identification of those who are more in need of either attention (because of being undernourished) or protection (because of being at a higher risk). The problem of community diagnosis was dealt with in Chapter 6. Our concern here is to identify at an early stage those who are either at risk or who are already affected, in order to make sure that the right measures are eventually applied to the right children. Since resources are scarce, selective coverage of those most in need is imperative. But, as we have seen, selection should be based on risk, and not on the fact of living near the clinic, as too often happens. Selection of children for preventive action ought to be epidemiological, not geographical. The concept of 'at risk', as developed by Stanfield[3] has proved very practical, because it does point to those most in need of attention and because it helps to define priorities. On the other hand, it has generally been used with reference to already undernourished children, while this reviewer uses the term 'risk' in a stricter epidemiological sense, that is as an expression of probability. A child, it is felt, can be at high risk, and yet be perfectly normal at the same time. Since the risk is more a characteristic of the family than of the child, preference should be given to the concept of the 'risk family'. Identifying such families, and assisting and educating them, is one of the key components of community nutrition (Chapter 8).

Family risk factors will vary from one place to the other. The presence of a malnourished child in a family is a key and universal risk factor.[1] Other factors would relate to education of parents, income, housing, sanitary conditions etc. (Chapter 7).

The purpose, then, of early detection is:

(a) Selection of 'risk families', in order to apply to them measures of 'specific protection' such as nutrition education, supplementary feeding, prevention of infectious diseases, medical care, etc. as well as through community action to allieviate the social and economic problems of the family.

(b) Management of those who are undernourished, involving the mother, whenever possible in the home.

(c) Referral of selected patients to a more complex centre or level of attention. If an adequate referral system does not exist, it has to be created. An example of how to refer cases is given in Figure 1. It shows how, in a given environment, Northeast Brazil, the risk family would come under some kind of action.[1]

(d) Classification of cases of malnutrition, for the purpose of evaluation, general information, and further planning.

(e) Surveillance of the community's nutritional status through the collecting and reporting of a minimum of statistical information. This would allow for monitoring change, and also serve as an early warning device in the case of an abrupt worsening of the situation.

Detection of undernourished children or of children or families at risk can be either passive, by weighing all those who come to the clinic, or active, by visiting the homes, or by calling the children to a central weighing place, etc. But, to be effective, active detection must ensure wide coverage.

Let us now assume that some mechanism for detection is operating effectively, and turn to the problem of the diagnosis of undernutrition.

AFFECTED FAMILY

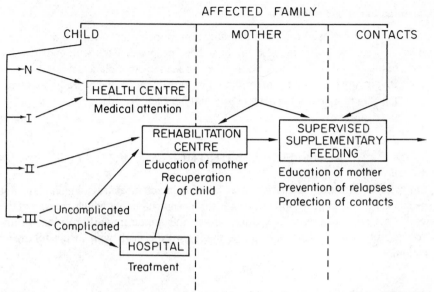

FIGURE 1. Flow of members of an affected family through a comprehensive nutritional rehabilitation and educational programme: example from Northeast Brazil. The signs N. I, II, and III refer to normal children, and children with first, second, or third degree of undernutrition, respectively (Reproduced with permission from I. D. Beghin, in Proceedings of the Western Hemisphere Nutrition Congress III, Bal Harbour, Florida, 1971, American Medical Association, Dearborn, Illinois, 1972

Diagnosis of undernutrition

The degree of accuracy of the diagnosis of the undernourished child will depend on the type of resources and the personnel available in the community. Diagnosis starts with measuring weight and height, particularly weight. Next in importance comes the dietetic history of the child, which should be at least semi-quantitative. It takes a little time and patience to question the mother or the childminder, but the value of the information is highly rewarding. Unfortunately, this essential part of the diagnosis is the one most neglected by doctors and other health workers.

Other elements of a good diagnosis are the clinical and personal histories of the child *and* its family; record of birth weight; physical examination, even if limited to only a few key signs (key signs in that particular region or country); and at least haemoglobin or haematocrit determination.

The diagnosis should never be a nutritional diagnosis alone: nutritional signs and symptoms are only part of a comprehensive, even if summary, medical diagnosis which includes other conditions such as the infections which are almost consistently present, and it should extend to the whole family. Deficiencies other than protein–energy malnutrition should be carefully looked for an specialized nutrition consultations are to be avoided.

Classification of undernutrition

There is a great need for good classification models, and a variety of systems, tables, scores, composite indices, etc. have been proposed, each with considerable merit, but also with serious drawbacks when applied to other places. What is important is that in any one country there should be agreement on one overall system, for the benefit of comparison between places and between periods.

NON-SPECIFIC NUTRITION ACTIVITIES

Non-specific nutrition activities are health-related measures which are not specifically aimed at preventing or treating undernutrition, but which are part of the general attention to the child and its mother and are particularly relevant to improving nutrition. *Specific* nutrition activities will be dealt with in the following section.

Management and prevention of other diseases

The strong correlation between poor nutritional status and the presence of other pathological conditions was stressed earlier in this chapter. Such synergism affects both mortality and morbidity. Comprehensive action is therefore required both for treatment and for prevention. In Candelaria, Colombia, for example, a significant reduction in the prevalence of malnutrition was achieved through control of infections and adequate medical care, without the administration of a dietary supplement.[4] From the viewpoint of the community health workers, a few priorities for action can be almost universally put forward.[5,6,7] They respond to the double criteria of reducing morbidity and mortality, and of being applicable even at a simple, unsophisticated level of care. Both the epidemiology of illness and death in the young child and recent experience suggest that the minimum health measures to be taken to improve nutrition, besides those we will call 'specific' in the next section, would be as listed below:

(a) Immunization against infectious diseases: measles in the first place, then tuberculosis (BCG) and whooping cough. Other vaccines such as polio and smallpox will be administered as well, but they bear little, if at all, on nutrition.

(b) Control of diarrhoeal disease through minimal health education (washing of hands, avoiding restrictive diet in case of gastroenteritis, early consultation), adequate early rehydration, and dietary management.[8]

(c) Control of respiratory infections, mainly through a wise, restrained, but energetic use of antibiotics or sulphonamides.

(d) Referral to a more qualified person or service. This point is often either missing altogether or inadequately complied with. A place with higher quality and sophistication of care should exist and be within reach; but the community worker ought to be trained in knowing when to refer a child.

Experience shows that the four types of responsibility outlined above can be adequately met by people with a limited level of formal education. Even illiterate or almost illiterate persons can function provided they are guided and supervised. In areas where malaria is endemic chemoprophylaxis and treatment would be on top of this list. Systematic deworming of children under surveillance has been advocated in hyperendemic areas. We feel that the nutritional benefits of such a procedure have not been fully demonstrated.

Family planning, health education and environmental sanitation

These three measures are important for the long-range improvement of nutrition. Family planning, through its effect on spacing of children, increase in the lactation period, improvement of nutritional status of the mother, the economics of having fewer children, etc. affects the health and well-being of the family to an extent which is not always fully appreciated. Family planning, in addition, is a fundamental component of any comprehensive mother and child health-care programme.

Health education is mentioned here because of the unfortunate divorce between nutrition education and health education. The former is part of the latter, and at this point in the book it should now be clear why there is no sense in isolated nutrition education.

Diarrhoea and undernutrition are the two great killers of young children, particularly when they associate their effects on the same victim: environmental sanitation, therefore, will go hand in hand with nutrition improvement measures. Here is a field of action particularly sensitive to community action. Each nutrition worker, from the specialized doctor to the community volunteer or committee member, must convert himself into an active propagandist for clean water supply, latrines and the use of latrines, and personal hygiene.

SPECIFIC NUTRITION ACTIVITIES

At the level of the community, health-related measures specifically aimed at either preventing or correcting undernutrition belong to any of the three following broad categories: management of the undernourished child, use of food supplements and food mixtures (Chapter 16), and nutrition education (Chapter 21). Nutritional rehabilitation centres belong, although with different degrees, to all three categories, and therefore will receive special treatment.

Management of the undernourished child

Whether the undernourished child is treated in the hospital, in a semi-ambulatory facility such as a nutritional rehabilitation centre, or as an out-patient, the same general rules apply. In the first place one should speak more of the management of the undernourished child than of treatment. Care in handling, warmth and affection are almost as necessary for the nutritional and social rehabilitation of the child as diet and drugs, but they are frequently overlooked. Stimulation and personalized attention help in improving the behaviour of the child, and facilitate the re-establishing of the all too frequently impaired mother–child relationship.

The basis of treatment is a good diet. It is not vitamin pills, protein isolates, amino-acid mixtures, hormones, stimulators of appetite, or other costly and often harmful products. Besides providing a good diet and affection, one must at the same time take care of other diseases such as infections, intestinal worms, malaria, etc. and carry out immediate immunizations in susceptible children. Measles vaccine, particularly, should be high on the list, since it has been shown to be both effective and innocuous, even in severe cases of malnutrition (Chapter 10). Lastly, there is good evidence that physical exercise helps to accelerate the recovery, together with mental stimulation, speech exercises and games (Chapter 11).

Very few places indeed respect *all* of the above rules. Their enforcement certainly offers a wide field for community action, particularly with reference to the non-medical aspects of the cure. An adequate reference system to a hospital, or from the hospital to the rehabilitation centre, or between the latter and the community at large, can often be established through organized community efforts. The same can be said of the follow-up of children after discharge from treatment.

(a) *Management of the severely undernourished child in the hospital.*

The severely undernourished child is a very ill patient, with a high risk of dying, even after the initial acute period. He not only is at risk of losing his life, but is also suffering and deprived. He is, by all standards, a top-priority patient.

Complicated severe malnutrition means hospitalization. Uncomplicated cases, however severe, should as a rule not be sent to the hospital.[9] Even third-degree malnutrition and overt cases of marasmus and kwashiorkor are managed successfully in semi-ambulatory facilities or in the home, all over the world. But whenever there is, or appears to be, a complication, the child must be admitted and dealt with as an emergency.

Two major complications, which are often combined, justify most of the admissions of undernourished children into the hospitals. They are water and electrolyte imbalance (due mainly to diarrhoea) and severe infection (such as bronchopneumonia, otitis media, urinary infections, and others) besides the already mentioned gastroenteritis. Early recognition of these in the home or the clinic is essential for the survival of the child, and in that respect there is much an organized community can do.

Management of the condition is divided into an acute phase and a long-term recovery phase. The acute phase is the province of the clinician. There are good specialized reviews of the subject.[10]

Once the water and salt imbalance is corrected and/or the infection has come under control, the child enters the long-term recovery phase. The stay in the hospital must be reduced to the minimum, and the sooner the child passes to a regular but rich diet, the better. Community volunteers and parents should not only be allowed to, but should be invited to assist the doctors and nurses and aid in feeding the children. The community, therefore, can considerably assist the hospital management of undernourished children by involving the mother early in the recovery phase, by helping in feeding and in stimulating the children, and in ensuring adequate referral of the child to the rehabilitation centre, the out-patient clinic, or the home.

Cook has convincingly shown that the hospital should be avoided whenever possible.[9] When admission is inevitable, then the child must find care of the highest quality. Only then will the confidence of the community be gained, and this is important both for early detection and for gaining the active participation of the people in improving care.

If hospitalization can be avoided, the child should be handled either in a rehabilitation centre or in the home.

(b) Domiciliary management of the undernourished child

When possible, treatment should be conducted in the home[11] to avoid further changes in psychological environment, prevent cross-infections, reduce the cost, and above all involve the whole family, and possibly the community, in getting the child back to normal nutrition. Therapeutic action should be extended to the other members of the family, mainly through education of the mother and protection of the contacts. Practically, this amounts to surveillance and/or management of the other young children and pregnant women in the family.

In some places nutritional recuperation has been achieved in the home, without donation of a food supplement, by the provision of adequate medical care, nutrition and health education, and close supervision through home visits. The use of a food supplement covering about 30 per cent of the recommended allowance for both protein and energy, and as close as possible to 100 per cent of the allowance for other nutrients, is the most effective therapy.[12] Milk should be a component whenever possible, but it can in part be replaced by a vegetable blend. Energy should be provided in the form of cereals, tuber flour, sugar, oil, etc. The other siblings and any pregnant or lactating mother in the family should also receive the supplement, as a protective measure (see section on supervised supplementary feeding).

Nutritional rehabilitation centres

A nutritional rehabilitation centre (NRC) is, in the original concept of Bengoa[13] a day-care centre for undernourished children, which is used both for treating the child and for educating its mother 'through the child's recuperation'. Only local foods are used, and the operation is kept at the lowest possible cost. The mother participates at periodic intervals in the operation of the centre: buying and preparing the food, serving the meals, and taking care of the children. The active participation of the mother is the main learning process, which may be reinforced by more formal educational activities.

The greatest advantage of the NRCs is their low cost.[14] In well-operated NRCs about 70–80 per cent of the children recuperate in less than 3–4 months, at a cost which is, on a daily basis, almost 10 times less than treatment in the hospital, and without the drawbacks and risks of hospitalization emphasized by Cook. NRCs admit children between 1–5 years, with uncomplicated but severe undernutrition. Frank kwashiorkor, severe marasmus, and third-degree malnutrition are successfully treated, as long as there is no complication at admission. Long-term results have not been adequately assessed, although all available evidence suggests results far superior to those of hospital treatment.[9,14] However, NRCs have some serious drawbacks, which should not be overlooked. Their major limitation is their narrow scope. In the first place their coverage extends only to a small geographical area, and this makes them useful only in densely populated areas or urban settings. Secondly they have usually not been applied to children below 10–12 months of age, nor do they reach the other children in the family, the 'contacts'.* Another drawback is that they seem to be extremely dependent on the personal characteristics of the person in charge and on the quality and frequency of supervision, both often unsatisfactory, as experience has shown. On the other hand, if those limitations are acknowledged, and if a few, but essential, conditions are met, then NRCs unquestionably represent an extremely useful weapon in our combat against undernutrition.[15] Among the conditions for success are the following.

(a) The whole family should be covered by preventive and/or therapeutic care, even if minimal. This may include immunizations, health education, supplementary feeding, medical care, etc.

(b) Nutritional rehabilitation should be understood in a broad sense, and should encompass speech, motricity, mental development and social reintegration.

(c) A few basic operational rules must be strictly respected, and frequent and adequate supervision ensured (some basic operational rules are suggested in Table 3).

(d) Due emphasis should be given to the education of the mother.

(e) Evaluation has to be built in, before starting.

(f) The community should be genuinely involved, in the whole operation, *after having participated in the decision to open or not to open a centre.*

More detailed discussions on NRCs can be found in recent reviews by Beghin and Viteri[14] and Beaudry-Darismé and Latham.[16]

The important point to keep in mind is that, in Bengoa's words, the NRC is only a link in a chain, and that from the community standpoint one must consider the chain first, that is, a comprehensive nutritional and mother-and-child health programme involving close to 100 per cent of the children affected or at risk. In this respect the linking of an NRC with a hospital, as successfully achieved in Uganda, seems well worth applying elsewhere.[17]

Supervised supplementary feeding

Food supplementation is a valuable component of community nutrition if it is intended either to (i) treat undernourished children, (ii) to protect families at risk, or

*Editor's note: The success of this approach in infants has yet to be demonstrated.

Table 3. Recommendations for the general operation of Nutritional Rehabilitation Centre of the day care type

Number of children	30–35
Admission criteria	Uncomplicated 2nd and 3rd degree malnutrition
Age of the children	1–4 years
Hours of operation	Approximately 8:00 am–5:00 pm, including Saturday
Personnel	One person in charge One maid Three mothers
Food	Exclusively food that can be bought locally
Menus	Must follow local habits and provide 100% of recommended dietary allowances
Medical supervision	Physician per child per day—1 min
Deparasitization, immunizations, etc.	Yes, but after recuperation
Discharge criteria	4 Months stay, or complete recuperation and/or satisfactory education of the mother

Remember: the purpose of the Centre is to educate the mother!
From reference 15

(iii) to be used as a vehicle of nutrition education. As a means of treatment it is, as we have seen, an indispensable component of the domiciliary management of undernutrition. It is a very effective protection device for the risk families, since it prevents undernutrition and its consequences among contacts, at a very low cost, as this reviewer and others have shown in Northeast Brazil.[12] Also, it can always serve as a pretext and an opportunity for nutrition education.

But food supplementation, except for emergency situations, has never been shown to improve the nutritional status of the population in any significant way, in spite of the claims of the large and powerful organizations involved in surplus food distribution. On the contrary, in a number of instances, it has been argued convincingly that large-scale food supplementation has done more harm than good.[18]

Table 4 is an attempt to compare the characteristics of many of the ongoing programmes with what an 'ideal' programme should look like. A sober analysis of the second column would lay the basis of such a programme, once clear objectives have been defined: treatment, specific protection, and/or education. The importance of supervising the use of the supplement, of strictly limiting the duration of feeding to avoid social dependence, and the need for a supplement that meets the actual deficit in the diet cannot be overemphasized.

If supervised supplementary feeding is seen in that light, it becomes another link in the chain we referred to in the previous section, i.e. an essential component of the programme. The responsibility to operate it rests on the community and on the

Table 4. Characteristics of programmes for distribution of food supplements

	Existing programmes	Proposed programme
Selection of beneficiaries	Characterized by few selection criteria: do not have effect on group most exposed to risk;	Selection based on medical criteria: most vulnerable group: children of pre-school age; only malnourished children (and their contacts);
	do not necessarily have effect upon those within the group who are of major priority;	
	pastor, social worker, etc. do the selection;	selection made only by a doctor or his assistant;
	no systematic protection of the contacts;	contacts are automatically included in the programme;
	philanthropic basis of selection	selection is based upon epidemiology
Nature of supplementation	supplementation does not always correspond to nutritional needs;	supplement satisfies nutritional needs;
	supplement is frequently viewed as charity;	supplement is viewed as a treatment and as an educational vehicle
	supplementation is often done with foods not available on the retail market	supplementation is based upon foods sold locally
Distribution	variable duration of supplementation, often indefinite	supplementation over a strictly limited time-period;
	lack of regular utilization;	rigorous control of utilization (weighings; required attendance by the mothers; imperative participation by the mothers; automatic health care to children who do not improve);
	supplementation often uncoordinated with other health activities	supplementation is always part of a health programme
Educational aspects	nonexistent, or limited merely to the preparation of the supplement	use of supplementation as a vehicle for nutrition education
Evaluation	evaluation is rarely made; when made it rarely demonstrates nutritional improvement	evaluation is a part of the programme: nutritional improvement ought to be achieved
Social aspects	often create dependency;	does not create dependency;
	palliative, resolve nothing	more than merely palliative, it has an educational role

From reference 12

CHAPTER 16

Role of Food Mixtures in Combating Childhood Malnutrition

PETER L. PELLET

INTRODUCTION

Soon after World War II awareness of the prevalence of protein–energy malnutrition (PEM) resulted in massive research activity in all areas related to protein. With the increasing availability of amino-acid analytical data and biological methods for the assay of protein quality the concepts of supplementation, complementation and amino-acid fortification became increasing widely known as the development of protein-rich food mixtures grew to be one of the major thrusts in the attempts to alleviate the scourge of PEM. The projects carried considerable prestige and high-level support and funding became widely available. Later it became almost mandatory for any nutrition research unit working on the problems of the developing world to have its own mixture. With hindsight it is easy to see that the enthusiasm may have been misplaced; complex problems do not usually have simple solutions and the problems of malnutrition are overwhelmingly complex (Chapter 7). For too long an implicit assumption has been that malnutrition was caused by ignorance and that scientific methodology would, when effectively marshalled, overcome it. A corollary of this viewpoint was that malnutrition was primarily food-and nutrient-related. We now realize that malnutrition, especially infantile malnutrition, may be more related to the absence of clean water than to low protein quality and more dependent upon flies and infection than protein intake. The solutions moreover are in the areas of preventive rather than curative medicine, in economics rather than in nutrition, and in land reform rather than in food technology.

All this is not to say that Food Mixtures do not have a place: with the recent realization that world energy (fossil fuel) supplies and food production are highly interrelated and not independent, their place may become more important. Within this review, I will discuss the rationale behind and history of food mixtures, their current status, some reasons for success or failure and their possible future role in a world of limited energy, limited food and ever-increasing population.

BACKGROUND

While the concept of complementation of proteins has only received scientific explanation since amino-acid data have become available, the principle has been traditional in the dietary habits of most peoples of the world since antiquity.[1] Just as soybean and rice have been part of the Far Eastern dietary pattern, wheat bread with legumes has been a hallmark of the Middle Eastern diets.[2]

The development of food mixtures has, throughout its history, had close association with several U.N. Agencies, notably WHO, FAO, UNICEF, and has led to the development of the Protein Advisory Group (PAG) (Chapter 24). Brief histories of the development of protein foods and the involvement of the U.N. Agencies have recently been given.[3,4] A series of statements and guidelines relevant to food mixtures have been made by the PAG, and extensive reviews and critiques of the whole field have appeared recently.[5-9]

In this context, food mixtures are considered as being a manufactured product. An alternative approach, advocated by many over a long period and recently discussed in detail by Cameron and Hofvander,[5] lies in the home mixing of components so as to produce more balanced mixtures for the feeding of infants and young children. While this is much more in the domain of infant feeding practice than in food mixture technology the approach is highly relevant and eliminates many of the limitations and dangers inherent in the food mixture approach as discussed by Popkin and Latham.[6]

AVAILABLE SOURCES OF VEGETABLE PROTEIN

Some 70 per cent of the world's supply of edible protein comes from plant sources of which nearly 70 per cent again is from cereals and 18 per cent from grain legumes. In the developing regions of the world a rather larger proportion of total protein comes from plant sources and most is directly consumed by humans. In the rich regions of North America, Europe and USSR, however, a major part of the cereals (except wheat and rice) and almost all of the grain legumes are used as animal feed.

The cereals have, in general, low protein quality and quantity, being generally low in lysine and tryptophan. Rice, however, while having a lower content of total protein has a better balanced amino-acid pattern than wheat and corn. The legumes, cotton-seed flour and milk, all have high levels of lysine and rather low levels of sulphur amino acids. Groundnut is an exception, while having a moderate level of protein (25 per cent), it has a poor content of essential amino acids. The other legumes, however, seem almost designed by nature to supplement cereals since they have higher protein content, either high or adequate levels of lysine and are themselves limited by sulphur amino acids which are present in moderate levels in cereals.

Despite the relatively low protein quality and quantity in cereals such as wheat, calculations appear to show that a child's protein requirement[7] *should* be met by cereal diets provided that sufficient of the diet could be consumed to meet energy needs. Whitehead[8] has shown indeed that children can grow, albeit slowly, on diets with a protein–energy ratio of only 0.078 (Pcal per cent = 7.8). However, in practice, diets would frequently be so bulky that insufficient could be consumed.[9] Hegsted and Nef[10] have argued that the methods in current use for the determination of protein quality such as net protein utilization (n.p.u.) have an inherent error when used to determine the quality of poor proteins such as cereals and will thus *overestimate* the true quality. Hegsted has shown further that protein requirement of the cebus monkey[11] is underestimated by the factorial method and claims that if quality is determined by a slope-ratio technique then predications of utilizable protein agree more with the growth obtained.

Whatever the reasons for these discrepancies, i.e. bulk, protein quality or even palatibility, it would appear that cereal alone cannot meet protein needs and that either amino-acid fortification, the improvement of quality by addition of the limiting amino acids *or* complementation, the mixing of other proteins with cereal protein to improve both quality and quantity, are necessary especially for the infant whose needs are high. In the rich third of the world, animal proteins fulfil this role but are not available to the poor nations on economic grounds. This is not to agree with the hypothesis that a world protein shortage in fact exists. Many authors have in recent years questioned the 'impending world protein crisis' school of thought, claiming that a food crisis does indeed exist but that with the exception of those communities existing on very low protein staples such as cassava, protein needs would be met if energy needs were met (Chapter 3). The problem is compounded by the fact that at low energy intakes protein is diverted into energy pathways and is burnt as fuel.[12] Recent FAO data[13] tend to confirm this viewpoint. The shortfall of energy is far more obvious than that of protein, this appears true even for the developing countries as a whole where protein availability is 47 per cent above requirements while energy needs are barely met (Chapter 5). This trend appears to continue with the projections for 1980. For the high-income countries, protein availability is 129 per cent above needs while energy is 21 per cent in excess. These values, however, have only an *indirect* relation to the incidence of PEM where the cause lies much more in maldistribution of protein within the family and it is here that the protein-rich foods may play a role.

Animal protein foods are expensive, partly because of the inefficiencies of the conversion of feed protein into protein for human consumption. This efficiency may range from about 24 per cent for eggs to less than 5 per cent for beef and veal (Chapter 4). This can be put another way in relation to the total energy subsidy invoked for 1 calorie (4.2 joules) of food output, the more energy needed in general the more expensive the product. Thus animal protein will be much more expensive than vegetable protein. There are of course differences in protein quality between these products. Legumes and cereals have n.p.u. = 0.40 and meat products n.p.u. = 0.75; however, protein mixtures of legumes and cereals can reach n.p.u. = 0.65 or above. These considerations give sound economic reasons for the value of protein food mixtures.

While legumes and cotton-seed protein products are ideal as complementary protein sources there are antinutritional factors which may be present, such as trypsin inhibitors, haemaglutinins and anticoagulant factors in legumes and gossypol in cotton seed (Chapter 12). Vegetable protein concentrates are excellent natural media for the growth of micro-organisms. Toxic aflatoxins were shown to be produced by *Aspergillus flavus* in peanut flour and this directly led to the demise of one protein mixture in Africa. A full discussion of these effects with many references to original work is given by Bressani and Elias[14] who also discuss the various technological advances which have solved many of the problems, allowing these protein sources to make a contribution to human diets.

COMPLEMENTARY PROTEIN MIXTURES

The mixing of two or more proteins does not always lead to complementation. Four types of effect have been described.[14] Only when the quality of the mixture is better than either of the components alone can true complementation be said to occur. Then essential amino acids of one protein source complement very closely the essential amino acids of the other, such complementation usually involving cereal–legume combinations. Mixtures giving maximum protein quality would range between 60:40 to 50:50 for proportions of cereal protein to legume protein. These would correspond to about 70:30 proportions by weight of, for example, wheat and chickpea or corn and beans. Other mixtures can show improved quality but the maximum quality of the mixture will slope to that of the better quality component, as for example with corn and cotton seed. If there is a common limiting amino acid at a similar level in both components, as with corn and groundnuts, which are both limited by lysine, no complementation can occur and the protein quality remains constant for all mixtures. It must be emphasized that considerations here are those of protein quality alone and the highest protein quality mixture is not necessarily the best supplement to a poor diet.

For complementation to occur and to give the maximum response, higher proportions of the non-cereal component are required than are present in the normal diet pattern of the region. However, if a mixture is consumed as a dietary supplement along with the staple diet of the region, whether it be corn or wheat, it can be seen that the effect of the legume will be much less in terms of the diet as a whole because of the further dilution of the legume with the cereal product. Only additions of high-protein products such as fish protein concentrate, skim milk powder, the limiting amino acid or even the legume alone would be expected greatly to affect the overall protein value. This means that the use of vegetable protein mixtures has extreme limitations when confronted with the unbalanced dietary patterns consumed in the real world. However, where a weaning mixture can replace the normal weaning food, theoretical benefits could follow provided that the hygienic environment is satisfactory and that because of cost considerations a net decrease in protein and energy cost is not caused.[6]

TESTING OF FOOD MIXTURES

While the early food mixtures were tested during their development by a variety of methods a set of guidelines has been developed by the Protein Advisory Group for the use of investigators so that all products could undergo similar evaluation. For those concerned with the development of food mixtures guidelines numbers 6, 7 and 8 are the most relevant. PAG Guideline No. 6[15] on pre-clinical testing is intended as a series of general recommendations rather than mandatory procedures, and the objective is to ensure the safety of any new product for human consumption. Consideration is given in the document to the testing of the nutritional value of the new product, using animal and chemical assays for protein quality and for amino-acid content and availability. Other criteria considered are toxicity tests with animals and the full microbiological evaluation of the product from production through to consumer packaging. Further details of sanitary production and use of dry protein foods are given in Guideline No. 11.[16]

Human testing of supplementary food mixtures follows from this point (Guideline No. 7[17]). The methods recommended are described as extensive but flexible so that the fewest number of subjects possible can be used to obtain significant data. The document outlines methods for the determination of product acceptability and tolerance, detailing such considerations as age and number of subjects, duration of the experiment, method of food preparation and the level of protein and energy in the test diets. Criteria are also suggested for the observations that should be made and how tolerance to the product should be judged. Growth and nitrogen balance studies are described with the precautions necessary for accurate determinations. New methods, however, are now being recommended for human determinations of protein quality using a variation of the slope-ratio assay technique.[18] Mention is also made of other measurements such as serum albumin, creatinine-height index and plasma amino-acid and enzyme levels which may be useful in assessing the value of certain food mixtures. Two categories of product are suggested.

1. Products requiring full testing procedures, both pre-clinical and clinical are:

   (a) Processed or non-processed protein-containing foods which have not previously been considered in WHO/FAO/UNICEF programmes;
   (b) Products, previously considered as suitable, which have been subjected to different processing conditions which may raise questions regarding their nutritional or toxicological properties.

2. Products requiring only limited clinical testing (acceptability/tolerance only) are staples and protein sources which are well-known or have been considered suitable in WHO/FAO/UNICEF programmes and have not been subjected to processing which could cast doubts on their safety.

Guideline No. 8[19] is a recommendation on the composition of supplementary foods considering both the physical characteristics, i.e. flavour, taste and packaging requirements, and also specifications for the levels of protein, energy, fats, minerals and vitamins. With regard to the quantity of protein the recommendations are that with protein of quality equivalent to cow's milk (n.p.u. = 0.80) the level of protein should be at least 150 g/kg on a dry weight basis. With n.p.u. less than 0.80, the quantity of protein should be increased pro rata to 200 g/kg at n.p.u. = 0.60. It is further recommended that no products should have an n.p.u. below 0.60 approximately equivalent to a PER of 2.1.

After satisfactory passing of the tests outlined in Guidelines 6 and 7 and meeting the composition standards of Guideline No. 8, marketing tests would follow. Guideline No. 10[20] is an extensive monograph on the marketing of protein-rich foods in developing countries. Consideration is given to the new protein food programme as part of a country's total nutrition system, project planning, technical and economic feasibility studies, project implementation and programme evaluation. The emphasis of the last few years has been placed more and more on the need for marketing studies as a prerequisite for support of a project under the FAO/WHO/UNICEF protein food programme.

NUTRITIVE VALUE

An extensive literature exists of chemical analyses, animal feeding trials and human feeding experiments. Examples are for Latin America and the early testing of Incaparina vegetable protein mixtures[14] for India[21] and for the Middle East.[2,22] The book *Protein-enriched Cereal Foods for World Needs*[23] also contains many references to testing and developmental experiments throughout the world. A recent report[24] discusses the nutritional effectiveness of soy-cereal foods in undernourished infants and concludes that a variety of cereal soy foods can be the major or only source of protein in the diet of growing infants and children. A series of papers[25] report on the use of legumes and green leafy vegetables in the feeding of young children and several papers consider the nutritional aspects.

Thus, the vast majority of the products have high nutritive value, the protein quality being usually close to that of casein, and feeding trials with human subjects showed high nitrogen retentions with both normal and malnourished children. It has, however, been reported[26] that while short-time experiments showed little difference when the protein source was milk or a variety of vegetable proteins or protein mixtures, in longer term experiments, the weight gain was less regular on vegetable protein mixtures than on milk even though the total gain was similar.

No explanation of the irregularities in growth was given, however, and it was also observed, again without discussion, that the percentage of nitrogen excreted as urea was lower in all babies fed vegetable proteins as compared to those fed milk.

It is thus in most cases not a question of praising or condemning products on the basis of their nutritive value but reporting on success or failure of the products on the basis of marketing acceptability and of considering their potential on economic criteria. It must be emphasized that this approval is for products which have been developed following the general PAG Guidelines[15,17] outlined earlier. The guidelines are reasonable and sensible and products which survive the test procedures are likely to be beneficial unless, and unfortunately this is a large reservation, they may encourage even more the abandonment of breast-feeding.[27]

PROTEIN FOOD MIXTURES

A wide range of products has been developed over the years in many countries. Cereal–legume mixtures predominate as the major components and are mainly proposed as weaning foods or gruels. Some other mixtures of higher protein content, composed of legume and milk or mixtures of legume were designed as protein supplements. A list of many such mixtures is shown in Table 1. Details are given of the components used for the formulation together with the proportions when known, the protein–energy concentration of the final product, costs both per kilogram and per kg protein, the main use and the current status with regard to production. Most, if not all, of the products listed include additional vitamins and minerals.

Recently, 69 schemes, originating from 36 countries, have been evaluated.[28] Nearly half of the schemes were from Central and South America (324 million population) while only 19 schemes were from Asia, with a population of nearly 2000 million. This bears no relation to the incidence of PEM[29] and probably reflects the fact that the initial development of these products came from INCAP.

It is obvious that products which have been developed, irrespective of their nutritional value and impeccable testing history, can have no effect on the incidence of malnutrition unless they are produced and consumed on a wide scale. It is thus salutary to examine in some detail the history of some of the products to ascertain reasons for success or failure and the degree of impact, if any, that these schemes have had on the world incidence of PEM. The excellent monograph by Elizabeth Orr[28] is recommended reading on the evaluation of protein food mixtures.

PRODUCT HISTORIES

The development of the various Incaparina formulations has been described[14] but before the product could be offered to responsible food industry companies, the consumer acceptability and marketability had to be demonstrated.[30] Field acceptability trials and market testing were carried out in several Central American countries during 1959–1960. Production commenced in early 1961 in Guatemala by Cerveceria Centro American SA, the principal Guatemalan brewer and soft drink producer, a company which was known to wish to diversify into food production. It is of interest that a Guatemalan affiliate of a large U.S. concern which had handled the market testing for INCAP was initially offered the long-term exclusive authorization. The parent company, however, was not prepared to make an adequate investment in the project and INCAP then sought another producer. Sales were slow to develop, partly as a result of the initial distribution which was undertaken by the drivers of the company's beer trucks. In 1964, special vans and wholesalers were used and in 1969 a separate sales organization and increased

Table 1. Composition, country of origin, price, use and current status of some protein-rich food mixtures

Product	Country	Composition[a]	Protein-energy ratio[b]	Price/kg U.S. $[c]	Price/kg protein U.S. $	Main use[d]	Current status[e]
Amama	Nigeria	Groundnut, casein	(0.51)	0.93	1.82	P	C
Arlac	Nigeria	Groundnut(75), DSM(25)	0.43	0.34	0.81	P	C
Bal-Ahar[f](A)	India	Groundnut(25), Wheat(65), Chickpea(10)	0.22	—	—	W	A
Bal-Amul	India	Soya(20–25), Cereal(25), Legume(20), DSM(15)	0.25	1.44	5.50	W	A
Cerealina	Brazil	Soya, DSM, Maize	0.19	0.63	3.12	G	A
Colambiharina	Colombia	Soya(30), Rice(20)	0.20	0.21	1.17	G	A
Conasupo	Mexico	Soya(30), Kidney bean(70)	(0.31)	0.27	0.86	P	IP
CSM	USA	Soya(25), DSM(5), Maize(68)	(0.20)	—	—	G	A
Duryea	Colombia	Soya, DSM, Maize	0.33	0.59	2.08	W	A
Faffa(SM)	Ethiopia	Soya(18), DSM(5), Legume(10), Teff(57) (Wheat from 1969)	(0.20)	0.30	1.64	W	A
Fortifex	Brazil	Soya(48), Maize(46)	0.33	0.64	2.14	P	IP
Incaparina	Brazil	Soya(38), Maize(58)	0.30	—	—	G	C
Incaparina	Colombia	Soya(21), Cotton seed(20), Maize(58)	0.30	0.21	0.76	G	A
Incaparina	El Salvador	Cotton seed(38), Maize(58)	0.30	—	—	G	C
Incaparina	Guatemala	Cotton seed(38), Maize(58)	0.30	0.53	1.94	G	A
Incaparina	Nicaragua	Cotton seed(38), Maize(58)	0.30	—	—	G	C
Incaparina	Panama	Cotton seed(38), Maize(58)	0.30	0.67	2.42	G	C
Incaparina	Venezuela	Soya(19), Cotton seed(19), Maize(58)	0.30	0.45	1.60	G	C
Kupangi Biscuits	South Africa	Soya, DSM, Wheat	(0.08)	0.25	—	B	A
Ladylac	Senegal	Groundnut(15), DSM(20), Millet(45)	(0.19)	—	—	W	C
Laubina	Lebanon	Chickpea(28), DSM(10), Wheat(60)	0.17	—	—	W	E
Leche Alim	Chile	Sunflower seed flour, DSM, Fish protein concentrate	(0.27)	—	—	D	E

Name	Country	Composition[a]					
Macaroni (Golden Elbow)	Brazil	Soya (30), Maize (60), Wheat (10)	0.23	0.80[g]	4.00	P	A
Milk Biscuit	Zambia	Soya (7), Maize (13), Wheat (27)	0.17	—	—	B	A
MPF	India	Groundnut (75), Chickpea (25)	(0.42)	0.72	1.71	P	A
Nutro Biscuit	India	Groundnut (25), Wheat (40)	(0.17)	0.69	4.19	B	A
Peruvita (sweet)	Peru	Cotton seed (47), DSM (4), Quinoa (23)	0.33	0.84	2.79	P	C
Peruvita (savoury)	Peru	Cotton seed (52), DSM (4), Quinoa (28)	0.41	—	—	P	C
Protamin	India	Groundnut (75), Chickpea (25)	(0.45)	0.33	0.73	P	A
Pronutro	South Africa	Soya, Groundnut, DSM, Maize	0.21	0.84	3.80	CS	A
Sekmama	Turkey	Soya (20), DSM (10), Chickpea (20), Wheat (40)	(0.25)	—	—	W	A
Solein	Brazil	Soya, DSM	0.28	0.53	1.60	G	IP
Simba	Kenya	Maize (85), DSM (15)	(0.12)	0.23	1.83	G	A
Superamine	Algeria	Wheat (28), Chickpea (38), Lentils (19), SMP (10)	0.20	0.54	2.69	W	A
Super Maeu	Mozambique	Soya (10), DSM (8), Maize (61)	0.27	0.39	—	D	A
Supro	Kenya	Cereal (50), DSM (15), Yeast (25)	0.25	—	—	G	A
Weaning Food	Egypt	Wheat (25), Chickpea (25), Broad Beans (25), DSM (10)	(0.20)	—	—	W	NK
Weaning Food	Madagascar	Soya (38), DSM (5), Rice (40)	—	—	—	W	NK
Soya Porridge	Uganda	Soya (38), DSM (5), Maize (42)	(0.21)	—	—	G	A

[a] Approximate percentage composition is given when known. Almost all include vitamin and mineral supplements, in addition some may have small amounts of flavouring.

[b] Values in brackets have been estimated from protein content assuming 400 kcal/100 g. (1670 KJ/100 g.)

[c] Prices mainly 1970 retail from Orr.[28]

[d] Major intended use: P = Protein supplement; B = Biscuit/Cookie; G = Gruel; W = Weaning food; D = Drink.

[e] Production status: A = Active production; IP = Intermittent production; E = Experimental; C = Ceased production; NK = Not known.

[f] Several alternative formulations exist.

[g] Estimated price—said to be comparable to U.S. retail price for normal macaroni.

promotion began. Initially, production was in a corner of the parent company's brewery with manual filling of the packages, in 1968 a factory solely for the production of Incaparina products was built with a capacity of nearly 8 tons per 8-hour working day. These improvements allowed sales to increase from 228 tons in 1965 to 1284 tons in 1970. Increases in sales allowed a 20 per cent reduction in price in 1966, and in 1967 an addition of synthetic L-lysine to the product to improve nutritional value was possible without a price increase.

From Table 1 it can be seen that Incaparina was introduced into several Latin American countries but that production has ceased in many of them. The experience of Incaparina in Venezuela is of interest, showing how failure can occur despite the involvement of a highly financed international company with a considerable degree of expertise in production and marketing. Incaparina was launched in Venezuela in the provincial city of Valencia by Productos Quaker de Venezuela C.A. but under INCAP supervision. Initial publicity was well-planned and stimulated high demand for the product. INCAP, however, had given permission to only one private enterprise company to manufacture and market the product and no direct support could be given by the government. At the same time, USAID-donated milk powder was available free for governmental feeding programmes. Sales soon slumped, fell further when the price was raised, and ceased the following year. The product did not appeal to Venezuelan culinary habits which call for a thicker 'atole' than could be made from Incaparina. A further deterrent to sales may have been the name since in the same city there was a large manufacturer of animal foods whose product names mostly ended in the suffix 'ina'.

The *Peruvita* enterprise in Peru was launched by the local Nestlé associate and had considerable government involvement together with that of several U.N. Agencies. Planning and publicity once again led to good initial sales, but was followed by no second purchases. Initial consumer testing had been extremely poor since the produce appeared to be completely unacceptable in taste, colour and smell. A major factor was the use of quinoa, a cereal-like product which was used for feeding chickens and pets and regarded at best as a poor man's food.

If the Peruvita enterprise could be described as a debacle, the Fortifex project also launched in 1963 by a Nestlé associate in Brazil was merely a failure. There were again initially good sales but demand declined and except for batches made for institutions, production ceased in 1966; the probable major reason was non-acceptability of the product. Repeat sales are usually only generated when a product is liked, not because it has high nutritional value. It is not surprising that a two-year informal involvement between Nestlé organization and the American University of Beirut for the proposed commercial production and marketing of Laubina never got beyond some minor changes in the formulation and very small-scale pilot production.

From Africa can be cited moderate success stories for *Faffa* in Ethiopia and *Pronutro* in South Africa and failures for *Amama* in Nigeria and *Ladylac* in Senegal. *Amama* was produced by the U.K. pharmaceutical company, Glaxo, and was one of the earliest protein food schemes in operation; its composition was mainly groundnut with some milk protein. It was designed as an additive and the approach was more towards its role as a medicine rather than a food. Sales were already declining but production ceased in 1961 after the presence of aflatoxin in groundnut meal was discovered. A rather similar product, *Arlac,* began production in Northern Nigeria in 1963 with both government and UNICEF support, production continued for some five years and final closure was precipitated by political problems in the area and withdrawal of UNICEF support.

Ladylac was also produced with government involvement and U.N. assistance in the planning stages, however, production ceased within six months. The main reasons given for failure were the high costs of the product in relation to local wages. It was estimated that the minimum economic scale for production was over 200 tons per year while the prospective market was less than 20 tons per year. The introduction of a convenience-type food within the cultural pattern of Senegal may well have been before its time.

Pronutro had estimated sales in 1967 of about 7000 tons and a quote from the company that 'Sales of product are beyond expectations and have led to capacity problems' is cited by Orr.[28] This would lead to expectations of further increases in production. The product has been promoted as a separate dietary item as a breakfast food and also flavoured as a soup mixture and it is claimed that more than half of the total production is to the local African population. As a 'spin-off' from the project, production of soybeans was stimulated in the area, and while initially all beans used were imported now only locally grown beans are used for its production.

Faffa is manufactured by the Ethiopian Nutrition Institute which is jointly sponsored by the Ethiopian and Swedish governments.[31] Sales commenced in 1968 and had risen to some 400 tons by mid-1971. Throughout the development of the project market research has been an integral component. A change in formulation to improve the 'image' was made with wheat replacing teff as the cereal when the product was marketed in the lowlands. The consultant involved throughout the project is Dr. B. Wickström, author of the recent PAG Guideline on the marketing of protein-rich food in developing countries.[20] The problems to be overcome are those of low income, lack of the concept of the needs for special foods for children, lack of the habit of buying packaged foods and a distribution network of a multitude of small stores with a passive retailer attitude. About 1000 tons per year will be needed for the project to be self-supporting on a non-profit basis (Chapter 27).

The introduction of *Superamine* in Algeria was widely assisted by the U.N. Agencies, followed closely most of the PAG Guidelines and took into account many of the lessons of the past.[3] The World Food Programme donated skim milk powder and sugar to the project until 1975, thus giving some degree of subsidy. In 1970 some 75 per cent of total production (523 tons) was purchased by the government for direct free distribution to malnourished children in institutions and in the lower socio-economic groups. It is believed, however, that a new retail market will need to be developed so that the product can establish itself as part of a normal feeding pattern for the weaning of infants. Plant capacity has recently been increased for the free distribution programme but the development of a retail market remains disappointing. Expansion of Superamine into the Egyptian and Tunisian markets has recently taken place.

In India some of the world's largest quantities of food mixtures have been produced, for example 26,500 tons of *Bal-Ahar* (Hindi for child's food) were produced in 1969 and in 1970 it constituted two-thirds of all the special foods produced in low-income countries. Production in 1973 was programmed for 50,000 tons and future production was projected upwards. Bal-Ahar has been manufactured by the Food Corporation of India since 1967. Several different formulations exist besides the example shown in Table 1, for example groundnut could be replaced with cotton seed or soya flour, wheat with maize and there are formulations with dried skim milk.

The product has been designed to protect the health of children in famine and has also been used in school feeding programmes. The development of these and other products has been reviewed.[32] A continuing problem has been the potential presence of aflatoxins in groundnut flour. Techniques have been developed to eliminate or reduce the hazard by fumigation in the field immediately after harvesting and by adequate sorting of the nuts or even by direct removal of the toxin.[32]

The development of *Bal Amul* has involved Government, USAID and U.N. Agencies, with particular care being given to marketing aspects as in the Faffa project in Ethiopia. The product has been on sale since 1970 and production expansion is programmed to 6000 tons per year. The cost is extremely high compared to other similar products but is still below proprietary baby foods. Much of the high cost is in the packaging which is still reported to be in cans.

The product at present can only appeal to upper- and middle-income groups and thus cannot have much impact on infantile malnutrition, unless the price can be reduced.

An alternative product designed primarily as food supplement called *Multipurpose Food* (*MPF*), consisting of 75 per cent low-fat edible grade peanut flour and 25 per cent chickpea flour, was also developed in India some years ago. It had the great advantage of supplying the largest amount of protein per unit cost[32] but overall cost has been greatly affected by packaging in cans. There are several production plants in the country, including the Central Food Technological Research Institute. The major part of production has been used by the Government for institutional use and for famine relief and the retail use has been small. *Protamin* is essentially the same formulation but the price is considerably less.[28]

OTHER PRODUCTS

So far consideration has only been given to the dry food mixes designed to be used as gruels or weaning foods. However, an increasing number of beverages are being produced. They are not complementary protein mixtures as have been discussed above, but are usually soya-based and take advantage of the desire for soft drinks throughout the world. Their relevance to PEM is that they *do* contain protein and they are in direct competition with products such as Coca-Cola and Pepsi-Cola and their worldwide imitations which contain no protein whatsoever (Table 2). By far

Table 2. Country of origin and composition of some protein beverages

Product	Country	Ingredients	Comments
Beanvit	Singapore and Malaysia	Soya milk	Produced since early 1950s
Milpro	India	Animal milk groundnut isolate and vegetable oil	Marketed in Bombay, 1970
Mil-Tone	India	Buffalo milk, groundnut isolate, glucose, minerals and vitamins	Total production about 365,000 litres per year. Two varieties— one primarily for child feeding, the other flavoured for use as commercial beverage
Poluk milk	Thailand	Soya milk, DSM and butterfat	Sold since 1964; 400,000 bottles per year, but production not increasing. Very highly competitive market in soft drinks in Thailand
Puma	Guyana	Soya isolate with banana flavour	Produced since 1967. High concern with marketing—image of 'vigour'. Retail sales in excess of 29,000 bottles per year
Saci	Brazil	Soya milk, vitamins and minerals with flavouring	Test marketed in 1968, by Coca Cola Company. High concern with marketing—image of 'health'. Test marketing does not appear successful. Protein content = 3.0 per cent
Samson	Puerto Rico	Milk whey, vitamins and minerals	Dry powder for home reconstitution. A product of the same name also marketed in Surinam since 1970. Experimental marketing only
Vitabean	Singapore and Malaysia	Soya milk	An improved version of Beanvit with minerals and vitamins. Satisfactory sales, expansion planned
Vitasoy	Hong Kong	Soya milk	Production commenced in 1940 and recommended in 1945. Sales initially poor, product and 'image' improved. Plant capacity trebled over years. Sales now in excess of 120 million bottles per year. Most successful of all protein beverages, protein content = 3 per cent
Yoo Hoo	USA and Iran	DSM, whey chocolate flavour, minerals and vitamins, may also contain vegetable protein	Produced under licence in Iran— sales satisfactory and expansion planned. Protein content = 3.5 per cent

the most successful is Vitasoy in Hong Kong with sales of over 120 million bottles per year. The reasons for this success have been discussed.[28] The product is sold both cold and hot, thus extending the season. The promotion now emphasizes the 'thirst-quenching' properties of the drink rather than the child-feeding aspects. Undoubtedly, however, successful sales are due to the provision of a product that meets consumer needs. It seems unfortunate but true, as with the powdered products, that marketing appeal based on the 'it's good for you' approach is rarely successful.

HOME-MADE FEEDING MIXTURES

Protein complementation can of course occur when protein sources are mixed together by the mother, just as well as by a manufacturer, generally at much lower cost. While the consideration of home-made feeding mixtures is more properly the province of infant-feeding practice and nutrition education rather than of food science and technology it is important that some mention be made here of this very relevant approach. While the concept is not new and much has appeared in the literature, a recent manual by Cameron and Hofvander[5] on feeding infants and young children puts much of the information together in one place. This manual is designed to give comprehensive information on the preparation of home-made weaning foods so that more efficient use can be made of the locally available staples. Based on relevant nutritional composition data, recipes are given for double, triple and multi-mixes to be produced from the most important local staple together with other cereals, roots, legumes, dried milk and/or other protein sources so that the resultant product has high nutritional value and utilizes the available proteins in the most efficient manner.

The manual in its present form is intended primarily for professional groups with some basic knowledge of nutrition but simplified versions, using local products and the local language, could be easily prepared and made available to nutrition aides who could then educate mothers in making the mixes.

The problems of implementing such a programme on a scale large enough to be effective should not be underestimated. However, the major advantages lie in costs. Even cheap food mixtures are relatively expensive and can sometimes reduce nutrient availability on a fixed income. Education, in mixing normally available foods, allows high quality at minimal cost and eliminates many of the limitations and dangers inherent in the food mixture approach.[6]

CONCLUSIONS

Much emphasis has been placed by nutrition scientists, by U.N. Agencies and by governments on low-cost nutritious foods to solve world malnutrition. The scientific interest has been understandable if only for the fact that a considerable armoury of methodology can be brought to bear on the problem. The interest of governments and U.N. Agencies is also understandable: protein complementation has the element of 'two plus two equals five.' In order to evaluate the situation, two major questions need to be asked: (i) Assuming the emphasis to have been correct, do these products still show promise in the fight against world malnutrition? (ii) Has the whole emphasis been based on misconceptions and are programmes perhaps producing harmful consequences?

It is unfortunately true to say in terms of alleviating malnutrition, even under limited objectives, the actual effects have not been great. An evaluation of experience with protein-rich food mixtures[28] concludes 'that a rough calculation of the potential production of protein-rich foods, if available capacity were fully utilized, indicates that in global terms, and even if all that could be produced with present capacity was in fact consumed by the primary target group, the nutritional impact which could be made is small'. Vitasoy is usually cited as a success story and the production of 120 million bottles per year seems remarkable; however, to put this in perspective with a population of 3.5 million in Hong Kong, this represents only 4 g of protein per individual, per week. In the highly unlikely event of the whole production being consumed by the very young, this would still not exceed 40 g of protein per week. This assumes further that money spent on Vitasoy would not have been spent on some other food product—if Vitasoy replaces Cola there is net increase, albeit small in protein intake, if it replaces bread, it is another story.* With Incaparina in Guatemala, surveys[30] showed wide knowledge of the product and favourable opinions on the price and its acceptability. Despite this the overall consumption per family was low, only some 3 kg per family per year[20] and the use was primarily that of a 'family' product rather than specifically for children. When extrapolation is made from 1970 production of 1184 tons using the INCAP recommended consumption of 75 g per child per day, this represents consumption by only 8 per cent of the population of children between 1–3 years.[28] If it could be assumed that the individuals most in need received the product then this would be of value, however it was shown that only 29 per cent of Incaparina consumers were in the lowest income level of under $20.00 per annum.[32]

With the Faffa project in Ethiopia the nutritional goal was to supplement the ordinary diet of an undernourished child with about 100 g Faffa per day: some 20 g of protein. Market surveys[20] have shown that Faffa products were used irregularly and much below the prescribed quantities, averaging only 3 servings per month. A review on the nutrition protection given to vulnerable groups through protein-rich mixtures also concludes that the impact has not been great.[33]

On the other hand, technology has proved that products of high nutritive value can be made from vegetable materials and that they can be cheap, though perhaps not cheap enough. In overall economic and energy balance terms, the advantage of mixing vegetable proteins together is real, protein that would have been wasted both directly and also in physiological utilization, is saved: this is a real net gain.

The developed world has been as wasteful in its energy use in food production and distribution as it has been with its personal transport. Yields in farm production in relation to energy input have probably decreased in the U.S. since 1945[34] and

*Editor's note: PEM is now rare in Hong Kong, not as a result of Vitasoy.

further a tremendous shift has occurred in historical development of agriculture. 'Primitive' cultures could obtain yields of 5–50 food calories for each calorie of energy invested while current industrialized systems require 5–10 calories of fuel to obtain 1 food calorie[35],[36] The implications of this are that if energy costs continue to rise, the price differentials between animal protein foods and vegetable products will increase and the need for food mixtures which can give good quality protein from low-energy-intensive products may well increase.

A further set of advantages are indirect; for example, the production of soybeans in areas where they were not produced before and publicity about protein-rich foods may have influenced overall nutrition to a greater extent than sales figures would indicate.[28]

The rationale for the the development of protein-rich foods originated in the period when it was heresy to question the reality of the 'impending world protein crisis'. As has been discussed earlier (Chapter 3) the protein gap is probably a myth but we are left with a massive investment in protein-rich food schemes. These products have been termed 'commerciogenic nutritious foods' by Popkin and Latham,[6] who believe that 'the limitations and potential dangers of relying on commercially produced, low cost nutritious foods to reduce or eliminate malnutrition have neither been adequately investigated nor put in perspective'. The burden of their criticism is upon the place of these foods in a market economy rather than on the foods themselves. They believe that commercially processed foods are not appropriate for the very poor and can in fact contribute to a deterioration rather than an improvement in nutritional status. Energy in some of these foods can cost 8–40 times its cost in the normal diet and protein may be 3–18 times as expensive. Similar values were reported from Lebanon[37] where commercial weaning foods could cost 20 times as much for energy and 43 times as much for protein as home-produced weaning foods. Popkin and Latham[6] demonstrate that *replacement* of standard dietary items by certain commercial products may have disastrous effects on an individual of fixed purchasing power in that both protein and energy intakes could be reduced. This is not even to consider the other disastrous effects when breast-feeding is replaced by artificial feeding in an unhygienic environment (Chapter 8). With both these aspects the role of advertising is paramount, even fully honest advertising can pull in the wrong direction, dishonest advertising in these circumstances is criminal.

A further major problem lies in the political implications; one does not have to be a cynic to read the salesmanship behind the altruism. The connection between the development of a 'protein-rich food, containing soybeans, the support of USAID and the potential market for U.S. soy exports' is not entirely coincidental. Nor is the wish of the giant international food companies, whose annual turnover is frequently greater than the G.N.P. of many developing nations,[38] to be able to supply baby foods in the underdeveloped world entirely without thought of a future blossoming retail food marketing system. Blind faith in big business is not necessarily the best route to a solution of world protein–energy malnutrition.

Perhaps the resources and efforts, which have been massive and expert, that have been devoted to the developing and marketing of these products, with their in-built subsidies to the rich while supposedly benefiting the poor, would have been better directed toward the transforming of the agricultural and social structures of the developing world. Nutritional advances can only be made when it is realized that solutions based on food and nutrients will never work by themselves but that improvement must come in the wider, controversial and potentially dangerous contexts of economics, politics and national development.

REFERENCES

1. Tannahill, R. *Food in History,* New York, Stein & Day, 1973.
2. Cowan, J. W. and P. L. Pellett. The development of 'Laubina'—infant food mixtures for the Middle East, in *Protein-Enriched Cereal Foods for World Needs,* Max Milner (Ed.), The American Association of Cereal Chemists, 1969, p. 305.
3. Kapsiotis, G. D. History and status of specific protein-rich foods: FAO/WHO/UNICEF protein food protein and products, in *Protein-Enriched Cereal Foods for World Needs,* Max Milner (Ed.), The American Association of Cereal Chemists, 1969, p. 255.
4. van Veen, A. G. and M. L. Scott van Veen. Pioneer work on protein foods, *Nutrition Newsletter,* **11,** No. 4, Oct.–Dec., 1973.
5. Cameron, M. and Y. Hofvander, *Manual on Feeding Infants and Young Children,* Protein Advisory Group of the United Nations System, PAG Document 1.12/26, 1971.
6. Popkin, B. M. and M. C. Latham. The limitations and dangers of commerciogenic nutritious foods. *Am. J. Clin. Nutr.,* **26,** 1015 (1973).
7. FAO/WHO 1973. Energy and protein requirements, FAO Nutrition Report Series No. 52, Food and Agricultural Organization, Rome, 1973.
8. Whitehead, R. G. The protein needs of malnourished children, in *Proteins in Human Nutrition,* Porter, J. W. C. and B. A. Rolls (Eds.), London and New York, Academic Press, 1973, p. 103.
9. Nicol, B. M. Protein and calorie concentration. *Nutr. Revs.,* **29,** 83 (1971).
10. Hegsted, D. M. and R. Neff. Efficiency of protein utilization in young rats at various levels of intake, *J. Nutr.,* **100,** 1173 (1970).
11. Samonds, K. W. and D. M. Hegsted. Protein requirements of young cebus monkeys, *Am. J. Clin. Nutr.,* **26,** 30 (1973).
12. Miller, D. S. and P. R. Payne. Problems in the prediction of protein values of diets: Caloric restriction, *J. Nutr.,* **75,** 225 (1961).
13. FAO Agricultural Commodity Projections 1970–80. Vols. I and II. Food and Agricultural Organization of the United Nations, Rome, 1971.
14. Bressani, R. and L. G. Elias. Processed vegetable protein mixtures for human consumption in developing countries, *Adv. Food Res.,* **16,** 1 (1968).
15. FAO/WHO/UNICEF Protein Advisory Group. PAG Guideline on preclinical testing of novel sources of protein. (PAG Guideline No. 6, 1972).
16. FAO/WHO/UNICEF Protein Advisory Group. PAG Guideline on human testing of supplementary food mixtures. (PAG Guideline No. 11, 1972.)
17. FAO/WHO/UNICEF Protein Advisory Group. PAG Guideline on sanitary production and use of dry protein foods. (PAG Guideline No. 7, 1972.)
18. Anonymous. Evaluation of Protein Quality. A revised edition of NAS-NRC Publication No. 1100 by a joint committee of FNB/PAG/IUNS. In press.
19. FAO/WHO/UNICEF Protein Advisory Group. PAG Guideline on protein-rich mixtures for use as weaning foods. (PAG Guideline No. 8, 1972.)

202

20. FAO/WHO/UNICEF Protein Advisory Group. PAG Guideline on marketing of protein-rich foods in developing countries (PAG Guideline No. 10, 1971).
21. Chandrasekhara, M. R., S. R. Shurpalekar, B. N. S. Rao, S. Kurien and K. S. Shurpalekar. Development of infant foods based on soy bean, *J. Food Sci. Technol.*, **3**, 94 (1966).
22. Asfour, R. Y., R. I. Tannous, Z. I. Sabry and J. W. Cowan. Protein-rich food mixtures for feeding infants and young children in the Middle East. II. Preliminary Clinical Evaluation with Laubina mixtures. *Am. J. Clin. Nutr.*, **17**, 148 (1965).
23. Milner, M. (Ed.). *Protein-Enriched Cereal Foods for World Needs*, The American Association of Cereal Chemists, 1969.
24. Graham, G. C. and J. M. Baertl. Nutritional effectiveness of soy cereal foods in undernourished infants, *J. Am. Oil Chemists, Soc.*, **51**, 152A (1974).
25. Anonymous. Symposium on legumes and green leafy vegetables in the nutrition of the infant and young child. PAG Bulletin, **3**, No. 2, 1973.
26. Knapp, J., L. A. Barness, L. L. Hill, R. Kaye, R. Blattner and J. M. Sloan. Growth and nitrogen balance in infants fed cereal proteins, *Am. J. Clin. Nutr.*, **26**, 586 (1973).
27. Wade, N. Bottle feeding: Adverse effects of a western technology. *Science*, **184**, 45 (1974).
28. Orr, E. The use of protein-rich foods for the relief of malnutrition in developing countries: An analysis of experience. Tropical Products Institute, No. G.73, London, 1972.
29. Bengoa, J. M. and G. Donoso. Prevalence of protein-calorie malnutrition. *PAG Bulletin*, **4**, No. 1, 24 (1974).
30. Shaw, R. L. Incaparina in Central America, in *Protein-Enriched Cereal Foods for World Needs*, M. Milner (Ed.). Part VIII, The American Association of Cereal Chemists, 1969, p. 320.
31. Agren, G., Y. Hofvander, R. Selinus and B. Vahlquist. Faffa: A supplementary cereal-based weaning food mixtures in Ethiopia. In *Protein-Enriched Cereal Foods for World Needs*, M. Milner (Ed.). The American Association of Cereal Chemists, 1969, p. 278.
32. Parpia, H. A. B. Protein foods of India based on cereals, legumes, and oilseed meals. In: *Protein-Enriched Cereal Foods for World Needs*, M. Milner (Ed.), The American Association of Cereal Chemists, 1969, p. 129.
33. Wickström, B. Marketing of protein-rich foods to vulnerable groups. In: *Nutrition—a priority in African development*, B. Vahlquist (Ed.). Dag Hammarskjöld Foundation, Stockholm, Almquist & Wiksell, 1972, p. 97.
34. Cordaro, D. B. and D. L. Call. Nutritional protection of vulnerable groups through protein-rich mixtures: a critical review. In: *Prox. IX, Intern. Nutr. Congr.*, Mexico City, 1972, in press.
35. Pimentel, D., L. E. Hurd, A. C. Bellotti, M. J. Forster, I. N. Oka, O. D. Sholes and R. J. Whitman. Food production and the energy crisis, *Science*, **182**, 443 (1973).
36. Steinhart, J. S. and C. E. Steinhart. Energy use in the U.S. food system. *Science*, **184**, 307 (1974).
37. Pellet, P. L. and L. McGregor. Food as a cause of childhood malnutrition. *Proc. 6th Symp. Nutri. Hlth. Near East*, American University of Beirut, 1971, p. 53.
38. Berg, A. Industry's struggle with world malnutrition. *Harvard Business Review*, Jan. 1972, p. 130.

CHAPTER 17

Food Fortification

D. M. HEGSTED

The addition of essential nutrients to foods to control deficiency diseases has become possible and a logical tool in public health as (i) the essential nutrients for man have been identified, (ii) reasonable estimates of the requirements and toxicity of the essential nutrients have been developed, and (iii) they have become available commercially at a reasonable price. The first recommendations of this kind were for the addition of iodine compounds to salt for the control of endemic goitre.[1] Early in this century vitamin A concentrates were added to certain foods for the control of xerophthalmia, and somewhat later additional vitamin D was provided in selected foods at first by irradiation and then by the addition of concentrates or the pure vitamin. At the time of World War II the addition of certain B vitamins, iron and sometimes calcium to certain products was begun.

A joint FAO/WHO Expert Committee on Nutrition considered this topic in considerable detail in 1971.[2] Only a limited review and discussion are possible here.

Several terms have been used to describe the addition of nutrients to foods. In the United States the term 'enrichment' has been applied to describe the addition of nutrients in conformity with certain government standards: enriched bread, for example. 'Restoration' has been suggested as the appropriate term for the addition of nutrients to replace those removed during processing and some have thought that the term 'fortification' should be limited to additions of nutrients not originally in foods or to additions of amounts greater than occur in the original foods. The utility of these and other such distinctions can be debated and in this discussion fortification is used as a general term for the deliberate addition of nutrients to foods for nutritional purposes.

The general philosophy which has been used to support fortification schemes was reasonably well expressed by the Council on Foods and Nutrition of the American Medical Association in 1954[3] as follows:

With carefully defined limitations, the principle of the addition of specific nutrients to certain staple foods is endorsed for purposes of maintaining good nutrition as well as correcting deficiencies in the diets of the general population or of a significant segment of the population. The requirements for endorsement of the addition of a particular nutrient or a particular food include (a) clear indications of probable advantage from increased intake of the nutrient, (b) assurance that the food item concerned would be an effective vehicle for distribution of the nutrient added and (c) evidence that such addition would not be prejudicial to the achievement of good health in other respects.

In a more recent statement[4] the Food and Nutrition Board of the National Research Council–National Academy of Sciences expanded on this and endorsed the addition of nutrients to foods . . . when all of the following conditions are met:

1. The intake of the nutrient(s) is below the desirable level in the diets of a significant number of people;
·2. The food(s) used to supply the nutrient(s) is likely to be consumed in quantities that will make a significant contribution to the diet of the population in need;
3. The addition of the nutrient(s) is not likely to create a dietary imbalance;
4. The nutrient(s) added is stable under customary conditions of storage and use;
5. The nutrient(s) is physiologically available from the food;
6. The enhanced levels attained in the total diet will not be harmfully excessive for those who may employ the foods in varying patterns of use; and
7. The additional cost is reasonable for the intended consumer.

The following practices for the United States were specifically endorsed:

The enrichment of flour, bread, degerminated corn meal, corn grits, whole grain corn meal, white rice and certain other cereal grain products with thiamin, roboflavin, niacin and iron; the addition of vitamin D to milk, fluid skim milk, and nonfat dry milk; the addition of vitamin A to margarine, fluid skim milk, and nonfat dry milk; and the addition of iodine to table salt. The protective action of fluoride against dental caries is recognized and the standardized addition of fluoride to water in areas in which the water supply has a low fluoride content is endorsed.

It is important to understand that these principles or guidelines have clear public health objectives. It is assumed that there is some reasonable evidence of need in the population whether this be based upon estimated intakes relative to estimated need, or biochemical or clinical evidence of deficiency. One then searches for an effective vehicle to distribute the needed nutrient to the population or the segment of the population in need. The reasonableness of utilizing salt to distribute iodine is clear since this is a universal food and in many instances the only suitable commercial vehicle to which the addition can be made, supervised and controlled. The appropriateness of milk and milk products for the distribution of vitamins A and D to infants and young children is self-evident in many parts of the world. The selection of bread, flour and other cereal products for the distribution of certain B vitamins and iron can be similarly defended in that these are nearly universal foods in many populations, low in cost and thus generally eaten by the segment of the population most in need, and usually subject to reasonable control. The latter is, of course, not true in areas of the world where rice or other cereal products are milled at home or in village operations. The question has recently been raised as to whether bread is an appropriate vehicle in the United States since the consumption of bread and cereals has fallen substantially over the years and especially in certain segments of the population.

Recent developments in the food industry and in the nature of the food supply in many countries raise entirely different issues from those indicated above. Many new processed foods are now being produced and marketed. In the United States, for example, a rather large proportion of the total food supply now consists of so-called 'convenience foods', partially or completely prepared for consumption when sold. An increasing amount of food is consumed outside the home. Some of these new foods are simple mixtures of familiar ingredients and may be presumed to be nutritionally similar to familiar foods but many others are not. With increasing sophistication of the food industry it can be expected that the trend will be away from simple mixtures and the use of unfamiliar materials. At the extreme, for example, meat substitutes made from vegetable protein sources are now appearing on the market.

If, as may be expected, the proportion of the total food supply moves toward these kinds of products, the 'conventional wisdom' which has allowed people to obtain reasonably satisfactory diets with only a minimum of nutritional knowledge will no longer suffice. The housewife or whoever prepares food has less control over, and less capability of evaluating, the nutritional quality of the diet. It would seem certain that unless specific attention is paid to the matter the nutritional quality of diets will tend to fall. The food industry must assume more responsibility, some controls may be required, and there must be increased efforts to educate the consumer.

With regard to such foods the Food and Nutrition Board of the National Research Council–National Academy of Sciences of the United States recently recommended that: 'their nutritional value should be at least equal to the foods replaced' and

> The composition of a new or formulated food becomes especially important when an average serving of the product it imitates or replaces contributes 5 per cent or more of the recommended daily allowance (RDA) of any essential nutrient or energy. The formulated food should contain on a calorie basis at least the variety and the amounts of important nutrients provided by the food it replaces. Exceptions should, of course, be made for foods intended for therapeutic or modified diets in which the nutrient content is deliberately modified quantitatively or qualitatively. A product designed primarily as a meal replacer should provide in the portion designated as a 'meal' 25 to 50 per cent of the RDA or, for those essential nutrients for which the RDA had not been established, 25 to 50 per cent of the estimated requirement. Caloric value of such products will depend upon recommended use.

Many of these points must be the subject of continuing debate and consideration. Although it is suggested that fortification will be of special importance when a new food provides 5 per cent of the energy, it is not clear how this will be determined.

Average values are not very useful. Some people may consume large amounts of a product even though the average consumption is low. Another major problem is the definition of 'nutritional equivalence'. Is it safe to define such equivalence only in terms of those nutrients for which requirements or recommended intakes are commonly available or does one attempt to add all essential nutrients? In meat analogues, for example, should potassium, sodium, phosphorus and trace elements be added at the levels found in meat products? If so, what levels can be suggested for essential nutrients such as selenium, the requirements for which are poorly defined and which is toxic at intakes not much above requirement levels?

It should also be emphasized that it is becoming increasingly clear that the definition of a nutritionally adequate diet on the basis of essential nutrients alone is not possible. The relationships between dietary fat and hypercholesterolaemia and cardiovascular disease: between diet and dental caries; the possible relationships between dietary fibre and colonic cancer, diverticulosis, and possibly other diseases emphasize that adequate nutrition is not ensured by attention to essential nutrients alone (Chapter 9).

Just how these questions will ultimately be resolved is unknown. On the one hand, we must be aware of the limitations of our knowledge and not be lulled into a false sense of security. On the other, the talents and capabilities of the food industry to improve the nutritional quality of the food supply must not be unduly restricted.

PRIOR EXPERIENCE WITH FORTIFICATION PROGRAMMES

The relationships between classical nutritional deficiency diseases and the corresponding essential nutrients leave no doubt as to the central role played by the essential nutrients. It is somewhat surprising, therefore, that the benefits derived from fortification programmes are not, in most instances, very clear.

There is unequivocal evidence that the fortification of salt with iodides is effective against goitre due to iodine deficiency and that the fluoridation of water supplies is effective in reducing dental caries. The latter does not, of course, eliminate dental caries but a reduction of approximately 50 per cent or more is the common experience when fluoride is added to water supplies low in fluoride.

The direct results of other fortification programmes have been much more difficult to ascertain. The introduction of irradiated and vitamin D fortified milk, for example, occurred at a time when the nutritional needs of infants were being better recognized and preventive paediatric care was being developed. The prevalence of rickets undoubtedly fell to very low levels but the specific role of food fortification cannot be clearly determined. It may be noted, however, that recent findings in Canada[5] suggest an increase in the incidence of rickets probably related to the lack of availability of fortified milk.

Similarly, the virtual disappearance of pellagra in the southern United States cannot be clearly related to food fortification since the fall in the incidence of pellagra ante-dated widespread food fortification. The late 1930s was a time in which the economic conditions were improving in many areas of the country, considerable effort was made to improve nutrition through home gardens and general education, and the relationship between nutrition and pellagra and the value of materials like brewer's yeast were becoming much better understood by physicians and others. No doubt all of these contributed to the reduction in pellagra (Chapter 3).

The nutrition survey in Newfoundland in 1945[6] demonstrated deficiencies of vitamin A, the B vitamins and iron. A general fortification programme was begun, including the fortification of bread with thiamine, riboflavin, niacin, iron and calcium as well as the fortication of margarine with vitamin A. A resurvey in 1948[7] indicated substantial improvement. However, the intervening period was one of economic growth, an improvement in the variety of the food supply, distribution of skim milk to schools and cod liver oil to expectant mothers and infants, and general efforts in nutrition education.

The work done in the Philippines[8] appeared to demonstrate the need for and the effectiveness of thiamine fortification of rice. However, general fortification of rice was never achieved. Nevertheless, the prevalence of beriberi has fallen in the Philippines and in many other countries from pre-war levels.

It is somewhat disappointing that we do not have hard data to prove the efficacy of most fortification programmes. This must not, however, be interpreted to mean that the programmes were ineffective. Data are not available to demonstrate what might have happened if fortification had not been practised. Provided the vehicle is appropriate and the costs are low, one may expect that fortification will be an effective way of reaching the part of the population most in need and least likely to be reached by other approaches such as education, medical care, etc. If costs are sufficiently low, certain fortification programmes may be justified purely as insurance. However, as indicated in the next section, some degree of surveillance should be undertaken to ensure that the benefits expected are indeed derived from the programme.

SPECIAL PROBLEMS WITH FORTIFICATION PROGRAMMES

The outbreak of hypercalcaemia in infants in the United Kingdom[9] and some other countries during the 1950s was apparently due to excessive fortification of national dried milk and perhaps other materials with vitamin D. The toxicity of vitamin D had long been recognized, but the likelihood that fortification schemes would be hazardous had been discounted prior to that time. In 1957 the Ministry of Health in the United Kingdom recommended that the levels of vitamin D in the national milk, in infant cereals and in cod liver oil preparations be reduced. The prevalence of hypercalcaemia has apparently fallen to very low levels since that time. It is interesting that although hypercalcaemia constituted a serious problem, the number of infants affected was small compared to the large numbers who must have consumed excessive vitamin D. Presumably, there are large differences in individual susceptibility.

Arneil[10] states that in Glasgow it is likely that some 50 per cent of infants suffered from rickets in 1920. This incidence had fallen to something of the order of 20 per cent by 1940 and with the provision of fortified national milk fell to very low levels by 1950. Data from the Royal Hospital for Sick Children in Glasgow indicate only one or two children per year with rickets from 1953–1958. With the modifications recommended due to concern over hypercalcaemia, admissions to the same hospital with rickets ranged from 4–24 between 1962 and 1966. The provision of a completely safe yet effective level is apparently not easy to achieve.*

The provision of iron by the fortification of cereals seems an eminently logical step in a population in which iron deficiency occurs. There is accumulating evidence, however, that the fortification of bread, flour and some other products has not been as successful as was anticipated. Low or moderately low haemoglobin values are prevalent in the United States and clinical evidence of iron deficiency is common 30 years after cereal fortification was begun.[11,12] Obviously, the problem might be worse at this time if fortification had not been practised. Nevertheless, it would appear that (i) insufficient iron might have been used; (ii) the consumption of bread and other fortified materials might have fallen in the susceptible population; or (iii) that the form of iron used in the fortification programme was unavailable or relatively unavailable.

No doubt all three of these possibilities contribute. Cereal consumption has fallen to relatively low levels in the United States and especially in some women, and poorly utilizable forms of iron have been used in the fortification mixtures. However, the availability of iron depends not only upon the form of iron in the food but also upon the nature of the diet with which it is consumed,[13,14] and individual differences in iron requirements are large.[11] Knowledge of the iron content of a diet may be a relatively poor indicator of nutritional 'adequacy' or 'inadequacy'. The clinical significance of moderate iron deficiency and the most rational public health measures which might be used to combat it are a matter of continuing debate.[15]

Although the prevalence of classical nutritional deficiency diseases is low in most of the developed nations, there is often a significant problem among the destitute and alcoholics. Among the latter it appears that the brain damage due to cerebral beriberi is largely irreversible. The total costs of patients with permanent disabilities are very high, even though the numbers may not appear to be large. Thus, it may be worthwhile to explore special fortification methods to reach the very small groups who are most susceptible.

Considerable interest has been generated in the possible use of amino-acid fortification of cereals as a means of increasing the amounts of available protein.[2,16] The advantage of amino-acid fortification, as opposed to other methods of increasing the availability of protein, would be that such fortification would not require the modification of the usual food pattern. It can be readily demonstrated under laboratory conditions that the proteins of cereals can be improved by amino-acid additions. However, the aetiology of protein–energy malnutrition is complex (Chapter 7) and there is, as yet, no satisfactory evidence that the addition of either

*Editor's note: See Chapter 30, reference 15.

amino acids or protein to the usual diets in those areas where protein–energy malnutrition occurs has measurable beneficial effects. Amino-acid fortification is relatively expensive and costs are borne, directly or indirectly, by the consumer. Any increase in the costs of basic foods in developing countries may accentuate malnutrition. The case for amino acid fortification has not yet been made.

In conclusion, fortification of foods with nutrients is a logical tool for the control of malnutrition and undoubtedly fortification will increase in the future. The major and unresolved problem for the immediate future, considering our fragmentary knowledge of the nutritional needs of man, is to develop a rational policy that prevents over-reliance on fortification.

Experience demonstrates that, depending upon the nutrient involved, fortification may not be as effective as anticipated and may not be without risk. Rational surveillance systems should be an inherent part of all fortification programmes to determine compliance, effectiveness, and risk of undesirable effects. The cost of both the fortification programme and the surveillance systems as well as prior experience will, however, determine the degree of surveillance that is justified.

REFERENCES

1. World Health Organization, *Endemic Goiter,* WHO Monograph Series No. 44, Geneva, 1960.
2. World Health Organization, *Joint FAO/WHO Expert Committee on Nutrition,* 8th Report, WHO Technical Report Series No. 477, Geneva, 1971.
3. Council on Foods and Nutrition, *J. Amer. Med. Assoc.,* **154,** 145 (1954).
4. Food and Nutrition Board, *General Policies in Regard to Development of Nutritive Quality of Foods,* National Academy of Sciences–National Research Council, Washington, D.C., 1973.
5. Barsky, P. *Canad. J. Public Health,* **60,** 29 (1969).
6. Adamson, J. D., N. Jolliffe, H. D. Kruse, O. H. Lowry, P. E. Moore, B. S. Platt, W. H. Sebrell, J. W. Tice, F. F. Tisdall, P. M. Wilder and P. C. Zamecnik, *Canad. Med. Assoc. J.,* **52,** 227 (1945).
7. Aykroyd, W. R., N. Jolliffe, O. H. Lowry, P. E. Moore, W. H. Sebrell, R. E. Shank, F. F. Tisdall, P. M. Wilder and P. C. Zamecnik. *Canad. Med. Assoc. J.,* **60,** 329 (1949).
8. Food and Agriculture Organization, *Rice Enrichment in the Philippines,* FAO Nutritional Study No. 12, Rome, 1954.
9. British Paediatric Association Committee Report, *Brit. Med. J.,* **2,** 149 (1956).
10. Arneil, G. C. *World Rev. Nutr. Dietet.,* **10,** 239 (1969).
11. Council on Foods and Nutrition, Committee on Iron Deficiency, *J. Amer. Med. Assoc.,* **203,** 407 (1968).
12. Center for Disease Control, *Ten State Nutrition Survey* 1968–1970, *Biochemical,* Vol. IV, Department of Health, Education and Welfare, Atlanta, Georgia, 1972.
13. Layrisse, M., J. D. Cook, C. Martinez-Torres, M. Roche, I. N. Kuhn, R. B. Walker and C. A. Finch. *Blood,* **33,** 430 (1969).
14. Cook, J. D., V. Minnich, C. V. Moore, A. Rasmussen, W. B. Bradley and C. A. Finch. *Amer. J. Clin. Nutr.,* **26,** 861 (1973).
15. Elwood, P. C. *Iron in Flour,* Reports on Public Health and Medical Subjects No. 117, Her Majesty's Stationery Office, London, 1968.
16. FAO/WHO/UNICEF Protein Advisory Group, *PAG Statement on Amino Acid Fortification of Foods,* United Nations, New York, 1970.

CHAPTER 18

Group Feeding in Normal and Emergency Situations

Roy E. Brown

There are many factors to be considered when managing to feed groups of people, the first being the determination of whether it is a normal or an emergency situation. Similarities within the two situations will be apparent to the reader, but here each will be dealt with separately.

NORMAL SITUATIONS

Group feeding in normal situations would apply when dealing with populations in such institutions as schools, hospitals, prisons, camps of various sorts, and military or other gatherings. At the start, it must be determined how many meals each week would be provided. Would this be a short- or long-time situation, and are snack foods to be included for the group? There exists a variety of 'cycle menus' that have been developed not only to provide the full nutritional requirements for the group, but also a changing selection of foods. It clearly would be important to distinguish the provision of school lunches five days a week as contrasted with three meals a day for a group attending a one-week conference or with the provision of food for a military base or patients in a hospital.

There are certain groups that may have special requirements that must be considered. These include infants and growing children who might require artificial formula or vitamin supplementation, pregnant or lactating women with additional vitamin or mineral requirements, elderly persons, and those with special medical problems requiring dietary management. The need for a nutrition specialist for consultation in such circumstances would be essential.

Attention mut be given to the logistics of various aspects of group feeding. The ordering of local foods as well as those that must be brought in from outside the immediate region may definitely be influenced by the provisions available for storage and refrigeration as well as by the available budget for food purchasing. Both the preparation of the meals and the distribution to the recipients may constitute significant logistical considerations. A balance must be achieved between nutritional requirements and the convenience of various types of delivery systems of meals.

When one is involved in the provision of food for a group, the opportunity for introducing nutrition education to the group should be taken. As a first step, it is important to determine what constitutes the 'ordinary' or 'usual' diet of the group. The so-called 'balanced' diet is generally aimed at the provision of daily requirements of energy, protein, vitamins and minerals, with requirements for special cases being considered as indicated above. The introduction of new foods, along with an extension of the accepted cultural foods, can become a very important aspect of group feeding.

If one is concerned with the provision of food for a group during a specific period of time, or with only a fraction of the individual's overall food intake, there may be an identifiable need to attempt to influence either subsequent diets or the diet provided at home. For example, five mid-day meals for the school child may very well be developed in such a way as to have a definite influence on the remaining food habits of the family. One approach that has been used to great advantage, especially with children, is to involve the recipients in both the selection and preparation of foods.

It becomes essential to make a 'good' diet both interesting and pleasurable. The foods and the mealtimes should be organized in such a fashion as to be as pleasant as possible, served in quiet and non-disruptive surroundings, with comfortable tables and chairs and a generally attractive atmosphere. Food exploration should be encouraged so that individuals extend their food preferences. With a rotating or cyclic menu, the boredom of having the same sort of meals over and over again can be avoided, but it is important to take advantage of local produce and products as well as to be fully aware of cultural preferences in both the types of food and their preparation.

Another important aspect of the programme is the evaluation of the group feeding from an objective as well as from a subjective point of view. The usual approach is to estimate how much wastage there is by inspection of the disposed food, and this provides a ready means of learning which foods are desirable and which are not. More objectively, one can evaluate the growth records of children to determine whether height and weight for age or other such anthropometric measurements are acceptable according to reference standards. Menu evaluation can be easily achieved, but this will serve no purpose if a large proportion of the food is not ingested for one reason or another. Whoever is in charge of the overall group feeding should take advantage of consultation of others more familiar with the various aspects of such a programme described above.

GROUP FEEDING IN EMERGENCY SITUATIONS

As with the normal situations, provision of food for groups under emergency conditions necessitates the consideration of various factors. It might be important to identify the high-risk or most vulnerable sub-groups in order to determine who the priority recipients should be. It is usually predictable that infants and growing children, along with pregnant and lactating women, the elderly and sick or disabled persons are the most vulnerable and therefore constitute individuals with special requirements. It is necessary to set priorities early in the programme and also to develop and implement a system of evaluation.

The factors which influence nutritional status go far beyond dietary intake. Infectious diseases often have a negative effect on nitrogen balance and therefore on nutrition. Contributory is the anorexia which is associated with any infectious process.[1] Especially when the nutritional status is borderline, any contagious disease causes the nutritional imbalance to become more severe and significant complications may arise of synergistic origin.[2,3] Intestinal parasitic infestations of roundworms and hookworms and even such relatively minor skin problems as impetigo or scabies can negatively alter nitrogen balance (Chapter 10).

The recommendations which follow deal with both health and nutritional considerations. The programme could easily be conducted by supervised paramedical personnel, would be easy to administer, and would be both inexpensive and implementable. Many of the paramedicals may be recruited from within the camp itself.

Mass campaigns can be organized for feeding the large numbers of people, with orientation towards correcting the specific conditions that were highly prevalent among them. A number of fundamental questions must be asked: Does the provided foodstuff have to represent a complete diet or will it be supplementing the available local diet? Are there other sources of local foodstuffs? Can the people fish, is farming a possibility, and are there milk-producing animals in the region? Other questions that must be considered include: Are there facilities for the group to do its own cooking, and are food and water available along with pots, pans, cups, plates and so forth? Are there strong local food preferences characterized by a long-standing staple diet, and can such a diet be achieved under existing conditions?

There may be present other medical problems in the group, and early in the programme the overall and specific nutritional needs should be determined by some sort of survey technique.[4] There may be long-standing nutritional problems among certain members of the group, and in most instances there will be a need for incorporating a medical programme along with the provision of food. What are the immediate and long-standing health problems and should special consideration be given to the rehabilitation of certain group members?

Superimposed on the base of undernutrition, there may be found certain medical problems. Anaemias, respiratory conditions including tuberculosis, gastroenteritis and dehydration, malaria, infectious diseases, especially measles and chicken pox, skin conditions including septic sores and scabies, and helminthiases, especially hookworm and roundworm infestations, constitute the common medical problems in emergency situations.

Severe malnutrition will reduce an individual's resistance, especially of the young child, making him more susceptible to certain diseases such as measles and tuberculosis and the complications of many infections. A number of factors combine to produce anaemia, such as iron deficiency, poor protein intake, malaria, and hookworm parasites, along with other infectious processes. Anaemia may be severe in many cases, and there may be the need for a massive public health campaign specifically developed to attack this problem.

Although the anaemia may have multiple causes, it may be presumed that iron-deficiency anaemia will be widespread. Therefore, some form of iron medication, either as tablet or liquid, should be distributed once a week or once a fortnight to supplement whatever iron is present in the diet.

If malaria is identified as a significant problem, mass prophylaxis with chloroquine could be introduced. With a jet injection apparatus in the field, 1000 people per hour can be given mass immunizations.[5] We strongly recommend that all children be given triple vaccine (DPT) fo protection against diphtheria, pertussis and tetanus and that all be vaccinated with BCG against tuberculosis.[6,7] Given the crowded living conditions, the psychological problems and the duress associated with the emergency situation and the fact that malnutrition is extremely common, it can be assumed that there will be large numbers of individuals with active and highly contagious tuberculosis.

Young children with severe malnutrition often have advanced forms of tuberculosis, the type that is generally found in the adult, with cavitation and positive sputum tests replacing the more commonly found primary type of tuberculosis among better-nourished children. When considering the aetiology of diarrhoeal diseases, in addition to the generally prevalent infections associated with enteropathic organisms including typhoid and cholera, there must be considered other possibilities such as lactase deficiency and milk intolerance that may be found among children with severe malnutrition.

Vaccination against smallpox can easily be administered on a mass scale with the pedojet apparatus. Mass treatment for scabies and other skin infections is advisable during the times that people wait in line for food distribution.

It is easier to conduct mass programmes such as these with large numbers gathered together in feeding programmes than in an ordinary community. They can be administered easily if planned in terms of the logistics of the group, the availability of paramedical personnel and of medications that are not expensive and are extremely easy to administer. Other mass campaigns which may be indicated can be undertaken in parallel fashion.

It is well known that starting prophylactic measures early will help to forestall complications and later mortality. One can apply a crude cost of accounting to the health circumstances in such emergencies. For instance, within the intestinal tracts of the numbers of people under consideration, roundworms are cumulatively stealing tons of protein from ingested food sources. Similarly, uncountable litres of red blood cells are passing from the intestinal capillaries into the bodies of millions of hookworms.

It is not suggested that the proposed remedial approaches will cure either the individual or the large groups. It must be pointed out that such prophylactic medicinal campaigns, when carried out in conjunction with the mass feeding programmes for the high-risk categories, can help keep the balance of borderline nutritional status from tipping over into overt deficiency diseases.

In order to arrive at the ideal mechanism for food distribution, it is important to evaluate the kind of organized groupings that exist. Often such groupings may facilitate the logistics of such a situation. For example, in refugee camps, there may be separately organized sub-groupings or communities, and this may facilitate the distribution of supplies. There may have been schools organized, hospitals or field clinics or outlying villages and towns that may easily lend themselves to various distribution processes.

One must be aware not only of the need for food and medicine, but, in addition, of the specific problems of logistics and distribution. There obviously is a need for fuel, spare parts for vehicles, equipment for administration of drugs and vaccines, provision of refrigeration where electricity may be unreliable, outside advisers in certain fields, as well as training of teams of locally recruited paramedical personnel. Methods of drug administration must be designed so that non-professional personnel can be usefully employed. For example, basic schedules of drug dosages using safe drugs with a high therapeutic index must be devised. Therapeutics must be simplified for mass distribution with a very limited number of items that can be prepared in a pre-packaged form.

A set of simplified guidelines for the management of common medical conditions is needed. A standard and uniform approach to the management and therapy of different illnesses is essential. The guidelines should emphasize simplicity rather than medical sophistication.

Part of a standardized approach to therapy should be a limited number of medications. Furthermore, it must be borne in mind that individuals suffering from malnutrition often have altered metabolic pathways and abnormal levels of enzymes so that the utilization and detoxification of various drugs may be unpredictable, making it vital that extreme care be used in treatment. Only restricted medications should be carefully employed. A separate set of guidelines and listing of drugs should be developed for paediatric problems.

Where indicated, entire groups could be given such items as iron, anti-worm medications or skin treatments, if these conditions were found to be particularly prevalent. Using this approach, one could see large numbers of patients and treat them at the same time as food is being distributed, with each member of the paraprofessional team carrying out a single task under close supervision.

A 'triage' approach (sorting according to quality) to the medical problems found should be developed. This must be directed to the identification of those conditions that can be easily remedied, as distinguished from those that need more intensive care and possible referrals.

Such matters as communication and transportation must be taken into consideration in relation to available medical and nutrition supplies. Are personnel available, either locally or from outside the group, to serve as administrators, managers, organizers and supervisors? There may be the availability of trained personnel in the medical, nursing, engineering or construction fields who could provide immediate services as well as develop training programmes to organize members of the group for the provision of such services. There will clearly be a need for cooks, aides, as well as assistants in various aspects of the nutrition and medical programmes. Whether the people are basically farmers, fishermen or herdsmen may be important.

Training courses for young men and women must be developed in all long-standing emergency situations. High-school students can be easily trained to identify children suffering from severe malnutrition and to bring the identified children for medical attention. In addition, there may be the need for conducting first aid courses so that there will be other trained personnel to assist the professionals when indicated.

Training courses for these workers should be of several days' duration, conducted on the spot where clinical material is readily accessible, and taught in conjunction with a simply written training manual.

To cover medical facilities adequately and to provide assistance for such large numbers of people, a step-wise progression should be planned, so arranged that a more experienced level of medical personnel is made responsible for training the next level of individuals, and so on down the line. For example, the physician might train the nurses and paramedical personnel and these, in turn, would assist with the training of the volunteer personnel.

At every level there must be provision for continuing supervision. This would represent an in-service surveillance system, a responsibility of the supervisory physicians. Personnel working in the feeding programmes, including cooks and food handlers, should receive some minimal instruction on sanitation and in the recognition of obvious signs of clinical malnutrition.

Despite the difficulties involved with medical management of large numbers, emergencies afford a unique opportunity for medical students, physicians in training, nursing and other medical personnel to gain first-hand knowledge in the management of catastrophic medical problems. Rotation of students, physicians and nurses could be organized and systematized so that various regional medical and nursing schools could provide adequate coverage at the same time as field training is developed.

The training manuals and courses should concentrate on a limited number of severe medical conditions—those that are not only common but can be readily diagnosed clinically without aid of laboratory or X-ray facilities. These conditions include:

1. Severe clinical malnutrition, particularly kwashiorkor, marasmus and marasmic-kwashiorkor.
2. Lesser signs of malnutrition such as hair and skin changes, oedema, wasting, gum bleeding.
3. Severe anaemia, as shown by pallor of tongue, mucous membranes conjunctiva, palms and nail beds.
4. Severe dehydration associated with gastroenteritis.
5. Respiratory infections. Recognition of:

   (a) bronchopneumonia with fever, shortness of breath and retractions;
   (b) chronic cough, productive of sputum;
   (c) cyanosis and extreme distress.

6. Common skin conditions:

   (a) scabies;
   (b) infections such as impetigo or pyoderma;
   (c) common rashes of infectious diseases such as measles, chicken pox and certainly smallpox.

Under conditions associated with mass feeding programmes, there may be the need to develop related preventive medicine campaigns. There is general agreement that mass immunization campaigns will have a positive nutritional advantage particularly when people are living under conditions of crowded and insanitary housing and when there is need for additional protection for high-risk individuals. Similarly, there is justification for campaigns for the detection and treatment of individuals with tuberculosis, as well as for spraying the houses against malaria-carrying mosquitoes, if that happens to be an endemic consideration.

In addition to personnel, consideration must be given to the identification of available resources, including housing, vehicles for transportation and all-weather roads, and to the enumeration of foodstuffs that are available in the region. It is obviously important to make maximum use of indigenous foods, but at the same time to be concerned with the nutritional status of the people living in the sourrounding area. The customary food habits must be of great concern, along with what foods are available through the assistance of international agencies that may be asked to donate food. Both storage and preparation facilities must be developed and incorporated into the system of distribution. In some instances, with the availability of ovens, special bread can be baked into which such items can be incorporated as skimmed milk, vitamins and iron.

Environmental sanitation and personal hygiene must represent a major concern, and it may be possible to organize working groups from among the local population to be responsible for these aspects. Periodic general 'clean-up' campaigns are recommended both to provide necessary occupation for the campaign members as well as to improve the sanitary conditions under which people will have to live. Supplies of water must be identified and may have to be chlorinated in order to provide adequate purification. Where refuse disposal is inefficient or where surrounding bushes are used instead of latrines, a high incidence of diarrhoeal diseases can be anticipated. Breeding of flies and contamination of food are predictably higher under such conditions than normally. There may be greater risk of contamination of the water supply due to faecal disposal and unhygienic conditions, and this may be more of a problem during certain seasons of the year. Dysentery may represent a major consideration and so there is an indication for the introduction of certain basic measures of community hygiene. When measles, chicken pox, whooping cough, tuberculosis and dysentery are superimposed upon already existing undernutrition, there may be a marked increase in morbidity and mortality, particularly among the very young and the elderly because a negative nitrogen balance will result in susceptible individuals. Nothing can be taken for granted and resources such as pumps for water, tools for farming, equipment for preparation of meals, as well as medical supplies, equipment and drugs, must be organized. It is recommended that a limited number of essential medications be developed that will provide adequate care but not excessive selection.

The training programmes for nutrition, health and preventive medicine personnel must be developed early. It should be determined what cultural advantages exist in the area and what trained personnel might be willing to participate in such programmes. The particular organization of the family groups may represent an important advantage in that in some regions women may be encouraged to provide breast milk for infants in addition to their own, and other women without nursing infants of their own may be induced to lactate, if this were an accepted cultural norm.

Among the lowest socio-economic groups, the infant who cannot be provided with mother's milk is in serious jeopardy of succumbing early in life to either malnutrition or recurrent and fatal gastroenteritis. When a mother has died or become seriously ill or run away, female relatives may undertake to breast-feed the infant until he is able to accept another diet. This process is relatively simple if the woman serving as a wet nurse has had a recent birth and is lactating adequately. However, as has been described in both Asia and Africa, women who are not lactating, such as young grandmothers and/or aunts of the infant, can be induced to lactate if they have the interest and desire to do so.[8] Induced lactation has been reported in nulliparous women as well as in nulliparous experimental animals.[9,10]

Individuals living in circumstances of emergencies become very pragmatic. If they can be convinced that a certain process works to their benefit, they will fully accept it. Obviously, every nursing woman must be adequately fed. It is simpler and cheaper to provide an adult-type ration which will satisfactorily nourish a lactating mother, than it is to provide either a formula or a weanling diet to an infant.

An essential aspect of induced lactation requires a positive desire on the part of the mother or other woman to be a breast-feeder. The use of small doses of thorazine orally (Largactyl, 100 mg) three times daily for 10 days is helpful, both as a lactogenic agent and as a 'quasi-placebo'.[11] Both the physician and nurse must express an absolute belief that the particular 'special' medicine being given will actually stimulate and increase the flow of breast milk.

Adequate quantities of breast milk for the infant up to the age of 4–6 months, and for the older infant as supplemental protein, present a distinct improvement over artificial formulae. Refrigeration may be absent and the water supply, not always pure, can contaminate artificial formulae. Providing adequate supplies of milk powder or liquid for infant feedings is always difficult, and in addition there is the major problem of properly preparing formulae by a population that may have a high illiteracy rate.

Giving to the mothers a more adequate nutritional intake can obviate the need of sending in milk for artificial feedings in enormous quantities, importing countless feeding bottles which cannot be adequately sterilized, and attempting, with almost no facilities, to help thousands of women prepare the formulae after the milk powder or liquid has been distributed.

In contrast, a mass educational programme could reasonably be undertaken to convince women individually that a 'special and powerful medication' will stimulate an adequate flow of breast milk. If this were successful, the children would be provided with innumerable litres of breast milk, high in protein, free of contamination, and readily available to nourish the large numbers of infants under the age of 2–3 years. This sort of programme has never been attempted on a mass scale in the past, but there seems to be no reason why, with careful planning, it could not be successfully managed.

Consultation with the group leaders would be important in order to help with the selection of supervisors and other individuals who could be trained for specific jobs. The availability of knowledgeable administrators is a vital resource and the identification of an overall programme director of critical importance. Information would be necessary to arrive at the type of diet that is culturally acceptable within the limitations imposed by available food, budget and cooking facilities.

Nutritional considerations are so intimately linked with medical concerns that it is impossible to separate completely these two aspects of the programme. It is necessary to have a full descriptive report of the situation periodically in order to arrive at reasonable evaluation procedures. The basic need in a demographic report would be of numbers of people, morbidity and mortality figures, as well as additions through new births or new arrivals. A very simple system for medical and nutritional evaluation should be introduced early in the programme so that periodic determinations can be easily made. In addition to growth measurements for young children, the simple determination of prevalence rates of anaemia, positive skin tests for tuberculosis, and the prevalence of skin or eye conditions or intestinal parasitism could serve as important measurements of the status of the population.

There is a definite need for periodic and repeated evaluation of both the medical and nutritional status. This could be done with sub-samples of the population. Because young children are the most sensitive to deficiencies, the nutritional sub-sampling is best directed toward the under-5 age group. Periodic evaluations of a reasonable number would make it feasible to detect changes with time, and also permit comparisons among various groups. In the absence of such objective measurements there are no means by which those furnishing relief can determine how the overall programmes are benefiting the nutritional status of the population. Table 1 presents a simplified form, to be used by a team of evaluators with minimal training on sample groups of children under 5 years of age.[12]

There would have to be provision for rapid processing of such data and for overall summarizing or scoring of the individual evaluations and for compiling group evaluations. Such nutritional and health scoring appraisals, carried out at periodic intervals of perhaps 4–8 weeks, would be extremely useful in conjunction with the vital statistics that are available.

Without accurate census data, it is impossible to prepare either morbidity or mortality rates. Nevertheless, records should be collated which cite and compare the actual numbers of various diseases being identified, and of the numbers and causes of death according to age and sex. In addition, simple maps are needed which indicate the locations of living quarters, the feeding centres, the centres for medical treatment of both out-patient and in-patient types, and the locations of schools, markets, ration and bread distribution centres, and other points of health and nutrition interest. Finally, it should be pointed out that groups that are gathered together for the purposes of feeding can easily be organized for the application of various mass medical procedures, such as prophylactic immunizations, tuberculin skin testing and screening for anaemia and parasites as well as for mass therapy for those conditions that have been identified. It is a well-known fact that a synergism exists between certain infectious disease processes and malnutrition, so that their treatment becomes an integral part of the provision of food for the group. It would be completely justified to treat for hookworm at the same time as providing a diet that is high in iron, with both procedures aimed at eradication of the anaemia. The provision of good nutrition will in most instances improve the resistance of the individual to various infections, and the elimination of various infections will influence the nutritional status of the individual.

Table 1. Proposed form for evaluation of the nutritional status of children under 5 years of age

1. **Demographic information** Such as name, identification number, age, and sex

2. **Minimal anthropometric measurements** It is recommended that height, weight and mid-left-arm circumference be recorded. With the possibility that only the approximate age can be noted, with the measurements indicated it will be feasible to calculate weights for height and arm circumference for height, in lieu of an exact age

3. **Obvious severe clinical malnutrition** Should be noted and the child should be designated as suffering from:
   (a) Kwashiorkor;
   (b) Marasmus;
   (c) Marasmic-kwashiorkor

4. Five **nutritional signs** that are easily discernible and should be checked off as being present and to what degree:
   (a) Hair changes for colour, texture and sparseness;
   (b) Skin changes including 'crazy pavement', 'flaky paint' and scabies;
   (c) Eye signs including Bitot's spots, corneal xerosis and keratomalacia;
   (d) Clinical pallor according to the severity;
   (e) Description of the extremities for the presence and severity of oedema and wasting

For successful management of any of the conditions it is of paramount importance that the efforts by the various involved groups be coordinated. The importance of close communication and contact in the overall supervision of the health and nutrition problems cannot be overstressed. Even if sufficient medical and food supplies to care for the people were on hand, and even if the personnel to provide for the feeding programmes and medical management were sufficient, there would still remain the need for providing responsible and well-trained administrators. It is suggested that a 'Relief Dictator' be designated to be the overall supervisor in charge of massive programmes in times of catastrophe.[12]

Along with a group of central administrators, there must be dependable field administrators on site who will carry out the programmes as stipulated. None of the efforts in careful planning will come to fruition without the means and supervisory staff to take the programmes into the field. Emphasis must always be placed on simplicity and innovation in order to facilitate the programme management and to minimize the impediments resulting from bureaucratic obstruction. Finally, where not all of the above recommendations can be implemented, it is preferable to undertake those that can be capably performed, rather than to flounder and to be overwhelmed in an attempt to do too much.

REFERENCES

1. Frood, J. D. K., R. G. Whitehead and W. A. Coward. Relationship between pattern of infection and development of hypoalbuminaemia and hypo-beta lipoproteinaemia in rural Ugandan children, *Lancet*, **ii**, 1047 (1971).
2. Scrimshaw, N. S., M. A. Guzmán, M. Flores, *et al.* Nutrition and infection field study in Guatemalan villages, 1959–1964: 5. Disease incidence among pre-school children under natural village conditions, with improved diet and with medical and public health services, *Arch. Environ. Health*, **16**, 223 (1968).
3. Gordon, J. E., W. Ascoli, L. J. Mata, *et al.* Nutrition and infection field study in Guatemalan villages, 1959–1964: 6. Acute diarrheal disease incidence, *Arch. Environ. Health*, **16**, 424 (1968).
4. Christakis, G. (Ed.). Nutritional assessment in health programs, *Am. J. Pub. Health*, **63**, Nov. Supplement (1973).
5. Ifekwunigwe, A. E. A symposium of nutrition and relief operations in times of diasaster, *Famine*, Swedish Nutrition Foundation, Symposium IX, Uppsala, 1971, p. 144.
6. B.C.G. by Jet Injection. Editorial, *Brit. Med. J.*, **4**, 506, 1971.
7. Report from the Research Committee of the British Thoracic and Tuberculosis Association, *Tubercle*, **52**, 155 (1971).
8. Jelliffe, D. B. *Infant Nutrition in the Sub-tropics and Tropics, 2nd edition*, World Health Organization Monograph Series No. 29, Geneva, 1968.
9. Mead, M. *Sex and Temperament in Three Primitive Societies*, New York, Dell Publications, 1963, p. 186.
10. Newton, M. and N. Newton. The normal course and management of lactation, *Clin. Obst. Gynec.*, **5**, 44 (1962).
11. Brown, R. E. Nutritional considerations in times of major catastrophe, *Clin. Ped.*, **11**, 334 (1972).
12. Recommendations of the Symposium of the Swedish Nutrition Foundation IX, *Famine:* Nutrition and Relief Operations in Times of Disaster, G. Blix, Y. Hofvander and B. Vahlquist (Eds.), Uppsala, Almquist and Wiksell, 1971, p. 192.

RECOMMENDED READING

Famine, Nutrition and Relief Operations in Times of Disaster, Swedish Nutrition Foundation, 1971.

The Nutrition Factor, Alan Berg, Brookings Institution, 1973.

Nutritional Assessement of the Community, D. B. Jelliffe, World Health Organization Monograph Series, No. 53, 1966.

Nutritional Assessement in Health Programs, *American Journal of Public Health*, **63**, Supplement, Nov., 1973.

Medical Care in Developing Countries, Maurice King, Oxford University Press, 1966.

CHAPTER 19

Prevention of Atherosclerosis and Coronary Heart Disease

RICHARD W. D. TURNER

Atherosclerosis (atheroma) is a metabolic disorder of large and medium-sized arteries, narrowing and sometimes occluding the lumen and thus interfering with the nutrition of the tissues. It is a widespread but patchy condition, mainly affecting the heart, brain, kidneys, aorta and lower limbs.

Its chief clinical manifestations are sudden death, myocardial infarction, angina pectoris, cerebral infarction, aneurysmal dilatation of the aorta and ischaemia of the lower limbs, sometimes causing gangrene.

However, atherosclerosis is not primarily a degenerative disease nor an inevitable part of ageing. In some parts of the world, such as rural Asia and Africa, New Guinea and other Pacific islands, it is rare while in others, including most of the western world, it is almost invariable and frequently advanced before middle age. It is an active metabolic disorder basically of nutritional origin but with varying individual susceptibility influenced by a number of environmental factors.

Although coronary heart disease (CHD) is the most important target for preventive cardiology today because it is so common and so lethal, cerebral infarction is in some respects more tragic because many who survive the acute attack are severely handicapped and only too well aware of their disability and dependence, with years of disappointment and frustration after an active life.

Secondary prevention, that is in those who have already developed symptoms, is worthwhile and too often neglected, but clearly second best because the underlying arterial disease is often too advanced for much improvement to be possible. Clearly only primary prevention could be really effective and this means that advice must be given to, and accepted by, apparently healthy people.

Coronary heart disease is the most frequent clinical manifestation of atherosclerosis. It illustrates the interaction of inherited predisposition and environmental causes and, being related to the practical problems of nutrition and diet, will be described as a good example of a community disorder about which something can be done. It is the responsibility of many, including family doctors, paediatricians, general physicians, community nurses, health educationalists and other welfare workers, all of whom should see the situation in perspective and be aware of the facts and their implications for health authorities and governments.

The problem is not so much that of not knowing what to do but how best to do it and how to motivate the medical profession, not only to treat their patients with symptomatic disease more vigorously but to give advice on primary prevention against atherosclerotic disease to the apparently healthy at high risk. These include all with hypertension and diabetes, all with a strong family history of relevant disorders and all found on examination to have a combination of high-risk factors.

However, not until the surely sensible principle of regular health examinations is accepted will most of those at high risk be detected so that they can receive appropriate individual advice. Meanwhile, what can be done as regards the general population, many of whom are at high risk but unknown to their practitioners, is to give advice on preventing or reducing obesity and modifying general dietetic habits so as to lower plasma lipid levels.

There is at present some difference of opinion amongst experts and therefore confusion in the minds of non-experts as to what dietary recommendations should be made for the population as a whole on the one hand, and for coronary patients and those at high risk on the other. Having reviewed the evidence on this and on other coronary risk factors, firm recommendations are made on the grounds that the advice given is very likely to be beneficial, is unharmful and is acceptable to the majority.[1]

CORONARY HEART DISEASE

The fact that in most countries the incidence of CHD is increasing, especially in middle-aged and younger men, together with the geographical variation between countries and even different regions of the same country; the experience of migrants from poor to relatively affluent countries where they develop the disease, and the fall in incidence in food-deprived Europe during the war, all these suggest that the causes must largely be environmental. They are therefore potentially preventable. Certainly there will not be any spontaneous improvement.

In the United States 1 man in 5 is likely to develop symptoms of CHD by the age of 60[2] and in the United Kingdom by the age of 65.[3] Many die much younger than this, often suddenly. Sudden death is the first and consequently last manifestation of CHD in about 25 per cent of cases and of those who die about 60 per cent do so too rapidly for medical aid.

Coronary care units, coronary ambulances and coronary arterial surgery can do little to improve this situation because by the time symptoms first appear the underlying disease is usually far advanced. Although there are good reasons for believing that atherosclerosis is primarily a nutritional disorder, CHD is of multifactorial origin. Since the heart is a muscle and under nervous control, it is only to be expected that other important factors include physical inactivity, smoking and stress. The last two have a final common pathway in the excessive secretion of catecholamines (adrenaline and noradrenaline) which have many potentially adverse effects on the myocardium, the arterial walls and the blood. In addition, hypertension accelerates atherosclerosis.

Table 1. Coronary risk factors

Family history
Smoking
Hypertension
Hyperlipidaemia
Carbohydrate intolerance
Obesity
Physical inactivity
Stress

Atherosclerosis often starts in youth or earlier and the pathological changes increase with age. It follows that, to be really effective, prevention must start long before the condition can be detected clinically, and logically with appropriate feeding in childhood.

OVERNUTRITION

In many countries now it is overnutrition rather than undernutrition, in the conventional sense of a deficiency disorder, which is the major dietetic problem with resultant obesity, frequent post-prandial lipaemia and hyperlipidaemia. Impaired carbohydrate tolerance may be an important by-product.

Insurance companies have shown that obesity shortens life, mainly from cardiovascular and cerebrovascular disease. They are not philanthropic bodies but guided by acturial experience.[4] Policies are loaded in proportion to the degree of obesity, at least when above 20 per cent of what is considered healthy. They have also shown that life expectancy improves with its reduction. Nevertheless, the balance of evidence indicates that obesity itself is probably not a strong coronary risk factor. It may be that it is an association with hypertension and hyperlipidaemia which is causal. However, blood pressure and lipid levels fall with its reduction and this is likely to be beneficial.

In the latest report from the long-term community study in Framingham in the United States,[5] it was concluded that obesity itself does carry some measure of independent risk, although the mechanism is unclear, and that the additive effect of obesity to other risk factors is very important. There was a more striking relationship with sudden death and angina than with acute myocardial infarction.

At all events, obesity is the cause of much other preventable ill health and disability. It has adverse associations with diabetes, gallstones and gout, with chronic bronchitis and varicose veins, with orthopaedic disorders from excessive weight-bearing and in relation to accidents and operations. The presence of obesity, in some degree, in most coronary patients and in others at high risk is in a sense useful because it provides the opportunity to give advice on the quality of the diet so that plasma lipid levels are reduced. It also indicates a goal at which to aim.

It is an important factor that obesity is often associated with relative physical inactivity and there is evidence that this also is an important coronary risk factor.[6]

LIPIDS AND LIPOPROTEINS

The fats in the blood come from food and are known as lipids. They are insoluble in water but rendered soluble in the blood by chemical combination with proteins to form compounds known as lipoproteins. Lipoproteins vary in density and in surface electrical charge and hence can be differentiated by physical means. However, for most practical purposes only chemical measurement of the constituent lipids is required.

The two most important lipids concerned in atherosclerosis are cholesterol and triglyceride. Most fat in food is in the form of triglyceride, but the small amount of cholesterol is believed by some to be more important in causing atherosclerosis. Although most epidemiological studies have been in relation to cholesterol, triglycerides probably also play an independent role.

There is a continuous gradient of plasma lipid levels in the population, like those of blood pressure, and no sharp cut-off point between normal and abnormal. It is a mistake to assume that average levels in the western world are synonymous with normal or optimal. Healthy levels are likely to be those found in communities with a low incidence of atherosclerotic disease. The lipid content of the arterial wall and of atheromatous plaques is mainly derived from lipoproteins which infiltrate from the blood. This process is accelerated by an increase in blood pressure and facilitated by factors such as smoking which increase the permeability of the wall.

HYPERLIPIDAEMIA, ATHEROSCLEROSIS AND DIET

Population studies have shown that there are close links between diet, hyperlipidaemia, atherosclerosis and CHD.[7] Their interrelationships are complex and since there is considerable variation between individuals, other factors must be involved. However, the evidence suggests that the disorder is basically nutritional. There is also a vast amount of epidemiological, clinical, pathological and experimental work to indicate that hyperlipidaemia, influenced by inherited predisposition and habitual diet, has not only a high association and hence is a strong predictor, but is a causal factor in the aetiology of atherosclerosis and CHD.[8,9] Nevertheless, there are gaps in knowledge and the crucial evidence that the incidence, extent and mortality of CHD can with certainty be reduced by dietary means alone is not at present available. The trials which have been reported are promising but have imperfections of design and therefore are not accepted as conclusive.[10] Ideally they should begin in childhood before atherosclerosis is advanced, as it often is in middle age, but this would add to the difficulties referred to below.

The problems of carrying out dietary trials are immense. Recently it was estimated that a satisfactory full-scale trial would require between 24,000–115,000 participants, would need to last for 7–10 years and would cost between $500 million–$1000 million.[11] In addition, it was anticipated that there would be great problems on account of drop-outs, the fact that about 20 per cent of Americans change their place of living each year, that participants would probably be motivated to change other risk factors and controls to modify their habits owing to a change in the climate of opinion, and thus influence the study. Also the trial might never be finished and, if it were, the results might be inconclusive.

In the absence of proof and in such a serious situation, decisions must be made and advice given or withheld on the basis of probability. Paradoxically, far stronger evidence is often demanded for preventive measures than is ever considered necessary for giving drugs or advising surgical treatment. The evidence supporting a causal relationship between hyperlipidaemia and CHD, and hence justifying dietary advice, includes the following facts.

1. CHD is uncommon or non-existent in populations with low mean plasma cholesterol levels (below 180 mg/100 ml).
2. There is an almost linear relationship between plasma cholesterol levels above 200 mg/100 ml and the incidence of CHD.[12]
3. CHD at a relatively young age is common in patients with familial hyperlipidaemia.
4. The hallmark of the atheromatous plaque is the accumulation of cholesterol.
5. The concentration of cholesterol in the arterial wall is in proportion to that in the plasma.[13]
6. Plasma lipids are mainly derived from the food and can be raised or lowered by changing eating habits.

It has been repeatedly shown that atherosclerosis can be produced in many species by feeding a high-fat–high-cholesterol diet but, most impressively, in primates nearest to man atherosclerosis and its complications of myocardial infarction and peripheral gangrene have been induced by feeding a western-type diet.[14] Furthermore, the pathological changes in the arterial wall regress on changing back to a natural diet.[15] The clinical counterpart in man is regression in cutaneous manifestations of hypercholesterolaemia after treatment by diet or drugs.[16] Recent epidemiological studies have shown that hypertriglyceridaemia is probably an independent risk factor.[17]

Finally, as mentioned above, recent dietary trials in man are encouraging.[18]

Variation in plasma lipids

Although it is clear that atherosclerosis and plasma lipids are mainly nutritionally determined, lipid levels vary in populations and in individuals living on a similar diet and even between those kept on an identical diet in a metabolic unit. This reflects varying capacities to handle food constituents. Nevertheless, in everyone lipid levels are much influenced by diet. Not only is there considerable variation between individuals, but in the same individual from time to time and even day to day. The reasons for this are not fully understood but include dietary and non-dietary factors. Dietary factors include total calories, total fat, saturated and unsaturated fat, refined and unrefined carbohydrate, cholesterol, sugar and alcohol. Non-dietary factors include smoking, exercise, stress, season, posture, changes in weight, myocardial infarction and drugs.

DIET

Reduction in lipid levels is likely to have a favourable effect in all at high risk (Table 2) but most of such cases are unknown to their practitioners. Consequently it is reasonable to advise some modifications in diet for the population as a whole, many of whom have relatively high lipid levels by ideal standards, that is to say above those in countries with little or no atherosclerosis. If regular health examinations were accepted and lipid levels known, advice could be given on an individual basis. However, at best it will take some years before such routine screening can be introduced.

Table 2. High-risk groups

Patients
Coronary heart disease
Cerebrovascular disease
Peripheral vascular disease
Hypertension
Diabetes

First-degree relatives of patients
Family history of sudden death, hypertension, atherosclerotic disease, diabetes
Symptom-free individuals with combinations of high-risk factors

The principles of diet are not difficult to learn nor does adherence to them entail much hardship. Habits can often be changed if the reasons are appreciated. There need be no absolute taboos, and general rules can be forgotten when dining out or on other special occasions. In the obese energy restriction should include reduction in total fat and carbohydrate intake. Saturated fat, sugar and salt should be reduced, with a switch from saturated to polyunsaturated fat at table and in cooking. The same basic diet for lowering plasma lipids can be advised for all coronary patients and others at high risk, with modifications for particular circumstances.

Obesity, hypercholesterolaemia and hypertriglyceridaemia are undesirable. The aim should be to eliminate adiposity and maintain cholesterol and triglyceride levels in the lower physiological range. There is no evidence to suggest that excessively low levels can be induced. If cholesterol levels are inadequately lowered by the basic diet there must be greater emphasis on saturated fat and eggs, and if triglyceride levels are inadequately lowered, on sugar and alcohol. The benefits of increasing energy expenditure by regular exercise should also be explained. Should this regime be inadequate, the next step is to give clofibrate. This increases the excretion of cholesterol in the faeces and is tolerated by almost all without side-effects of any kind. Only a few require more detailed laboratory investigation of lipoprotein and individual drug therapy.

POST-PRANDIAL LIPAEMIA

Post-prandial lipaemia refers to visible cloudiness of the plasma which can be seen after a fat-rich meal and which is due to chylomicrons carrying triglycerides. Hypertriglyceridaemia refers to plasma in the fasting state, that is to say after abstinence for at least 10 hours.

If frequently repeated, post-prandial lipaemia could be an important coronary risk factor. Ancel Keys[19] put forward the hypothesis that atherosclerosis is basically due to an endless succession of fatty meals. Lipaemia is often prolonged in patients with CHD and in their relatives. It leads to increased viscosity and coagulability of the blood and to platelet aggregation. The capillary circulation is slow and myocardial oxygen extraction reduced. It is increased by smoking and reduced by exercise. It follows that an adverse combination of circumstances is sitting in a chair after a rich meal, smoking a cigarette and perhaps drinking further alcohol!

After heavy consumption of alcohol, enhanced triglyceridaemia may persist for many hours, a fact which should be remembered when taking a fasting blood specimen with a view to having this lipid measured.

Cholesterol

The average daily intake of cholesterol is about 500–700 mg. Egg yolk has by far the highest content of any food (200–250 mg) and it is for this reason that restriction is advisable for some. Most foods which are high in saturated fat (meat, milk, butter, cheese) also contain a fair amount of cholesterol but others with a relatively high content, such as shellfish, liver, kidney and sweetbread, are usually taken only infrequently and therefore need not be avoided on such occasions. For coronary patients and those at high risk, restriction in dairy products and butcher's meat has already been advised so that the only traditional item to be stressed is eggs, of which no more than 2–3 should be taken each week, including those used in cooking.

Sugar (sucrose)

In recent years there has been some controversy as to whether saturated fat or sugar is the more important dietary factor. Although almost all workers believe the evidence strongly favours fat as being dominant the argument is a sterile one for it is not a matter of 'either/or', but both.

Sugar does little to satisfy appetite, is an extra source of energy of no nutritional value, is metabolized into saturated fat and brings out an insulin response which some think may be atherogenic. Added sugar should be avoided at table and in cooking and the high sugar content of many purchased articles and restaurant meals remembered. For the man or woman accustomed to add 2 teaspoonsful of sugar to each cup of tea or other drink, the daily saving is likely to amount to more than 500 calories (2.1 MJ). Healthy children do not 'need' sugar because they are physically active and the 'sweet tooth' is to be discouraged if only because obesity and dental caries are so common.

Salt

There is some experimental evidence that dietary salt may be important in the pathogenesis of hypertension.[20] Severe salt restriction can reduce high blood pressure levels to normal, although in adults accustomed to adding salt to food this may be unacceptable. It is logical to advise salt restriction in all patients requiring treatment for hypertension, not only because this alone will reduce the blood pressure but because it permits a lower dose of antihypertensive drugs. This may be especially important in relation to oral diuretics because a smaller intake will result in less hypokalaemia and this might be an advantage over the years in those being treated on a long-term basis.

Alcohol

There is no evidence that alcohol is an independent risk factor, but it may contribute to excessive energy intake and hence to obesity and can increase hypertriglyceridaemia. Beer contains maltose which is a refined carbohydrate and hence, like sucrose, may be important. Alcohol before a meal stimulates appetite and during a meal tends to be associated with a higher intake of food. In the obese it must be 'watched' and when plasma triglycerides fail to fall with an appropriate diet, alcohol may be the cause.

Meals

When alternatives are available, choose fish, poultry or game, including rabbit, rather than butcher's meat (beef, mutton, pork) or organ meat (liver, kidney, sweetbread).

Select lean cuts and remove visible fat (including the skin).

Limit beef, mutton, pork and ham to four main meals each week, and eat only 2–3 eggs each week.

Take vegetables, salad and fruit in great abundance and variety.

Cream. icecream, top of milk and hard margarine should be avoided. Use only soft margarine and vegetable oils, labelled as being high in polyunsaturated fat, at table and in cooking.

Ordinary cheese can be taken in moderation but cottage cheese, which can be flavoured in many ways, in abundance.

Made-up dishes of uncertain composition, such as sausage rolls, pies, and the like should usually be avoided.

If obese, remember that bread, potatoes and cereals, pastries, puddings and pies, sweet biscuits, cake and sugar are all very fattening. Once the habits and arts are learned, meals can be very attractive and most soon come to regard rich, sweet and obviously fatty foods as undesirable.

Alcohol is high in energy, and beer also in sugar (maltose) and should therefore only be taken in moderation, counting the energy cost.

PREVENTION IN CHILDHOOD

The incubation period of CHD is long and the underlying pathological changes in the arteries often start in youth or even earlier. It should not be too difficult to bring up children virtually free from risk factors if they were sensibly fed, could be persuaded not to smoke and had regular health examinations, with appropriate advice, before leaving school and at regular intervals thereafter.

The first step in prevention lies with infant feeding. The advantages of breast-feeding include greater ease in avoiding obesity, which frequently precedes that in childhood and adult life. It is still the traditional 'bonny' baby who gets the prize rather than the parents who should be allotted the booby prize! Supplementary feeds are often given when unnecessary and of inappropriate strength, and solid foods started too young. Thirst may be mistaken for hunger, especially if the salt intake has been high. Babies vary in their requirements as do adults and excessive gain in weight should be immediately countered, as at any age.

There is evidence that the number of fat cells in adipose tissue is determined by the age of 12–18 months and may be stimulated by overfeeding.[21] Weight reduction may reduce the size of these adipocytes, but not their number, and later they are readily filled if energy balance is again disturbed.

Breast milk has been gradually developed towards perfection over millions of evolutionary years and for a normal baby born to a healthy mother is an all-sufficient food for the first few months. Cow's milk is unnatural, except for calves. It is more saturated than human milk and, in particular, contains less of the important polyunsaturated linoleic acid. It has been claimed that the major blood vessels of infants who have been bottle-fed may show intimal changes at an early age in contrast to those who have been breast-fed.[22] The sodium content of cow's milk is four times greater than breast milk. This could be an important factor in later hypertension especially as solid foods which are given to infants are also often high in sodium.

Recently it has been suggested that cow's milk (and especially heat-dried milk) has antigenic properties, and for some this could be a causal factor in atheroma.[23]

Antibodies to cow's milk are high in many patients with myocardial infarction and there is evidence that immunoglobulins may increase platelet aggregation and permeability of the arterial wall. Breast milk has no such antigenic properties and it is claimed that early breast-feeding is in some measure protective against the action of cow's milk after weaning.

Neonatal plasma cholesterol levels are under 100 mg/100 ml but in affluent populations, unlike poorer ones, they may double within two years.

Appropriate weaning should include the use of polyunsaturated fats and oils, at table and in cooking, and the avoidance of added sugar and salt. Good habits learned early are likely to be continued.

School meals also require review with the same principles in mind. It has been shown that plasma lipid levels even in childhood, although they vary between individuals, are often high and reflect social class and nutrition. There should be greater emphasis on poultry and fish than butcher's meat. Vegetables, salads and fruit should be offered in abundance and variety with relatively few eggs and no 'extra' milk. Health talks to children should include emphasis on food and alcohol as well as on exercise and smoking.

IMPLICATIONS

Changes in agricultural policy, in the food industry and in catering will be needed if the public are to be advised to reduce their consumption of saturated fat and increase that of polyunsaturated fat, but first they must be given encouragement to do so by governments. The special knowledge and expertise are available. Subsidies, such as for butter, must also be reconsidered. This should lead to a greater choice of food in restaurants, canteens and other public institutions. Hospitals should rationalize what is offered to patients. There are implications also as regards the clear labelling of foods with their constituents so that the public can make an intelligent choice.

Mothers require greater encouragement to breast-feed their infants and clearer advice not to overfeed when substitutes or supplements are given, and not to add sugar and salt. The manufacture of infant foods requires control. Child welfare clinics and schools should review their policies with the same principles in mind.

SUMMARY

Atherosclerosis accounts for more than half the deaths in the western world and coronary heart disease (CHD) for more than one-third of those under the age of 65. Most who die do so too quickly for medical aid and most who develop symptoms have advanced atherosclerosis. Consequently, secondary prevention is second-best and only primary prevention can have a major impact.

CHD occurs in adults but starts in childhood so that prevention must start early. The first logical step lies in infant feeding with breast milk followed by appropriate weaning and healthy meals for school children. Obesity should be countered at any age by a combination of diet and regular exercise.

High-risk individuals include coronary patients and their close relatives, all with a family history of atherosclerotic and hypertensive disease, and all with hypertension, diabetes, hyperlipidaemia or a combination of high-risk factors. However, most at high risk are free from symptoms and unknown to their doctors. It follows that they can only be detected by health examinations. Until this sensible principle is accepted and put into action, certain changes in the national diet are recommended for the population as a whole.

There should be reduction in energy for the obese by restricting total fat and carbohydrates and reductions for all in saturated fat with substitution of polyunsaturated fat, in sugar, in salt and, for some, in alcohol. For those at high risk there should be stricter adherence to the above regime and, in addition, restriction of eggs to 2–3 a week.

It would seem that a virtual revolution in our attitude to food is needed or perhaps it would be better to say a counter-revolution to more natural ways.

REFERENCES

1. Turner, R. and K. Ball. *Lancet*, **2**, 1137 (1973).
2. Stamler, J. *Brit. Heart J.*, **33**, supp., 145 (1971).
3. Morris, J. N. *Proc. Roy. Soc. Med.*, **66**, 5 (1973).
4. *Soc. Actuaries Build & Blood Pressure Study*, **1**, 17 (1959).
5. Gordon, T. and W. B. Kannel. *Geriatrics*, **28**, 80 (1973).
6. Metropolitan Life Ass. Co. Overweight, its prevention and significance, 1960.
7. Masironi, R. *Bull. Wld. Hlth. Org.*, **42**, 103 (1970).
8. Connor, W. E. and S. L. Connor. *Prev. Med.*, **1**, 49 (1972).
9. *Lectures in Preventive Cardiology*, New York, Stamler, J., 1967.
10. Stamler, J. *Geriatrics*, **57**, 5 (1973).
11. Nat. Heart Lung Inst. Task Force on arteriosclerosis, *Arteriosclerosis*, **1**, 17 (1971).
12. Kannel, W. B. and T. R. Dawber. *Heart & Lung*, **1**, 797 (1972).
13. Smith, E. B. and R. S. Slater. *Lancet*, **1**, 463 (1972).
14. Armstrong, M. L., E. D. Warner and W. E. Connor. *Circulation Res.*, **27**, 59 (1970).
15. Getz, G. S., D. Vesselinovitch and R. W. Wissler. *Amer. J. Med.*, **46**, 657 (1969).
16. Oliver, M. F. *Bull. N.Y. Acad. Med.*, **44**, 1021 (1968).
17. Miettinen, M., O. Turpeinen, M. J. Karvonen *et al. Lancet*, **2**, 835 (1972).
18. National Heart Foundation of New Zeland. *Coronary Heart Disease*, Dunedin, John McIndoe, 1971.
19. Keys, A., N. Kimura, A. Kusukawa, B. Bronte-Stewart, N. Larsen and M. K. Keys. *Ann. Int. Med.*, **48**, 83 (1958).
20. Dahl, L. K. *Amer. J. Clin, Nutr.*, **25**, 231 (1972).
21. Brook, C. G. D. *Brit. Med. J.*, **2**, 25 (1972).
22. Osborn, G. R. *The Incubation Period of Coronary Thrombosis*, London, Butterworths, 1963.
23. Davies, D. F. *Amer. Heart J.*, **81**, 289 (1971).

CHAPTER 20

Control of Obesity

W. H. SEBRELL

Obesity is one of the world's greatest problems in malnutrition (Chapter 9). There is a widespread misconception that obesity is primarily a problem in economically advanced countries and among the well-to-do. Epidemiological studies in the U.S.A. indicate that obesity is most prevalent among middle-aged economically deprived women and is related to income. As income decreases, there are more obese women and more thin men, as income increases, more women are lean and more men are obese. The explanation for this observation is obscure. Although no statistics are available, obese mothers may be seen accompanied by malnourished children. In all probability, obesity is a worldwide problem with a deep socio-economic, psychological and cultural background. There are genetic factors involved as well as a relationship to certain diseases, especially diabetes. It is also of significance whether obesity develops in the infant and small child, or whether onset is later in life. It has been well-established that most adipose tissue cells are formed in early life and the obese infant lays down more of these cells than the normal infant. Lifelong eating habits are established very early in life and the mother who uses food as a reward or creates a distorted place for food in the child's life by making it obese, is not only causing the child to form more adipose tissue cells, but is also creating an attitude toward food that is going to make obesity a lifelong problem. Childhood-onset obesity is more difficult to correct later in life than adult-onset obesity.

Obesity is primarily a psychological problem and nothing of permanent benefit can be done for the obese individual unless there is a strong internal motivation to lose weight and a willingness to make a permanent change in behaviour toward food. It is true, from a thermodynamic viewpoint, that in order to lose adipose tissue the food energy intake must be less than the energy expenditure. However, this approach cannot solve the problem of maintaining the weight loss unless there is also a psychological adaptation.

Starvation will cause any obese individual to lose adipose tissue, but such loss will be rapidly regained with perhaps even more adipose tissue as soon as the period of food deprivation ends unless there is strong motivation to restrict and change eating habits permanently.

This is why practically all reducing diets fail. Hundreds of special reducing diets have been proposed over the years and new ones as well as variants of the old ones keep appearing. All of them, if they create a deficit in food energy, will cause a loss in weight and many of them are nutritionally inadequate either in minerals, vitamins or other essential nutrients. It can be said with confidence that most individuals will regain the lost weight as soon as they give up the diet unless something has occurred which makes the individual adopt a permanent change in food habits.

No attempt will be made here to cover completely the very large number of weight-loss schemes that have been devised over many years. Most of them can be classified by type.

Low-carbohydrate diets

A large number of these have appeared from time to time. Some of these try to limit carbohydrate to 30–60 g a day, others try to eliminate it as completely as possible.

There are a number of problems involved with this type of diet. Some individuals develop symptoms of hypoglycaemia, much of the early weight loss is water, not adipose tissue, and discouraging plateaus of stationary weight occur. If carbohydrate is eliminated ketosis will occur. The weight loss is brought about by the restriction in energy that occur as a result of reducing the intake of sweets. Well-known examples of such diets are Dr. Yudkin's diet, the drinking man's diet, the Air Force diet.

High-protein diets

As the name implies, these require that you eat mostly foods that have a high content of protein. The metabolism of protein requires more water than other diets because of the formation of urea. Therefore, a large water intake should accompany a high-protein diet. Such diets are, of course, nutritionally unbalanced and require nutrient supplementation. They also present a heavy urea load to the kidney and they may result in ketosis and electrolyte imbalance.

As with other diets that greatly distort the normal eating pattern, they are likely to be abandoned and the weight loss regained. Examples are Dr. Stillman's diet, the Gaylord Hauser diet, the Petrie diet.

High-fat diets

This type of diet has been used for a long time and in modern times was popularized by Dr. Pennington and more recently as The Atkins Diet. Such diets are high in saturated fats and cholesterol and may present an added danger from coronary artery disease and atherosclerosis. They also produce ketosis.

Starvation diet

This is a severely limited diet in the range of 500–600 kcal (2.1–2.5 MJ) per day, or complete abstinence from food. Such a drastic regime should be done only under close medical supervision in a hospital. Symptoms of starvation occur, the relative loss of nitrogen is high and a few unexplained deaths have been reported.

Numerous other special food-reducing diets have been proposed such as the tomato and egg diet, the seafood diet, the grapefruit diet, the banana and milk diet, liquid mixture diets, the rice diet, etc.

All of these suffer from the same defects that doom them to eventual failure in maintaining a weight loss. They have multiple nutrient deficiencies and they represent such an abnormal way of eating that they are likely to be used only for a limited period of time. The individual then returns to his former eating habits and rapidly regains the lost weight while enjoying his release from an unpleasant food restriction. They all cause temporary loss of weight because of the limited food energy intake.

In most instances, the individual cannot distinguish between total weight loss and adipose tissue loss. A rapid and large loss of weight is very likely to be mostly water. Loss of adipose tissue with a minimum loss of nitrogen occurs much more slowly and therefore requires much more perserverence on the part of the individual for a long period of time. It cannot be done with short periods of severe food restriction.

HOW TO COMBAT OBESITY

A successful programme is one which enables the individual to attain a normal body adipose tissue content, remain healthy and make a permanent change in eating habits and attitude toward food so that the individual never becomes obese again and follows a healthful way of eating without the use of drugs, nutritional supplements or special dietetic foods.

This is difficult for a physician to do since it requires a great deal of individual attention as well as a considerable knowledge of the nutrient value of foods and how to apply this to a satisfying selection of foods and appetizing food preparation. It requires a professional team of an applied psychologist, a physician and a nutritionist dietitian.

Such a programme consists of three parts (i) psychological handling, (ii) physical activity and (iii) a food programme.

Psychological handling

The excessively obese individual always has a psychological problem involved with his attitude toward food. The recognition of this is one of the most important factors in handling obesity and it is the lack of a planned approach through the use of applied psychology that causes failure by many physicians in their attempts to treat the obese patient. It must be recognized that no programme can succeed unless the individual has a strong internal motivation to correct the condition. This motivation must be maintained and reinforced in every possible way. If the motivation is lost, the individual will immediately and rapidly regain his lost weight or even become fatter than before. Even after several years of maintaining a normal weight, any relaxation of the motivation will result in overeating and regaining weight. When motivation is temporarily relaxed as a result of an emotional disturbance such as loss of a job, death of a relative or a festive celebration, as much as 10 to 15 pounds can be regained over a period of a few days, which then can be lost only by weeks of controlled dietary restriction.

There is much research which indicates that the obese individual eats in response to external 'cues' in contrast to the normal individual who eats in response to an internal 'cue' called hunger. Obese individuals often do not recognize what 'hunger' is—they never experience it. They eat in response to the appearance, taste, smell and quantity of appetizing food and they seem to have no internal 'cut-off' mechanism. They eat until all of the food available is gone, and they stop simply because there is no more food in sight. Thus, they may eat an entire ham or a half-gallon of ice cream or an entire pie or cake. Therefore, one of the most important parts of the psychological approach must be to educate the individual to modify his behaviour toward food permanently, limit carefully the quantity of food eaten by the use of weighed and measured quantities and to adopt a new meal pattern.

The eating pattern of the obese individual is often one of no breakfast, a light lunch, a big dinner, much between-meal 'nibbling' and then late-night eating and drinking until bedtime. This pattern often is difficult to change and it requires strong motivation to get the obese individual to eat as much as one-quarter of his food supply for breakfast.

Excessively obese individuals are usually withdrawn, self-conscious, embarrassed, lonely and secret eaters. An attempt to get an accurate food intake history is practically impossible. Their motivation to reduce is often based on a desire to look like other people and to be accepted in their social group and less frequently for health reasons. It is therefore necessary to learn what reward the individual expects as a result of his deprivation and to reinforce his motivation by stressing the rewards, and also to prepare the individual for possible disappointment if his imagined rewards are not attained.

It has been found that group interaction is a powerful force for reinforcing motivation. A group of obese individuals is assembled under the leadership of a lecturer who has been obese and succeeded in attaining a goal weight. This leader is trained in the type of applied psychology to use. No one is allowed in the room except members of the group. The lecturer is able to speak from personal experience and encourages the members of the group to react, discuss their problems with food, their failures, their successes. She stresses rewards, recognition is given for progress in the form of applause, certificates, pins, etc. Teaching is done in detail on how to follow the programme exactly, how to combat temptation, how to eat with the family, go to parties, etc. without violating the rules of the programme, how to substitute other rewarding activities for eating and finally, but most importantly, the permanence of the new way of eating, the new behaviour toward food and how to enjoy food without becoming obese. All this leads to a new and rewarding mental attitude, a new and more satisfying personality which is required for success.

Physical activity

This is a very difficult but important part of a reducing programme. It is difficult for many reasons. The obese individual is inactive. This is seen even in children and adolescents. They expend less energy even when they are required to engage in physical activity. If they are excessively obese, they even have difficulty walking because of respiratory and circulatory problems. It has often been pointed out that it requires a great deal of physical work to offset the added energy of a relatively small amount of food.

However, exercise, if properly done, has many important advantages. The difference between obesity and normal weight is the result often of a small food energy surplus over a long period of time therefore exercise, even if the energy expenditure is small, if done every day can make an appreciable difference in a year. It also has many other beneficial effects. It takes the individual's mind off eating, it creates a feeling of well-being, it provides some circulatory stimulation, it increases muscle tone and helps the obese attain a better physical appearance, it improves joint motion and gives a feeling of accomplishment which results in a psychological improvement. The physical activity must be done regularly every day. It must not be done competitively and it must not exceed the individual's capability—a good rule is to do it easily and slowly with enjoyment. When the individual feels tired or when exercise is no longer being enjoyed, it should be stopped at once. If there is no contra-indication, an easy way is to walk and to keep increasing the distance as capability permits. Simple callisthenics can be added, jogging, swimming and other mild, non-competitive activities can be used to suit the individual's physical condition and motivation.

Food programme

Given suitable motivation, a properly designed food programme is the heart of successfully combating obesity. Many factors have to be taken into consideration.

The word 'diet' should never be used. This has a psychological impact as being something different from usual eating and implies that it is a food pattern that will some time be given up. The change in attitude must be that this is a food programme that is the best that can be devised. It is merely a careful selection and measurement of the foods that everyone is using. The food programme should consist of two important parts, first, the restricted programme in order to bring the obese to normal weight and second, a maintenance programme which will maintain normal weight and health for a lifetime and is the way everyone should eat to remain healthy. Therefore, extreme care has to be used to see that every possible nutritional need is met and maintained.

The selection of a goal weight is a very important consideration. Every obese individual wants to know what his normal weight should be and how long it is going to take him to reach it. This, therefore, becomes an important factor in motivation. The weight tables of the Metropolitan Life Insurance Company are widely used in the U.S.A. as desirable weights but these are very difficult to use because they give a relatively wide range of weights for height and sex based on three body-frame sizes. The application of these tables to the individual often results in a weight selection that finds the individual at goal weight when still fat, which creates emotional distress. Actually, it is adipose tissue content, not total body weight, that is the factor in obesity and every weight has to be individualized by inspection. An adaptation of the goal weights which can be used to establish a *provisional* goal weight for an obviously obese individual is given in Table 1.

Table 1. Provisional goal weights for obese adults (25 years and older). Height without shoes—weight in indoor clothing

Women		Men	
Ht. (cm)	Goal wt. (kg)	Ht. (cm)	Goal wt. (kg)
147	43.6–51.3	157	54.9–65.4
150	44.9–52.7	160	56.3–67.2
152	46.3–54.0	162	57.7–69.0
155	47.7–55.4	165	59.0–70.8
157	49.0–57.2	167	60.8–73.1
160	50.4–59.0	170	62.7–75.4
162	51.8–61.3	172	64.5–77.2
165	53.6–63.1	175	66.3–79.0
167	55.4–65.0	177	68.1–81.3
170	57.2–66.7	180	70.0–83.5
172	59.0–68.6	182	71.7–85.8
175	60.8–70.4	185	73.5–88.1

As an individual approaches this provisional goal weight, a personal goal weight for that individual should be established by observation, professional consultation and discussion with the person regarding a satisfactory weight that, in an adult, is to be maintained indefinitely by adjustments in the food intake. Skin-fold calipers can be used to make a rough estimate but adjustment of the final body weight is a matter of inspection and judgment. If skin-fold calipers are not available, the 'pinch test' can be used as a rough method for estimating adiposity. Since a large proportion of total body fat is located just under the skin, pinching a fold of skin on the posterior surface of the upper arm midway between the elbow or clavicle and estimating the amount of fat in the fold assists in judging the total degree of adiposity in the body. Emaciation and loss of muscle must be avoided in the strongly motivated individual who becomes obsessed with weight loss and doesn't want to stop losing weight after reaching a desirable goal. In the excessively obese, it is desirable to provide tentative goals in increments in order to help maintain motivation. An individual faced with a goal of a total weight loss of 50 kg, requiring about a year of adherence to the programme, may regard this as just too great a task. If told that his goal is a loss of 12 kg in 3 months, this may seem within reach and he may get a feeling of accomplishment from attaining it, which is then followed with more enthusiasm for a loss of a second 12 kg in another 3 months, and so on.

FOOD ENERGY

The most basic consideration in the food programme is that the food energy intake be less than the energy expenditure. This does not have to be individualized. An estimated deficit below that required for resting metabolism plus light exercise for the normal-weight individual will cause a weight loss in any obese individual. The more obese the individual, the more rapid will be the early weight loss because the deficit is greater. However, it is very important that the deficit should not be too great, for several reasons. A severely restricted diet such as one containing 600 kcal (2.52 MJ) per day should be used only under strict medical supervision. It cannot be made nutritionally adequate and nutrient supplementation is essential. Also, such a severely restricted diet results in a proportionately greater nitrogen loss while the objective is to maximize the loss of adipose tissue and minimize the loss of nitrogen. This severe restriction also results in the symptoms of semi-starvation such as irritation, inability to concentrate, mental slowness, decreased pulse rate, decreased blood pressure, decreased metabolic rate and lethargy. All of this helps to weaken the individual's motivation and his craving for food may cause him to give up the programme.

Thus, a slightly active adult woman of normal weight may maintain weight on about 2000 kcal (8.4 MJ). A reduction of 800 kcal (3.36 MJ) below this level to about 1200 kcal (5.04 MJ) is sufficient to produce a weight loss in the obese indiidual of 2–3 pounds (1–1.5 kg) a week and still permit a food intake in satisfying variety and amount and one which can contain all of the necessary nutrients in adequate amounts without the use of vitamin, mineral or other nutrient supplements, or special food preparations. This requires a wide selection of a broad variety of foods with energy control obtained by the restricted size of the serving. It is important from a motivational point of view to permit the individual to have a small amount of his favourite foods rather than to ban them completely, and it is just as important to have a list of foods that can be taken in unrestricted or large amounts as it is to have a list of foods which cannot be taken in any amount.

The distribution of the food energy intake between protein, fat and carbohydrate is also important. A desirable distribution is 25 per cent of the energy from protein, 35 per cent from fat and 40 per cent from carbohydrate.

Sucrose (either as white or brown cane or beet sugar) is one of the items which must be denied simply because it supplies food energy without appreciable amounts of other nutrients and makes it exceedingly difficult to make a diet of restricted food energy that is also nutritionally adequate. Therefore, although 40 per cent of the food energy is from carbohydrate, this must come from the sugars in fruits and vegetables and the starches in grains, beans and roots. Since obesity is so often associated either with overt diabetes or with an abnormal glucose-tolerance curve, the carbohydrate should be enough to make the food palatable, to ease the craving for sweetness and to prevent ketosis but still not excessive. Therefore, the carbohydrate food energy should not exceed 50 per cent or be less than 40 per cent of the total food energy.

The lipid content of the programme poses some difficult problems in that there is no established 'most desirable' recommended daily level for lipid intake and the kind of lipid is important (Chapter 19). Since lipids are the most concentrated sources of food energy (supplying weight for weight more than twice the energy of proteins and carbohydrates) the amount must be carefully controlled. The diets in countries where the mortality from atherosclerotic heart disease is highest all supply more than 40 per cent of the food energy from lipids and all contain a high proportion of animal fats rich in saturated fatty acids. There is much experimental evidence which shows that a diet not excessive in food energy with a restricted total lipid content and an increased amount of linoleic acid will lower the blood cholesterol level. There are human studies which suggest that a food regime of this type will decrease the incidence of coronary artery disease and epidemiological studies show that there is an association between obesity and the risk of coronary artery disease. The objective, therefore, is a diet programme of lipid food energy not above 35 per cent of the total and with a polyunsaturated–saturated fatty acid ratio of approximately one to one. From a practical point of view, this means that butter fat must be eliminated from the diet (except for a limited amount in cheese), the fat from mammalian sources such as beef and lamb must be restricted and the lipids in the diet be obtained from fish and vegetable oils. The usual vegetable oils such as soybean oil, corn oil, safflower oil, sunflower seed oil, etc. all contain relatively large amounts of linoleic acid. Olive oil and coconut oil contain oleic acid, which is not as unsaturated as linoleic acid, but they do not contain the undesired saturated fatty acids of animal fats. The fat of poultry, turkey, duck and geese is also permissible but the total of 35 per cent of the energy from lipid sources must not be exceeded. In many countries, the lipids (oils) are in short supply and the price may be high so that the quantity is limited by availability and economic factors and the lipid intake may normally be considerably less than the recommended 35 per cent. In this situation, the diet is usually distorted toward a high intake of carbohydrate from foods such as rice, millet, manioc, yams, plantains, potatoes, turnips, etc. These are always cheaper and more available than the high-protein foods and larger amounts are eaten, which gives a sense of fullness and satisfaction but does not give a desirable nutrient distribution. Every effort should be made to hold the total carbohydrate to not more than 50 per cent of the total energy and to keep the food lipid content to not less than 25 per cent of the energy, otherwise the diet tends to become unpalatable and it is difficult to prepare tasty meals. No butter, cream or solid fat can be used except liquid vegetable oil margarine.

The protein level at 25–30 per cent of the food energy appears to be high, but it is not high in the total weight of the protein being handled by the liver and kidneys.

Since the total food energy content is only approximately 1200 calories (5.04 MJ), 30 per cent of this is 360 kcal (1.51 MJ) which means only 90 g of protein. Many normal diets far exceed this total, and although this is considerably higher than the physiological need for protein of high biological value, this quantity allows for a mixed protein intake containing a considerable amount of protein of relatively low biological value from plant sources to supplement that from animal, fish and poultry.

It is essential, of course, that the food supply be adequate in all vitamins and minerals. The recommended daily allowance of these vary widely between different countries, for various reasons. The standard taken here is that of the U.S. National Academy of Sciences, National Research Council Food and Nutrition Board. It has been chosen because it represents the most complete listing of nutrients and gives in most instances the highest allowance which allows a greater margin of safety. This is particularly important in a restricted food supply under varying methods of preparation, preservation and handling and one which is going to be followed for a very long period of time. In order to attain these levels, certain categories of food selection are mandatory. A food pattern that will meet the necessary qualifications for an adult female based on U.S. and Western European food habits is given below.

The total amount of food should be taken in 3 or 4 meals with light between-meal snacks. Breakfast should approximate one-fourth of the total. No meal should ever be missed and late-night eating should be avoided.

Unlimited Foods: Clam juice, spices, herbs and other seasoning, tea, coffee, seaweed, water, lettuce, chives, chicory, celery, capers, parsley, watercress, radishes, pimentos, etc.

Limited: 3 bouillon cubes per day, 1 tablespoon unflavoured gelatin.

Fruit: Select 3 each day, oranges, grapefruit, papaya, strawberries (1 cup), tangerine, cantaloupe, honeydew or similar melon, ugli fruit, apricots, cranberries (1 cup), peach, pineapple (1 large slice), plums, apple, pear, etc. Once a week 1 banana, 1 cup grapes or $\frac{3}{4}$ cup of stoned cherries may be substituted for one of the above.

Vegatables: 1 vegetable (2 cups) from the group asparagus, cucumber, bean sprouts, green or wax beans, broccoli, cabbage, cauliflower, beet greens, egg plant, endive, mushrooms, kale, spinach, tomatoes, etc. A second vegetable: (4 ounces) from the group, beets, brussels sprouts, carrots, onions, peas, pumpkin, squash, etc.

Fish, meat and poultry: Use a 4-ounce serving for the midday meal and 6 ounces for the evening meal. Beef or lamb with all visible fat removed not oftener than three times per week. Chicken, capon, goat meat, rabbit, turkey, veal, etc. as often as desired to fit the programme.

Fish and seafood: Use at least five times a week in 4-ounce or 6-ounce serving at the midday or evening meal. Crabs, crayfish, lobster, mussels and shrimp should be used not oftener than once a week because of the high cholesterol content. Other fish and seafood: bass, carp, clams, cod, eel, flounder, sole, haddock, halibut, mackerel, finnan haddie, oysters, smelt, squid, turbot, tuna, etc. to fit the programme.

Bread and cereals: Bread should be made of enriched white flour or whole-wheat flour for its vitamin and mineral content and served in 1-ounce slices. Two slices per day. If neither enriched white flour nor whole-wheat flour is available, adequacy of thiamine, niacin, riboflavin and iron must be ensured from other sources. One ounce of breakfast cereal may be used (not pre-sweetened) with $\frac{1}{2}$ cup of skimmed milk.

Milk: Two servings of 8 ounces each of skimmed milk are required daily for adequate calcium, vitamins and protein.

Eggs: 4 eggs per week cooked in the shell or cooked without added fat are required for their iron content.

Liver: 1 serving per week of 6 or 8 ounces is required for its high nutrient and iron content. Both liver and egg yolk are high in cholesterol.

Cheese: May be used according to its fat content. Hard cheeses of 30 per cent fat may be used up to 4 ounces weekly. Softer cheeses of 20 per cent fat or 10 per cent fat or less may be used in correspondingly larger amounts.

Lipids: Are to be used at mealtime as 1 tablespoon of vegetable oil, mayonnaise or liquid vegetable oil margarine. No other lipids may be added.

For between-meal eating up to 12 ounces of tomato juice or mixed vegetable juice, coffee, tea, bouillon or broth may be used.

CHAPTER 21

Education to Combat Malnutrition

HELEN D. ULLRICH and GEORGE M. BRIGGS

Nutrition education has a vital role in all approaches towards obtaining an optimal nutritional status within any community. Before designing an education programme, the baseline data should include an assessment of the reasons for undernutrition and overnutrition within the community, the attitudes and beliefs of the population in relation to the foods available to them, and those foods which are needed to improve deficient diets. Imperative to any educational approaches to changes in food choices is personal involvement of the individual in the improvement of his life and that of his family.

By definition, nutrition education in the community is the application of the science of nutrition to the everyday lives of people. This means that education is related to the social, economic and cultural values of food in such a way that people are motivated to make food choices which will result in their optimal nutritional well-being.

Davey and McNaughton[1] pointed out that nutrition education should not be overlooked as a potential contribution to economic development. In addition to the increased work capacity of a better nourished worker, there is increased consumer demand for food which in turn calls for increased food production. These are factors that fit in the agricultural economic development plan of most countries.

The role of nutrition education is not specifically relegated to the nutritionist alone but is frequently touched upon by almost anyone having contact with the consumer, patient, farmer, school child, or family. Since nutrition education is an ongoing process, it must be considered in many different ways.

This chapter will discuss nutrition education in terms of how to assess the needs and develop approaches to affecting food habits of the target populations of the community. The training of some of the professional and paraprofessional personnel on the education team in the community will be touched on.

NUTRITION EDUCATION AS A PART OF HEALTH EDUCATION

Nutrition education by itself is not the solution to malnutrition. However, knowledge is a vital component of the complexity of factors essential for good health and good nutrition. It is essential when planning a community nutrition education programme to consider socio-economic and cultural conditions, communications networks, behavioural and motivational factors, sanitation, health, climate, population pressures, agricultural conditions, food availability and storage, and transportation facilities.

Nutrition education is an important segment of any total health education plan in the community. It is effectively incorporated in preventive medicine, health maintenance, and clinical therapy. The approaches would be somewhat different as the goals for the health programmes differ. Additionally, the individualized programme and the community-structured programme would require different approaches to the problems. For example, a health education programme on family planning, sanitation, or infant health would include certain nutrition information. Programmes for school lunches, supplemental feeding or agriculture would have somewhat different nutrition education components.

Whether the education programme is to be training for other professionals or paraprofessionals, a total coordinated community effort, or an individual project concentrating on a single target population group, the only way to be sure of the effectiveness of the programme is to have carefully thought-out objectives based on baseline data with built-in evaluation throughout the development and application of the programme.

EDUCATION IN THE COMMUNITY

In order to develop a nutrition education programme in the community, a baseline of information about the nutritional status and other relevant information about the community and the target audience should first be established. Then the concepts of what kinds of behaviour are to be modified should be outlined. Those groups or individuals who would be affected by nutrition education programmes should be identified and the appropriate approaches determined. Finally, ways in which the programme can be evaluated should be carefully outlined.

Baseline data

Gathering background data as it relates to an education programme must include:

A. A review of all assessments made of the nutritional status of the community;

B. Identification of which family members are most affected by nutritional and disease problems;

C. The mores, taboos, religious attitudes towards food and eating patterns of the family members and/or segments of the population;

D. An analysis of how people obtain food, e.g. from home gardens, communal farms, food vendors, traders or grocery stores;

E. An assessment of knowledge about food choices and level of interest in making a change:

F. An assessment of the availability and acceptability of foods which might improve the diet;

G. A review of the facilities available for storing, preparing and serving food in the home;

H. What changes in food use are economically feasible;

I. The sociology of the community such as who are the most influential persons to effect changes in food habits and who is the decision-maker within the family;

J. The resources for communication;

K. The sources of highest credibility to disseminate information;

L. The literacy level of the people to be reached:

Parlato[2] classifies the gathering of data as follows:

Nutrition	Socio-economic	Market ecology
Socio-economic factors	Education	Socio-economic factors
Method of food preparation	Income	Marketing channels
Eating habits	Spending patterns	Eating habits
Nutrition research findings	Information flow patterns	Government agricultural policy
Nutrition deficiencies	Adaption of change patterns	Climate
Available food	Media effectiveness	Geology
Food distribution within the family	Media exposure	Transportation links
Food beliefs and taboos	Aspirations Caste/religion	

Some of the background data can be found in existing records but other data must be gathered through field work. Observation in the field is important in understanding the interrelationships of all the factors affecting the community. Education is not effective until it is incorporated into the practices of the person to be educated.

An assessment of level of education is of importance in order to be effective in any educational approach. The decision as to whether a simple or complex idea can be effectively presented will depend upon the degree of education and sophistication of the community.[3]

Conceptual framework to bring about planned change

With the benefit of the baseline data a plan for the nutrition education programme can be developed around realistic concepts of behaviour to be modified, which will produce the desired change. These concepts should be listed in relation to the needs for change indicated in the baseline data. Concepts should be action-oriented statements such as 'to increase the feeding of pulses to weaned children,' 'to promote the practice of breast-feeding', or 'to increase the purchase of green vegetables in the grocery stores'. Concepts must be attainable within the context of the community for which they are planned. Knowledge does not change practice. There must be motivation to apply the information to change a practice.

Concepts should be planned for the specific target group of the population. The objectives of the concept should be measurable as a part of the evaluation of the programme.

Gifft, Washbon and Harrison[4] raise the important point about how planned change is related to values, attitudes and beliefs of the individual or community. There is a moral obligation on the educator to consider the total consequences of the change which will alter the values of the learner. Values, beliefs and attitudes control man's behaviour: the teacher's as well as the learner's. These are constantly shaped and changed as a part of learning. The teacher must be aware of his own value system as well as those of the learners in order to effect successful change and not just impart knowledge.

The developing of planned change could be described in a series of steps: **awareness**—the learner must be aware that there is a problem; **development of a receptive framework for learning**—an understanding that positive results are possible; **trial**—discovery through experience; **reinforcement**—an active give-and-take period between the learner and teacher; **adaptation**—developing a habit which fits into the learner's value system.

Concepts about food and nutrition as they relate to health are useful as a framework for developing the nutrition message. The following is one suggested framework.

Conceptual framework for nutrition education*

1. Nutrition is the process by which food and other substances eaten become part of you. The food we eat enables us to live, to grow, to keep healthy and well, and to get energy for work and play.

2. Food is made up of certain chemical substances that work together and interact with body chemicals to serve the needs of the body.

   (a) Each nutrient has specific uses in the body.
   (b) For the healthful individual the nutrients needed by the body are usually available through food.
   (c) Many kinds and combinations of food can lead to a well-balanced diet.
   (d) No natural food, by itself, has all the nutrients needed for full growth and health.

3. The way a food is treated influences the amount of nutrients in the food, its

---

*These concepts were recommended in the panel on Nutrition Education in Schools at the White House Conference on Food, Nutrition and Health, Washington, D.C., 1969.[5]

safety, appearance, taste and cost; treatment means everything that happens to food while it is being grown, processed, stored and prepared for eating.

4. All persons, throughout life, have need for the same nutrients, but in varying amounts.

(a) The amounts needed are influenced by age, sex, size, activity, specific conditions of growth and state of health—the amounts are altered somewhat by environmental stress.

(b) Suggestions for kinds and needed amounts of nutrients are made by scientists who continuously revise the suggestions in the light of the findings of new research.

(c) A daily food guide is helpful in translating the technical information into terms of everyday foods suitable for individuals and families.

5. Food use relates to the cultural, social, economic and psychological aspects of living as well as to the physiological.

(a) Food is culturally defined.

(b) Food selection is an individual act but is usually influenced by social and cultural sanctions.

(c) Food can be chosen to fulfil physiological needs and at the same time satisfy social, cultural and pyschological wants.

(d) Attitudes toward food are a culmination of many experiences, past and present.

6. The nutrients, singly and in combinations of chemical substances, simulating natural foods, are available in the market; these may vary widely in usefulness, safety and economy.

7. Food plays an important role in the physical and psychological health of a society or a nation just as it does for the individual and the family.

(a) The maintenance of good nutrition for the larger units of society involves many matters of public concern.

(b) Nutrition knowledge and social consciousness enables citizens to participate intelligently in the adoption of public policy affecting the nutrition of people around the world.

This framework, or one modified to suit the situation in a particular country, should be extremely useful to the nutrition educator in developing the overall concepts of nutrition information to be included in the programme. In addition, it will be necessary to interpret the guidelines to obtainable specific goals with defined behavioural changes to the intended target group for which a specific programme is planned.

Target audiences

The audience to be reached may be the whole community or very specific groups of people depending upon the concepts of behavioural changes desired. The message and approach will differ for each of several different target groups who are defined to be reached as a part of the programme. For example, if the intervention programme involves the necessity to produce a food not normally grown and eaten in the community, there would be a whole range of audiences to reach from the farmer to the change agent within the family. If there is to be a programme to change the practice of mothers from bottle-feeding to nursing their babies, there would also be a number of target groups to be considered besides the mother. If the value system of the community is not presently accepting the practice, policy developers within the community must be involved as well as the mothers and husbands. Careful attention must be given to determine the full range of audiences to be reached and then to determine the most effective approaches to bring about change.

Reaching large communities

Many developing countries are experiencing a movement of population from small, agricultural villages to large urban centres. The techniques for education must change also. It becomes more difficult in the urban setting to identify those within the neighbourhood who are change agents, such as the elders of the village or midwife nurses who are accepted by the village residents.

Health clinics, hospitals, day-care centres and schools are important focal points. Additionally, techniques of mass media must be employed wherever possible to create an awareness for the need to change and to inform people where they can get reliable information and assistance. The change agents in the urban areas are often government planners, social workers, food vendors and teachers in the schools and they should be involved in effective nutrition education.

The diet of migrants from rural to urban areas deteriorates for many reasons. The family is no longer able to grow and provide most of its food supply. Often the family is on a sub-marginal income and there is wide diversity of demand for the small amount of cash available. The wide range of motivational messages through word of mouth and mass media is very strong competition for often uncoordinated and hopelessly inadequate nutrition education approaches. In contrast, there are fewer competing factors in the rural areas, and small, informal meetings with villagers.

NUTRITION EDUCATION APPROACHES

The approaches used in nutrition education programmes in the community will vary with the magnitude of the problem, the composition of the community—whether it is mainly urban or rural, the kinds of education systems available, such as health clinics, day-care centres, schools and feeding programmes.

The following seven steps to health education were outlined by King et al.[6] These very basic steps were intended for rural communities in Africa but they could apply in almost any nutrition education programme. These steps are:

1. Learning about the people to be taught and making a community diagnosis.

2. Making a nutrition education plan. Trying to overcome blocks that are both important and easily removed. A nutrition education plan must be written down.
3. Making friends with the people to be taught.
4. Finding people's wants and making sure they are serious.
5. Showing people that there is a way out of their problems, and that they can have what they want. Teaching people only things that are possible for them to use.
6. Recording health education. Recording the lesson as well as what has been learned.
7. Evaluation. If the education is succeeding, then the families are doing what you tell them. If they are not, think carefully about what you are doing. Perhaps you should change the way in which you teach people, but do not get too impatient. People take a long time to change. In other words, in order to know if your education programme is working, you must go and see.

APPROACHES IN FORMAL SETTINGS

Person-to-person contact

Probably the most-used tactic and also one of the most expensive education techniques is the person-to-person contact. This approach would include the nutritionist, dietitian, health aide, physician or extension aide, working with individuals in clinics, private offices, homes or schools. However, through the personal contact, when a mother can show her teacher how she has learned to feed her child solid foods, she is more apt to keep up the practice.

The nutrition education component may be only one part of this type of contact. It can be interwoven with pre-natal or infant care consultation or in answer to a question on how to keep rice from being infested with bugs, for example.

Family contact

When the health or extension aide, social worker or nutritionist works directly with the family, there is an opportunity to assess the needs of the individual family. When the worker goes into the home, it is much easier to show the mother how to prepare different foods and see how well the mother is able to repeat what she has learned.

Small group contact

In all areas of the world, developing countries as well as developed countries, there have been educational attempts at reaching people on a group level. It is easier in the rural communities because of the closer interrelationships of people in small villages. However, even in urban areas there are often neighbourhood groups or voluntary groups such as churches or recreational groups. A variety of techniques have been worked out to reach people. A few suggestions include demonstrations, nutrition and health fairs, puppet shows, dramatic presentations, poster contests, field trips, cooking competitions.[7]

The mothercraft centre

One of the more successful nutrition education programmes being used in several areas of the world is the mothercraft community centre.[8-10] (Chapters 15 and 24).

Effective teachers in the non-classroom approach

Probably among the most useful purveyors of nutrition information at the community level are the 'nutrition aides' or lay-leaders who have had some personal nutrition experiences or informal training. Usually, whatever training in nutrition they receive is in-service training by a public health worker. Although these persons may not have had any formal schooling beyond elementary level, some may have completed the equivalent of high school or even college or university. Examples of these community workers would include:

1. **Paraprofessional aides**—extension or nutrition aides, health aides, nursery and day-care aides, teacher aides, midwives;
2. **Food service personnel**—schools, hospitals and nursing homes;
3. **Lay leaders (volunteer and paid)**—community service leaders, youth club leaders; and
4. **Food distribution personnel**—food store personnel and food vendors.

Paraprofessional training

Paraprofessional training is most frequently accomplished by an in-service approach. The paraprofessional working in the community on a one-to-one basis with a family or patient needs very specific kinds of training. This training would concentrate less on the basics of nutrition but more on the specific needs to ensure changes in the family eating patterns which might include specific foods in their diet and how to purchase, store and cook the foods in the home. This training should emphasize the techniques and approaches which will help the paraprofessional to be effective in teaching the patients or other clientele. The paraprofessional who is from the same village, neighbourhood or ethnic background can be very effective in understanding how to establish new eating patterns which will improve the nutritional status of the people being reached.

Semi-formal education

This means of in-service education is very effective. Behaviour studies have been conducted on the aides and cooperating families in the Expanded Food and Nutrition Education Program (EFNEP) of the Cooperative Extension Service in the U.S.[11] This programme concentrates on hiring and training aides who live in the neighbourhoods of the low-income areas. It has been found that the aides made the greatest strides in changing food habits because they have an opportunity to put into practice what they have learned by teaching others. For this reason, they were the most motivated persons contacted through EFNEP.

There are a number of handbooks written for the community worker in various areas of the world. Some of these handbooks are listed at the end of the chapter.

Classroom education in day-care centres and schools

Throughout the world there are programmes of feeding in day-care and school settings. It is one way in which children can be assured of at least a partially adequate diet. There should always be education accompanying feeding programmes.[12] The lunch room can serve as a learning laboratory. A training programme for the food handlers as well as the children should be included.

Nutrition education should also be an integral part of the total education programme being carried on in the day-care centres. In the centres, children begin to learn about food in relation to the world around them. It is at this time that food habits are forming and the understanding of simple food patterns can be established.

A sequential approach to the education programme in the school should be developed. This approach must be adapted to the food resources, social, economic and cultural needs of the community. Within the schools the elementary teacher can weave food choices into mathematics and reading, as well as science and health. Unfortunately, many teachers, whether at the elementary school level or the secondary level, do not feel secure in their own nutrition knowledge. For this reason, the nutrition education professional needs to carry out in-service training programmes and prepare curriculum guides for the teaching of nutrition. Often, health professionals, agriculturists and food processors can be called upon from within the community to contribute their know-how in the classroom. The school nurse has a special place in the school structure which makes her an excellent resource. Volunteer mothers can contribute specific projects such as preparing and serving new foods so that children can taste them. They can also help them to get interested in the selection of a wider variety of foods.

Teacher training

Teachers at nursery, elementary and secondary school levels are among the key persons to incorporate attitudes towards nutrition during the children's formative years. Special emphasis should be placed on incorporating nutrition into training programmes for teachers. The techniques for doing this will vary from country to country but, ideally, the subject of nutrition should be recognized as one of the science topics useful for certifying a teacher at the elementary level. Nutrition training should also be required of those teaching health, physical education and science courses. The professional nutrition educators in the community can be useful as teachers for in-service training of these educators.

Callahan[13] states that to promote interest in nutrition in the overcrowded school curricula takes genuine sales techniques. The in-service training of the professional must be action-oriented with behavioural objectives delineated which are relevant to the teaching situation.

Techniques and approaches in training community teachers

The trained nutritionist cannot be expected to train completely all those persons within the community who are to do some form of nutrition education. For this reason, a master plan must be developed and certain priorities established. The people with various abilities in nutrition education should be identified and utilized according to their special capabilities.

Audio-visual aids can be prepared on specific topics and made available to those who have received special training to teach others. The teachers in the schools would find curriculum guides prepared to meet local needs helpful in showing the ways nutrition can be incorporated in the various subjects such as mathematics, language or reading. Pre-packed sets of materials can be made up to fulfil a variety of needs. For example, pictures, posters, leaflets and simple filmstrips can be prepared by nutrition professionals to use in health and extension education programmes such as in health clinics, schools and lunch rooms.[14,15]

Mass communication as an educational approach

As the centres of population move from rural to village to large urban areas, it becomes increasingly difficult to reach individuals and to assist them on a person-to-person basis. For this reason, mass communication should be considered as a strong component of any educational programme within the community. In urbanized areas it may be the most important approach of all. Included in mass communication would be television, radio, newspapers, magazines, posters, calendars, and even newsletters, pamphlets and leaflets that are widely distributed.

The assessment of what is available and what people consider to be their sources of information is an important assessment which must be made before deciding how to focus a mass media programme. Mass education or mass communication should be considered to be a wide range of approaches which reaches population at all ages and levels of education and sophistication. The message to be communicated must be carefully thought out. The target groups to be reached must be identified and then those techniques by which each target group can best be reached should be used.

The use of television in nutrition education in developing countries is limited because there are countries where TV sets are not widely seen. Radio can be a very effective means of communication and a more generally available medium in most developing countries. In an article about communicating home economics information through the radio, Fewster[16] makes the following points: A programme should include teaching through listening, not simply preaching; the suggestion must seem rewarding enough to the listener to take the time and effort to listen and decide to act upon it; there should be a minimum of personal bias within the programme; knowing the audience is essential; the messages should be designed to be local, relevant, helpful and in a familiar language.

In a CARE-India report[17] of the application and extension of social action programmes it was pointed out that TV takes the last steps towards breaking down what was formerly a traditional society with reliance on the family and a close circle of friends. The introduction of information through that medium, it is felt, can do little more than present ideas and concepts and create at least a not-unfavourable attitude towards it.

A medium such as a poster can be effective. It has the potential to illustrate and to inform. It should be used carefully to spread ideas and make them well-known. Probably the most important function of mass media is the use of the trained person to disseminate information to large numbers of people. Manoff[18] feels that nutrition is a subject that can be adapted to the 'reach and frequency' technique of advertising, i.e. a short message frequently repeated.

The mass media audience is not a captive audience so techniques must be used to attract attention. Any campaign or programme must be based on research. Some of the questions which must be answered would be 'What is the nature of the problem?' 'Who are the target people?' 'Why are they targets?' For example, if they are not consuming adequate protein, what could they reasonably add to get enough? What would motivate them to change their behaviour? Manoff feels that this is the first step to take in research to clarify the problems which a mass media campaign could help to resolve.

It is of interest to note that Parlato[19] found in a marketing research approach with villages in India that there existed a gap between people's understanding and their attitudes towards new ideas. They understood the concepts but simply did not accept them. It was necessary to have face-to-face contact with an independently creditable person who would act as their reassuring agent.

In Korea, a national nutrition mass media programme[20] made use of the techniques of radio spot announcements, comic books and calendars. In the evaluation of this programme, it was found that the calendars were kept by the largest number of people and that the comic book actually achieved an impressive record of dissemination. However, again, it was pointed out that the mass media approach was better received by city dwellers than by the rural population.

EVALUATION AND RESEARCH

Essential to all nutrition education programmes is their evaluation, built into the original plan. Ritchie[21] suggests that some of the criteria or indicators for evaluation would include changes in morbidity and mortality rates; crop yields per acre; consumption levels of particular food; the proportion of local citizens or associates actively involved in programme activities; nutritionally important changes of behaviour observed in specific groups over stated periods of time.

Changes in people's behavioural practices are difficult to measure. Some of the techniques that have been tried include weighing and measuring the child and keeping records, measuring plate waste in the school lunch programme, pre- and post-testing of nutrition knowledge related to the programme, food consumption surveys, the increased purchasing of certain foods in the marketplace, increased growing of certain foods, and recording of resources where nutrition information is obtained as well as the informal reaction from the principals as to how they feel about what they have learned and how they feel they can make use of this information. Considerable research is still needed effectively to find ways to evaluate nutrition education.

In the Western Pacific World Health Organization Manual, *The Health Aspects of Food and Nutrition*,[22] the relative effectiveness of different types of learning experiences was related to the adoption of supplementary feeding practices. These were rated as follows, listed in decreasing order of effectiveness:

Direct purposeful experiences
Contrived experiences
Demonstrations
Field trips
Exhibits
Television
Motion pictures
Still pictures
Visual symbols
Lectures

SUMMARY

Nutrition education has a great potential which has thus far been generally limited to the pilot-testing dimension in most areas of the world. It must be a part of a carefully planned programme and have a vital role in any intervention programmes designed to improve the total nutritional health of the community.

Effective nutrition education as carried out in the community calls upon a wide range of people with an additionally wide range of information and nutrition knowledge. Before setting up a programme, one must assess the needs of the community, its resources, options for disseminating information, manpower available for teacher training and dissemination of knowledge, periods of human openness to change in the life span, and habits of communication within the community as well as the education resources.

REFERENCES

1. Davey, P. L. H. and J. W. McNaughton. Nutrition Education in Developing Countries, *FAO Newsletter*, **7**, 3, (1969).

2. Parlato, R. *Breaking the Communications Barrier,* CARE-India, Faridabad, Haryana, Thomson Press (India) Limited, India, 1972.
3. Fugelsang, A. Mass Communications Applied to Nutrition Education of Rural Populations: An Outline of Strategy, *PAG (Protein Advsory Group of UN) Bulletin,* **4,** (1), 7 (1974).
4. Gifft, H. H., M. B. Washbon and G. G. Harrison. *Nutrition, Behavior and Change,* Englewood Cliffs, N. J., Prentice-Hall, Inc., 1972, p. 254.
5. Ullrich, H. D. and G. M. Briggs. Chapter 17, The General Public, in *U.S. Nutrition Policies in the Seventies,* San Francisco, W. H. Freeman and Co., 1973, p. 185.
6. King, M. H., F. M. A. King, D. C. Morley, H. J. L. Burgess and A. P. Burgess. *Nutrition for Developing Countries,* Nairobi, Kenya, Oxford University Press, 1972, p. 103.
7. Devadas, R. P. and U. Chandrasekhar. Nutrition Education of Illiterate People, *J. Nut. Educ.,* **1,** 13 (1970).
8. *A Practical Guide to combating Malnutrition in the Preschool Child,* Nutritional Rehabilitation Through Maternal Education, New York, Appleton-Century-Crofts, 1970.
9. King, K. W. Mothercraft Centers Combine Nutrition and Social Sciences, *J. Nutr. Educ.,* **3,** 9 (1971).
10. Suter, C. B. Nutrition Education for Mothers of Filipino Preschool Children, *J. Nutr. Educ.,* **3,** 66 (1971).
11. Wang, V. L., L. W. Green and P. H. Ephross. *Not Forgotten but Still Poor,* Monograph 2, Cooperative Extension Service, University of Maryland, 1972, cited in *J. Nutr. Educ.,* **4,** 178 (1972).
12. Juhas, L., Nutrition Education and the Development of Language, *J. Nutr. Educ.,* **1,** 12, (1969).
13. Callahan, D. L. Inservice Teacher Workshops, *J. Nutr. Educ.,* **5,** 233 (1973). (1973).
14. Holmes, A. C. *Visual Aids in Nutrition Education,* A guide to Their Preparation and Use, Rome, FAO, 1968.
15. Fugelsang, A. *Applied Communications in Developing Countries,* Ideas and Observations, Uppsala, Sweden, The Dag Hammerskjöld Foundation, 1973.
16. Fewster, J. W. Communicating Home Economics Information, Reaching and Teaching Women by Radio, *FAO Newsletter,* **8,** 23 (1970).
17. CARE-India, *Planning for Nutrition Eucation,* The Application of Mass Media and Extension to Social Action Programmes, Delhi, India, 1973, p. 44.
18. Manoff, R. K., Potential Uses of Mass Media in Nutrition Programs, *J. Nutr. Educ.,* **5,** 125 (1973).
19. Parlato, R. Advertising and Mass Communications: A Model for Rural Nutrition Information Programs, *PAG (Protein Advisory Group of UN) Bulletin,* **4,** 17 (1974).
20. Higgins, M. and J. Montague. Nutrition Education Through the Mass Media in Korea, *J. Nutr. Educ.,* **4,** 58 (1972).
21. Ritchie, J. A. S. *Learning Better Nutrition,* FAO Nutritional Studies No. 20, Rome, FAO, 1967, p. 97.
22. *The Health Aspects of Food and Nutrition,* A Manual for Developing Countries in the Western Pacific Region of WHO, Western Pacific Region, Manila, WHO, 1969, p. 161.

SUGGESTED HANDBOOKS ON COMMUNITY NUTRITION EDUCATION

An Annotated International Bibliography of Nutrition Education: Materials, Resource Personnel, and Agencies, Taylor, C. M. and K. P. Riddle, 1971, Teachers College Press, 1234 Amsterdam Ave., New York, NY 10027.

258

Child Care: A Handbook for Village Workers and Leaders, Keister, M. E., 1967, Food and Agriculture Organization, available from UNIPUB, Inc., P.O. Box 433, New York, NY 10016.

Child Nutrition in Developing Countries, Jelliffe, D. B., 1968, U.S. Department of Health, Education, and Welfare, Public Health Service Publication No. 1822, available from U.S. Government Printing Office, Washington, DC 20402.

The Health Aspects of Food and Nutrition, World Health Organization, 1966.

Homemaking Handbook for Village Workers in Many Countries, Extension Service, USDA and AID, 1971, available from U.S. Government Printing Office, Washington, DC 20402.

Learning Better Nutrition: A Second Study of Approaches and Techniques, Ritchie, J. A. S., 1967, Food and Agriculture Organization of the United Nations, Rome, Italy.

Outlook on a National Nutrition Education Campaign, Fuglesang, A., 1971, The National Food and Nutrition Commission, Lusaka, Zambia.

Planning for Nutrition Education: The Application of Mass Media and Extension to Social Action Programmes, 1973, CARE-INDIA, B-28, Greater Kaillash-1, New Delhi-48, India.

Visual Aids in Nutrition Education: A Guide to Their Preparation and Use, Holmes, Alan C., 1968, FAO, Rome, Italy.

CHAPTER 22

Food Control

WAJIH N. SAWAYA

INTRODUCTION

With the advent of a modern industrial society, and the changes in mode of life associated with it, new trends in food production and utilization came into existence. At one time providing and preserving of food were the tasks of the individual and small communities were self-sufficient. Gradually this pattern changed. Factories and mills attracted and condensed big populations into small areas, which in time developed into big cities. Producers of the past became the consumers of today who go to the market to procure their daily necessities.

Centralization of food production, coupled with an increase in communal eating and an expansion in international trade, have changed the scope and increased the quantity of preserved foods, thus increasing the food-borne hazards. This has also put the consumer in the midst of a multitude of food items, making it very difficult for him to choose the most nutritious and at the same time the most economical product. The consumer thus became at a disadvantage and the need arose for a food-control system to protect him from health hazards, adulterations and deceptions.

Food control is a collective term comprising a whole set of food-control activities including laws and regulations, administrative service, inspection, laboratory analysis and consumer education. Due to space limitations, these subjects will be discussed separately but briefly.

FOOD LAW AND REGULATIONS

Food law is the framework of the food-control system, and embodies the whole set of legislation which deals with the production, sale and marketing of foods. The most important principle of the food law is the protection of the health of the consumer, the protection of the consumer from deceptions, including adulteration, and the ensuring of honesty in trade. The law states the administrative and legal machinery for supervision and supplements these basic rules with the necessary particular prescriptions with respect to additives, contaminants, etc. which are put in the form of regulations. While the food law contains the basic requirements for the protection of the consumer which are unlikely to change, regulations are set under the law for the reinforcement of these requirements by the necessary details, which can be regularly reviewed and updated. A modern food law should include the whole set of regulations for the protection of the consumer which cover the principal requirements set by law.

Protection of health

The health aspect is gradually becoming more important with the changes in living habits associated with the appearance of new food products in the market, and growing public awareness. The inherent risk in using more chemical substances in foods has increased the demand for stricter control measures in order to assure the consumer of the wholesomeness and the safety of the foods he eats. In addition, the increase in the number of instances of microbiological contamination of food, and the widespread contamination of foods due to environmental pollution, have strengthened this demand. The various elements involved in the protection of health are outlined below.

Food hygiene

The general principles of food hygiene are aimed at ensuring the fitness of food for human consumption. This is highly dependent on the different steps through which the food passes before it reaches the consumer. Food hygiene therefore requires the continual application of hygienic practices in the storage and handling of raw materials before and after harvesting and during processing. It also depends on the sanitary conditions of the water, equipment and utensils of processing plants, laboratory control, and general cleanliness of food handlers. Microbiological standards for perishable food items such as meat, milk, eggs, fish, etc. help in setting limits for microbial contamination. Hygiene codes and practice on the general principles of food hygiene, such as those of the Codex Alimentarius Commission of the United Nations, act as guidelines to assist governments in controlling problems of those food products which can present serious public health hazards. These codes have no statutory force, but are rather regarded as an interpretation of the requirements of the food hygiene regulations.

Food additives

The increased use of a wide number of chemicals in the food industry poses a big problem for the food-control authorities. Even though additives can contribute greatly to the preservation of food, especially in underdeveloped countries where adequate storage and facilities are lacking, their benefits should be weighed against the risks associated with their excessive use. National authorities in many countries, such as the United States and Canada, in addition to certain international organizations such as the Codex Alimentarius Commission and the European

Economic Committee, have done a large amount of research on the assessment of the safe use of a number of food additives, and have provided permitted lists of additives and the limits allowed to be used in foods. In addition to this, research has been going on for a long time to set specifications for the identity and purity of food additives that are allowed to be used in foods. Recent developments in toxicology, in the methods of testing for food additives, and in the increased awareness of the general public, food scientists, traders and legislators of the dangers of food additives, have contributed to an attempt to find a more effective way of control by governments although this is still far from being perfect and complete.

Food contaminants.

Food additives are those chemicals that are intentionally added to foods to aid in the processing, ensure good preservation and help improve the quality of the product, but contaminants get into food unintentionally. They include lubricants, packaging materials, traces of metals and plastics which get into food through machine handling, all of which are undesirable to both the consumer and the processor. The pollution of the environment presents a more serious potential hazard to human health. Such contaminants may arise from environmental and industrial pollution, e.g. as mercury, lead, arsenic and cadmium; from agricultural technology, e.g. pesticides and fertilizers; from food processing practices, e.g. nitrosamines and polynuclear hydrocarbons. In addition, some naturally occurring dietary toxins such as fungal toxins, pathogenic organisms and toxic components of food, may act as potential hazards.

Nutritional qualities

Food laws can serve as an instrument of nutritional policy by using the regulations to prescribe minimum nutritive levels of the common foods. This can be further extended to require certain foods to be fortified, e.g. flour with iron and vitamins, or to require the addition of certain substances for medical or therapeutic reasons, e.g. iodized salt (Chapter 17). In addition, the consumer needs to be protected from foods which are claimed to be nutritious, but are not as nutritious as they should be. The law should also ensure that a simulated food product which may resemble another food is not different in its nutritional quality from the original food, e.g. the substitution of saccharin, a non-nutritive sweetener, for sugar in a wide range of food products, or the removal of milk from liquid or dried milk, and the sale of separated or skimmed products. Food laws have a direct relationship with the socio-economic development of a country, and can be of great impact on the nutritional status of the population.

Protection against deception and adulteration

In order to ensure that the consumer is protected against adulteration, and gets his money's worth, food laws should contain provisions for the prohibition of sale of any adulterated food, and the stopping of all types of fraud, ranging from short measures to misconceptions about food products sold in the market, even though these may not affect the health of the consumer. This is done by regulating the quality of the composition of foods through standards for particular foods, and by setting standards for labelling.

Food composition

Food standards are essential means for the establishment of food regulations. Such standards in particular include definition of the food, its composition and its minimum quality requirements. Foods which do not comply with the set standards from chemical and bacteriological points of view should not be permitted to be sold on the market if locally produced and should be prevented from entering the country if they are imported. Food standards should be established in accordance with the development of the economy of a country, and only after serious consideration has been given to the relevant existing food practices.

National standards should be adopted only after the different parties involved, such as the food processors, manufacturers and consumers, have had the opportunity to comment on them.

Food labelling

It is not enough that the purchaser should be protected against adulteration, but he should also be safeguarded against buying food which is not what he expects it to be. Food laws therefore have to have clear labelling provisions so that misleading labels and advertisements are avoided. It is generally accepted that the more factual information that is given to the purchaser, the better he can use the label to evaluate the merits of competing products in the market. Recognizing this fact, information on the label should be required as mandatory, and should include the name of the product, compositional ingredients including food additives, the name of the packer, and its country of origin. Additional information such as the grade quality, or the nutritional and dietary value of the food can also be put on the label, as long as it is not misleading to the purchaser.

Honesty in trade

Food control can play an important role in the national planning of a country. The proper enforcement of the food laws has a direct impact on the socio-economic conditions of the entire population of a country and can help in the development of the food industry. Good quality control at the different levels of production and marketing of foods will ensure that the processed food is fit for human consumption and that it conforms to a specified acceptable standard. It can also aid in the provision of opportunities for the producers to obtain satisfactory prices for their products. In addition, high-quality standards enable foods to find their way to markets, thus increasing foreign trade and saving foreign exchange.

FOOD-CONTROL ADMINISTRATION

The food-control administration is the overall set up for the regulation of the different food-control activities in a country which are directed towards the protection of the consumer at the national level. In ideal circumstances, the food-control service comes under one administration, has its own budget, and is located in one ministry, usually the Ministry of Public Health, Agriculture or National Economy. Such an administration is responsible for setting policies, devising basic food laws and regulations including standards, for inspection of food production, processing and marketing, and for food analysis and research. In addition it will also be responsible for the implementation of the laws and regulations and for devising guidelines and procedures for rapid action against violations, either through voluntary action or legal proceedings. Rigorous enforcement should be directed in the first instance to hazardous or potentially hazardous areas, and to discouragement of fraudulent practices.

However, this should not be taken to mean that food control is a police action. It is rather a developmental action which is directed towards the socio-economic development of a country and should be adapted to the background and needs of the population.

FOOD INSPECTION

The importance of food inspection as part of the food-control system cannot be overemphasized. It is through inspection and monitoring that the consumer is continually assured of the wholesomeness and safety of the food he eats. Inspection should be performed by well-trained inspectors having a good knowledge of the foodstuffs they inspect, of the food law and regulations, and who are familiar with the basic principles of food science, hygiene and sanitation practices. It is also advantageous for a food inspector to be informed about pesticide residues, food additives and contaminants, packaging materials and food labelling regulations. Inspectors should test foods whether these come from local factories, shops, restaurants, catering establishments or whether they are imported. Samples should be periodically collected by them, and sent to the laboratory for chemical and/or bacteriological analysis, to ensure the safety of the food reaching the consumer and guarantee that its description and composition are as claimed.

Inspection should cover the sanitary conditions of food handlers, who are potential carriers of pathogenic organisms, and also the quality of water supply, state of cooking and eating utensils and food storage facilities. The food inspector can serve a double purpose in being an investigator in his control work as well as an educator acting as a consulting technician for food producers.

FOOD-CONTROL LABORATORY

A food-control laboratory plays an essential role in the food-control machinery, and is the complementary part of an effective food-inspection service. All food samples collected by the inspectors have to be analysed and verified by the laboratory before any suspected violators can be convicted. In many countries imported foods cannot be cleared through customs before chemical and/or bacteriological examinations have been run on them, in order to be sure that they conform to the standards set for consumption. In addition to this diagnostic work, a food-control laboratory can be very effective at the preventive level, in the monitoring and surveillance of public health practices and environmental contaminants which may be hazardous to health. It is an obvious fact that preventive measures should be an essential part of any food-control programme, because the primary concern should be to prevent food-borne diseases, not merely to diagnose them when they occur.

In order for a food-control laboratory to perform its task efficiently, it should be well-equipped and well-staffed. Equipment should be modern and adequate to enable the performance of all necessary analyses. The utilization of modern analytical techniques should be carried out by professional people, preferably university graduates in chemistry and microbiology, for proper laboratory operations. In addition the technical staff should be adequately trained in the use and maintenance of sophisticated instruments.

EDUCATION OF THE CONSUMER

Of the main aim of a government in setting up a food-control system in the country is to protect the consumer against health hazards and commercial fraud, then it is only fair that consumers should be informed about the nature and quality of the foods they eat, their composition, the standards governing their processing, and their nutritional and dietary value. Consumers should be informed about health hazards from bacteriological and chemical contamination, and of contamination from environmental pollution. The great range of food items in the market, and the increase in the number of similar foods of the same variety, have added to the confusion of the public about the quality and wholesomeness of the foods they buy.

Governments can play an important role in educating the public in this respect by encouraging advisory and educational programmes for consumers about food and nutrition. Advertisements about food should be strictly controlled and should be used as a medium for the education of the public.

Education of the consumer should be introduced into relevent school subjects, and more recognition of the consumer's voice should be created at governmental level. The promotion of voluntary actions, such as consumer protection societies, can assist to a great extent in creating more awareness among the general public. It can also aid the government in implementing the law, and in increasing the consciousness of the public towards the food sold in the market.

ROLE OF THE UNITED NATIONS AGENCIES (Chapter 24)

The United Nations Organizations, especially the Food and Agricultural Organization (FAO), and the world Health Organization (WHO), through their different activities in the field of food control have created a great awareness on the national as well as the international level. The Codex Alimentarius Commission on Food Standards has also been an encouraging step towards the harmonization of food standards of the world, and is of lasting value to all concerned with the international trade of food, whether they be producers, exporters, importers or consumers. The need today is greater than ever for governments to recognize the importance of food control, both for the protection of the consumer and the development of their trade.

FURTHER READING

World Health Organization, Food-Borne Diseases: Methods of Sampling and Examination in Surveillance Programmes, *World Health Organization Technical Series,* No. 543, Geneva, 1974.

World Health Organization, Microbiological Aspects of Food Hygiene, *World Health Organization Technical Series,* No. 399, Geneva, 1968.

FAO/WHO/UNICEF, *Proceedings of the Sub-Regional Seminar on Food Control,* Tehran, April 1972.

FAO/WHO/UNICEF, *Proceedings of the Sub-Regional Seminar on Food Control,* Beirut, March 1974 (in press).

FAO/WHO Expert Committee on Food Additives, General Principles Governing the Use of Food Additives, *FAO Nutrition Meetings Report Series,* No. 15 Rome, 1957.

FAO/WHO Expert Committee on Food Additives, Toxicological Evaluation of Certain Food Additives with a Review of General Principles and of Specifications, *WHO Technical Report Series,* No. 539, Geneva, 1973.

FAO/WHO Meeting on Pesticide Residues in Food, *WHO Technical Report Series,* No. 502, Geneva, 1971.

FAO/WHO Expert Committee on Food Additives, Specifications for the Identity and Purity of Food Additives and Their Toxicological Evaluation: Some Flavouring Substances, and Non-Nutritive Sweetening Agents, *FAO Nutrition Meetings Report Series,* No. 44, Geneva, 1967.

Special Reports, The use of chemicals in food production, processing and distribution, *Nutr. Revs.,* **191,** 31 (1973).

Codex Alimentarius Commission, Report of the Joint FAO/WHO Food Standards, Regional Conference For Africa, Nairobi, October, 1973.

Hobbs, B. and J. Christian. *The Microbiological Safety of Food,* London, Academic Press, 1973.

Herschdaerfer, S. M. *Quality Control in the Food Industry,* London, Academic Press, 1967.

Roe, Francis J. Metabolic Aspects of Food Safety, Oxford, Blackwell Scientific Publications, 1970.

Riemann, H. *Food-borne Infections and Intoxications,* New York, Academic Press, 1969.

Graham-Rack, B. and R. Binsted. *Hygiene in Food Manufacturing and Handling,* London, Food Trade Press, 1964.

SECTION IV

Role of Agencies

CHAPTER 23

Role of Government in Nutrition

J. P. GREAVES

INTRODUCTION

The duty of Government is to govern. At the very least, governments are expected to maintain law and order. Anarchy is unlikely to lead to improvement in nutrition—or in anything else.

The nutrition of a community is an index of its socio-economic condition. Under-nutrition is associated with poverty; overnutrition with wealth. But though affluence can hardly be regarded as a primary cause of overnutrition, poverty may readily be recognized as the basic cause of undernutrition. A government dedicated to the banishment of poverty is therefore, almost by definition, on the right track for dealing with undernutrition at its root (although all problems of undernutrition would not be solved even if poverty were abolished). Contrarywise, a government for which the abolition of poverty has a low priority will not, whatever its assertions, be doing anything of fundamental importance to relieve undernutrition.

These considerations lead inevitably to politics. The determination of priorities, and decisions about the allocation of resources to meet priorities, is the stuff of politics. Nutritional improvement cannot be divorced from politics.

This is a dogmatic statement. It may be objected that it is too dogmatic, too much of a generalization. Certain measures, it may be argued—such as the fortification of cereals, or of salt—may have little political implication, and can do much good. But even here there are likely to be problems of enforcement and control that could be at least partly political in nature. Also, more generally, such measures are likely to be relatively superficial, and to evade the real issues. Governments adopting them may be accused of fencing with the problem, not seriously tackling it head-on.

The extent to which it is thought proper for a government to intervene in the affairs of a nation is a political question. The governments of centrally planned societies, almost by definition, 'intervene' to a maximum extent. By contrast, Thomas Jefferson (for example) argued for a minimum of government intervention. Today, hardly a government in the world practices laissez-faire in its 19th-century harshness. The need for intervention, the need to plan, is commonly accepted. The debate, a political debate, is to what extent, by what means, and for what ends (Chapter 13).

The role of government in maintaining and improving nutrition is crucial and central. It is crucial because no other agency has the resources to deal with the problem. It is central because of the multi-factorial nature of nutrition: only government sits at the centre of that interlocking web of influences that together determine the nutrition of the community.

COMMITMENT

Study and analysis

Governments must have a commitment to study the nature of the nutrition problem in their own countries. Such a study will almost certainly require surveys to be done: surveys of nutritional status, of food production and distribution, of food consumption, of the prevalence and pattern of disease. Such surveys should seek as far as possible the reasons for the effects observed: the beliefs about food and feeding practices, and the causation of disease; the socio-economic conditions associated with malnutrition; the system of land inheritance; the facilities for marketing and credit, and for transportation of goods. Expenditure on such surveys should be regarded as an investment: they provide the information indispensable for intelligent planning. Without such information huge sums of money may be spent unproductively on programmes that are not able to come to grips with the real problems, because these have not been identified with sufficient precision.

Not infrequently governments feel a need to be seen to be taking rapid action on a large scale ('we are a big country, with big problems: we can't afford to waste time before tackling them in a big way')—often this arises from the pressures of short-term political commitments. But in the long-term such haste may be counter-productive. A commitment to study the problem implies of course the willingness and ability to provide sufficient staff and facilities for proper data gathering and analysis, yet it is not unknown for a decision to be made, in response to a sudden political demand, to initiate or expand the scope of a survey without sufficient regard being given to the availability of such resources.

Action and change

Study should lead to action, and here too governments must be committed. This particularly is where it can hurt. It is the nature of the nutrition problem that it is so often intimately bound up with the prevailing socio-economic stratification of society that action to make a substantial and sustained impact on the problem must as often aim to disturb that order. In other words, there should be a commitment to change. The fact that over the last couple of decades there has been little overall improvement in levels of nutrition in the world at large testifies to the difficulty in practice of a commitment of this sort. Yet, without it, no major improvement can be expected.

Where poverty is the manifest underlying cause of undernutrition a motley of feeding programmes, MCH and other medical services, and programmes of plant-breeding, fortification and education represent a series of skirmishes on the fringes of the battle: the major confrontation is being avoided. Or, to change the metaphor, such attempts to deal with the problem are like the efforts of a fire service to control a blazing building by directing the water hoses through the attic windows, when the fire is raging in the basement.

The point should not be pressed to an extreme. The kinds of programme mentioned above may well play an important role in particular situations, especially if they derive from a consistent national food and nutrition policy. For example, appropriate nutrition education is likely to be necessary at all levels of affluence: in particular, the nutrition of very young children is determined much more by the knowledge of mothers than by their wealth. Under-five clinics, or other forms of MCH service, may be the most effective means of showing and convincing mothers how they should feed their children. Feeding programmes may be a practical means of redistributing income. The provision of clean water can do much to reduce the precipitation of malnutrition. But where the basic problem is that too many people have insufficient money to enable them to purchase an adequate diet those who advocate such programmes should not delude themselves, or others, into supposing that they are thereby tackling the problem of malnutrition at its root. They are not.

Concern with the increase of the Gross National Product as the ultimate criterion of the economic growth and development of a nation is giving way to the recognition that improvement in the 'quality of life' of its members is the more fundamental objective, not so easily attained or evaluated: the GNP is too gross a measure. Questions arise as to how and to whom wealth should be redistributed; how and where new wealth should be created; who should benefit, to what extent, at the expense of whom, from what sorts of programme. These are political questions, and in seeking answers to them and in making decisions on investment policies and regional development programmes, etc. governments committed to improve nutrition should examine the likely impact of alternative proposals for economic development on the nutritional status of the people, as on other aspects of their life and environment.

COORDINATION

Because the activities of several departments of government have implications for nutrition, there is a need for coordination to ensure as far as possible that such activities are mutually consistent and complementary. This coordination must itself be an activity of government, but there is no standard pattern for how it should be done. Everyone agrees that coordination is a 'good thing', but in practice it seems extraordinarily difficult to achieve. Indeed, so difficult is it, that some people have argued that, however 'good' a thing in theory, it is wise to recognize its impracticability and therefore best to devise programmes that are self-contained within a given department so that the major intersectoral problems of coordination are avoided. This seems to be a counsel of desperation, if not despair. Nevertheless, in certain circumstances it may be expedient.

Local

There are several levels of coordination that should be considered. One is at the so-called 'grass roots' level: local-community level is what is often meant. This is characteristically a feature of the 'applied nutrition programmes' that have been attempted, often with support of U.N. agencies, in so many countries. Such programmes usually conceptualize coordinated action by field workers of two or more departments concerned with agriculture, health, education, social welfare and community development. Coordination is supposed to be attained by means of local committees at various levels on which are represented leaders of the community as well as officials such as agricultural extension officers and medical and education officers. But it is experience of difficulties of coordination that have been found in such programmes that has led to the 'counsel of desperation' referred to above.

Apart from isolated instances where magnificent coordination has been achieved because of outstanding leadership and qualities of dedicated service shown by individuals, it seems that effective coordination at this level cannot be attained unless it is also found at higher levels in the apparatus of government, up to the central ministries themselves, so that clear instructions are issued down the line of command. People have to be instructed to cooperate. A headmaster of a school is unlikely to cooperate enthusiastically with an agricultural extension officer about the introduction of school gardening unless the departments of education and agriculture have agreed on a joint programme and have instructed their staff accordingly. Nor will such a programme achieve its full potential unless some form of appropriate nutrition is included in the school curriculum, and this education should be consistent with, and supported by, the sort of education provided by medical and paramedical personnel at health centres and during home visits: the department of health is thus also immediately involved.

One could take another example: a feeding programme for pre-school children. Increasingly it is being recognized that such a programme is of limited value unless the beneficiaries also receive a modicum of health care, including immunization against prevalent diseases, and a safe source of drinking water. Those concerned with the total development of the child will also wish to see included some form of simple education or group care of the children, and also education of the mother in child feeding and other aspects of child care, in environmental hygiene, and family planning: the spacing of children, as well as control of family size. These problems of coordination have to be tackled at an early stage in the planning of the programme, so that the staff of the several departments involved in its execution are able to appreciate their role in relation to the whole, and are sufficiently motivated to do their bit, at the right time, in full cooperation with their colleagues.

It is of course obvious that problems of this sort are by no means unique to questions of nutritional improvement. Neil Armstrong would never have set foot on the moon when he did if exceedingly complex problems of logistics and coordination had not been grappled with and solved in a systematic and rigorous manner. What is essential is leadership, direction and . . . commitment.

However, community-level programmes for nutritional improvement have the added complication that for their long-term success they require changes, voluntarily utilisable forms of iron have been used in the fortification mixtures. However, the example, to ways in which mothers feed their children, or to the pattern of crops grown by subsistence farmers for home consumption, or to the ways in which such crops are stored and used, or to the attitude of the community to environmental sanitation. Such changes can rarely be imposed by decree from above. They are accepted only if they are recognized as conferring some clear benefit, and meet the needs of the people as they see these themselves. Therefore, details of such programmes and short-term objectives should be framed only after consultations at community level, in order to enlist maximum interest and participation. Yet such objectives must be accommodated within the framework of a programme agreed at central ministry level, if full resources are to be made available and maximum coordination between participating agencies achieved. This presents a special challenge to the planning process (Chapter 13).

The same challenge exists for all programmes of community development: how to get people involved in their own development—how to enlist community participation; how to ensure the delivery of a spectrum of services in a coordinated manner; how to promote economic growth of a community, of a region. Because of this similarity, and because programmes for nutritional improvement are but part of the more general question of rural development as a whole, many people argue for an integrated rural development approach, with one of its stated aims to be the improvement of nutrition. (Precisely the same could be said about integrated urban development.) 'Community development', in its early days, had a similar appeal, but latterly the term, if not the concept, has come into some disrepute, with departments of community development in a number of countries having only limited prestige and power. Yet the concept is admirable: what is needed, once more, is political commitment (Chapter 15).

Someone has to be the boss. A community development commissioner? Reporting to him administratively would be the local representatives of the various technical departments: agriculture, health, education, transportation . . .. If not coordination this way, then what way? It is of course impossible to dogmatize: countries differ so widely in their priorities and in their administration. Each government has to find *its* way.

The point here is that if the improvement of nutrition is to be one of the objectives of a local programme of integrated social and economic development there must be facilities (chiefly properly trained staff) for analysing the local implications for nutrition of proposed components of that programme. For example, the linking by road of a remote rural area to a township with good marketing facilities could have a profound impact on the nutrition of its inhabitants. Likewise, decisions on the nature of crops to be promoted; the arrangements for the provision of credit, or cooperative marketing; location of home industries; the siting and nature of health services; etc. Such decisions should be made only after the implications of the proposals for nutrition have been examined.

National

So, too, at the national level: what departments do, or do not do, can have either a positive or negative effect on nutrition. These effects can reinforce each other, or conflict. A policy to export red palm oil, for the manufacture of soap, conflicts with the aims of an educational campaign to increase home use of this rich source of carotene as a means of combating blindness due to vitamin A deficiency. The policies of agriculture and food departments with regard to the nature and level of price support (for example) may have been framed with the economic return to the producer in mind, but they are likely also to have a nutritional effect, good or bad, on the consumer. The propensity of the agricultural arrangements of the European Economic Community (at least as they existed in mid-1974) to create 'mountains' of butter or beef suggests that the consumer received little attention when these arrangements were made. This same propensity also illustrates an attitude that could, if it persists, have profound nutritional implications, not so much for those living in the Community itself as for the inhabitants of less developed countries. The diversion of grain from direct human use to the production of animal products in order to satisfy European palates (or for that matter those of the wealthy minority in poor countries themselves) may from some points of view be regarded as economically sound, but it may be quite inconsistent with a policy to raise minimum nutrition levels in a country. Textbooks of economics, discussing questions of choice of goals and allocation of resources, are wont to do so in terms of 'guns or butter'. They could in future use another slogan: 'beef for some, or bread for all'.

A further example: what do programmes of education—formal, non-formal, informal—say about food in relation to health? If they say anything, is it consistent with the realities of the market place? With the incentives before the farmer? With the instruction in medical colleges? How can it be made, or kept, consistent? These questions are particularly apposite to the training given to teachers, and the teachers of teachers. Some arrangements for training must already exist; they may have to be strengthtened or extended, and ways of ensuring the sort of coordination implied by such questions will probably have to be devised if the education ultimately given is to be as useful as it could be. Governments with scarce resources will be concerned that their expenditures *are* as useful as possible.

This last statement seems to be a perfectly obvious, in fact rather trite, remark. But as a statement of fact it would seem to be, not uncommonly, untrue. Of course, it depends on what one means by 'useful', and how one answers the question 'useful to whom': political matters again. 'Prestige projects' presumably are thought to have some political, if not personal, usefulness. These apart, governments may be concerned in practice to satisfy a maximum of competing claims by conceding a minimum of change in any one direction. In such a situation, who will represent the claims of better nutrition? It is one thing for the government as a whole to profess a commitment to a policy for better nutrition; it is quite another for the different departments of government to recognize explicitly the impact of their programmes on nutrition, and to agree to modify their programmes in ways that mutually complement and reinforce each other, or to devise new programmes, so that a maximum effect on the nutritional situation is obtained.

Research

A final example of coordination relates to the work of research institutes. These may be directly supported and controlled by government, or come under the aegis of a university or private foundation. They are likely to generate a great deal of information, much of which can be properly interpreted and fully utilized only if it is centrally collated. Too often research is conducted in an academic environment in which insufficient concern is shown about the utilization of its results. Research findings tend to be published in learned journals, and at that point responsibility ends. After all, a paper has been published: an academic reputation has been built, or strengthened. Coordination here has two aspects. On the one hand means should be found for ensuring that the sort of studies undertaken are in fact designed to find answers to practical problems of current and foreseen importance. These means should be consistent with principles of academic freedom, but the academic community should recognize that usefulness is no less valuable or prestigious than originality, and indeed can be fully consistent with it. On the other hand the results obtained should be applied with a minimum of delay in the formulation and execution of programmes. In a phrase, government has a coordinating role to ensure that research is relevant, and its findings used.

PROGRAMME FORMULATION AND IMPLEMENTATION

Government clearly has a unique responsibility for the formulation of policies and programmes concerning nutrition, and for their implementation (Chapter 13). The process of policy formulation should be systematic, starting with a full assessment of the situation, and leading to the specification of clear objectives. Such a procedure is likely to have a much greater impact than the adoption of a number of ad hoc measures which are generally thought to be 'good': let us have a school feeding programme, fortify wheat flour with fish protein concentrate, and mount a programme for 'nutrition education' (whatever that may mean) of the public through the mass media.

The systematic approach would begin by seeking answers to such questions as 'Who is malnourished?'; 'In what way, and to what extent?'; 'Where are they?' '*Why* are they malnourished?' The last question is of course particularly relevant to the business of finding appropriate solutions. Is the answer related primarily to a lack of sufficient purchasing power to enable enough food to be bought? To other characteristics of poverty: unhealthy environment and cultural apathy? To a lack of knowledge of how to prepare, or how to feed to young children, the food that is available? To a decline in breast-feeding? To an insufficient supply in certain areas of food rich in nutrients that may be lacking, even if money to purchase them is available? If the latter, is this because of poor distribution and marketing facilities? Or an inability or unwillingness of farmers to produce them locally? And *why* unable or unwilling?

Quite probably, each of these factors will be operative to varying degrees in different regions, both urban and rural, of a given country. Can one then identify bottlenecks, orders of priority and so arrive at objectives for action? These objectives, consistent with the social and economic goals of the government, will constitute the National Food and Nutrition Policy of the country, an integral part of its Economic and Social Development Plan (Chapter 13).

There is a complementary aspect to this process of policy formulation. As mentioned above, it consists in the analysis of ongoing and projected programmes of different departments of government to ascertain their likely impact on nutrition, with the object of then possibly modifying these programmes in order to improve their impact, or perhaps introducing complementary programmes to mitigate undesirable consequences. For example, some measures to improve agricultural production may benefit the more wealthy farmer because only he has the resources to enable him to take advantage of the improved technology; the small landowner or subsistence farmer may be relatively, if not absolutely, in a worse position. The 'green revolution' is a case in point. Should special credit facilities therefore be made available to the small farmer? Should the measures only be introduced concurrently with some programme of land reform? Should alternative employment opportunities be created?

This process should lead to a number of alternative proposals for action, each with an estimate of the costs that would be incurred and a statement of the benefits that could be expected. It may not be possible always to quantify the benefits in financial terms, nor is this strictly necessary: improvement in human well-being can be a sufficient justification. Choices would then have to be made, choices that will be influenced frequently by political considerations.

Implementation of the chosen programmes would then be a matter for the appropriate government departments: it is most unlikely that the need for a new arm of government to implement 'nutrition programmes' would be felt, since most of these would in fact be programmes of rural or urban development, delivery of health services, of agricultural production, etc., that have been formulated with nutritional objectives, amongst others, in mind.

Administration

What sort of administrative arrangements would be needed for a process such as this to take place? It is commonly argued that an essential feature would be a high-level inter-departmental committee, a national food and nutrition board, or its equivalent. Members of the committee would be senior representatives of all those government departments the activities of which impinge on nutrition. Their seniority would be such as to enable them to speak for their departments with authority.

The committee could meet only once or twice a year, to review the situation and make decisions on the choices put before it by its secretariat. The relation of the committee to the overall planning branch of the government would have to be made clear because, as pointed out earlier, the fundamental decisions will be of a political nature.

The chairman of the committee should be an influential member of the government, preferably not connected with any of the major implementing departments. The secretary of a Planning Commission, or the Prime Minister himself, would be particularly appropriate. The secretary of the committee should command respect both within and outside the government for his wide grasp of the multi-factorial nature of nutrition. He would be the head and technical director of its secretariat, and his role would be crucial to the success of the committee's work.

Some countries have set up national food and nutrition committees, but they have not been notably successful, and therefore their need has been seriously questioned, and some other administrative arrangement proposed, such as the delegation of policy and programme formulation to a food and nutrition institute, or the creation of a separate Ministry of Food and Nutrition. But the more likely truth is not that the committee approach has been tried and found wanting, but that it has not been tried properly at all. It is therefore probably premature to condemn it. What has usually happened is that the essential servicing aspect of the committee's work has been neglected, but this is of paramount importance. A national food and nutrition committee *by itself* is virtually impotent, but it is difficult to envisage how the sort of coordination discussed above can be achieved without such a body. Something of this kind would seem to be essential (would a separate ministry be able to impose its will on other departments?), but what is *also* essential is a technically competent multi-disciplinary secretariat, able to make the necessary analyses and prepare alternative strategies for action. Much of this work could be commissioned to outside research institutions or to relevant government departments, or to ad hoc working groups or sub-committees with specialist advisers, but the business of collation and preparation of the material would be the task of the secretariat itself. Where would this be situated? Preferably in some central department, such as a Planning Commission, or the office of the Prime Minister, but with close access to the planning sections of relevant government departments such as health and agriculture. Each government would of course have to find the particular administrative arrangements most appropriate to its own organization and method of work. There can be no universal prescription.

It has been the experience in many countries that advice offered to governments on food and nutrition policy from outside has seldom been effective. Those working in research institutes, for example, are often too remote from the day-to-day realities of government decision-making for their advice to be sufficiently relevant. Advice should be available within the government itself, both at the central coordinating and policy-making level in the manner discussed above, and also within those technical departments chiefly concerned with food and nutrition, such as agriculture, health, social welfare and education; preferably within their planning sections, perhaps with a supporting nutrition unit.

Monitoring and evaluation

The monitoring and evaluation of programmes is a related responsibility of government. Planning is a continuous process. Monitoring of a programme is most appropriately done by the department responsible for its implementation as a regular and routine means of programme management and improvement. Evaluation may also be done at periodic intervals by the concerned departments, to assess the extent to which the objectives of the programme have been realized, and at what cost; and to identify reasons for shortcomings. But a more objective evaluation is likely to be made under the aegis of the food and nutrition committee itself (or some other independent body), perhaps by commissioning an institute through its secretariat to do the work.

Trained personnel

Government has an important responsibility to ensure that people are properly trained to do the various jobs involved in programme formulation and implementation. A key position is that of the nutrition generalist, who may or may not be medically qualified, but who should have an awareness of planning techniques and management, and an understanding of economics and of the sociological and anthropological characteristics of his country. The secretary of the national food and nutrition committee should be such a person. Heads of nutrition units in different departments of government should have similar qualifications.

Government should ensure that appropriate training facilities are created, if they do not exist already. Recourse may be had to training facilities in other countries, perhaps through the offices of the international agencies. Training should include a strong practical component, part of which could be obtained while working in a particular job. Means should be found of breaking out of the closed circle that consists of requiring staff to have practical experience before employing them, thereby denying them the opportunity to gain the necessary experience. Some national and international agencies operate 'junior expert schemes' to get over this difficulty: advantage should be taken of them. Regular refresher training, and seminars to introduce and discuss new ideas, should be common practice.

Of equal importance is the responsibility of the government to ensure that those who are trained are properly used. If necessary, posts should be created and made sufficiently attractive to recruit and retain people of high calibre. Part of the attractiveness of the job will lie in the extent to which the person holding it is made aware of the importance of his or her own contribution. Seldom now does a medical doctor feel that specializing in nutrition will enhance his career. The role that dietitians can play in hospital management and public health programmes is frequently not recognized. Schools of home economics produce qualified graduates who, even when highly motivated, often have difficulty in finding suitable employment. Agriculturists trained in human nutrition are rare, and their potential usefulness seldom recognized. Governments have a role in ensuring that the assets to the country that such people represent are not wasted. There is a need for them both at the central planning level and at the periphery of programme implementation. Indeed, increased recognition is being given to the importance of continually modifying and adapting programmes conceived broadly on the grand scale to the particular needs and opportunities of the local situation—phrases such as 'planning from the bottom up' testify to this. Such a process of adaptation is particularly important in programmes designed to improve nutrition, since these so often depend for their success on persuading people to change their behaviour. (Not all nutrition programmes depend on this: many fortification programmes do not, for example, hence their potential power.) In this situation it becomes important for expert nutritional advice to be available at local level, in order that this adaptation be made wisely. Advice on food habits in programmes of nutrition education is an example. It is difficult to take seriously the intentions of a government to tackle the problems of nutrition in a concerted manner if it does not sanction posts for nutritionists at appropriate levels of the government structure.

CONTROL (Chapter 22)

Government has an obvious role in enacting necessary legislation to enable programmes to be effective: for example, legislation concerning food standards, including the fortification of certain foods with specified nutrients within stated limits, and governing the presence of adulterants. Concurrently it has a role in ensuring that appropriate inspection procedures are followed, and that laboratory facilities for the examination of suspected food samples are available. Penalties for infringement of the law should be sufficiently great to deter, and should be invoked fearlessly, and without undue delay.

DISASTERS AND EMERGENCIES (Chapter 18)

Earthquakes, floods, droughts and other disasters are sadly not uncommon in many countries of the world. Governments must recognize that though these may not be accurately predictable either in terms of scale or timing, in many countries it is virtually certain that over a period of years the rains (for example) *will* fail in one year. This fact must be taken account of in the planning process. Appropriate reserves of food and medical supplies should be maintained. Governments should ensure that their information system is such that they have as much warning as possible of an impending disaster, and are able to judge when the situation calls for emergency measures. Contingency plans should be prepared for such an eventuality, possibly involving the use of the armed forces for the rapid delivery of supplies. Such plans could include the basis of a rationing scheme.

The prospect of disasters should stimulate authorities both at central and local level to recognize the need for sensible food and nutrition policies, and for personnel trained to implement them, just as the disasters themselves can provide scope for practical experience in training programmes.

RELATION TO OTHER AGENCIES

In the international arena, governments have an obligation to be aware of the global food and nutrition situation, so that they can play a responsible role in the forums of the United Nations and its specialized agencies, and similar bodies (Chapter 24). The precarious nature of the world food situation is such that international action is likely to be needed increasingly in order to avert major disasters (Chapter 4).

Within their own countries, governments should be concerned to establish a climate in which non-government organizations are able to participate to a maximum extent in the types of programmes for which they are particularly suited. Voluntary and charitable organizations are often able to work with a rapidity denied to a large bureaucratic system (Chapter 25). Their members too are frequently highly motivated and dedicated, with an ability to gain the confidence of illiterate people and help them to improve their way of life. These characteristics of course are not confined to such groups: many government servants share them, but by the nature of things they tend to be more pronounced in the voluntary sector. There is great scope for government to enlist the participation of such organizations in its own programmes, perhaps on a selective basis (all may not be working towards the same goals), without destroying their independence. Tax concessions of various kinds could be used; facilities for training field workers could be strengthened; supplies and equipment could be provided; components of programmes could be delegated to their responsibility. At least, government should not attempt to compete with them. To build a government hospital across the road from a satisfactory private one providing the same, if not better, services—by no means unknown—is a sheer waste of resources. Cooperation, not competition, should be the guideline.

With regard to sources of external aid—bilateral donors or United Nations agencies—government's role will be, within the political framework of the country, to seek, again in cooperation, agreement about appropriate means of agency support. The government can help, or hinder, these agencies in doing their work. Naturally all governments wish to become independent of outside assistance as much as, and as soon as possible, but in this interdependent world, while help, technical or financial, is needed and is available, there is no shame in seeking it, in a spirit of friendly partnership and joint participation.

FURTHER READING

Berg, A., N. S. Scrimshaw and D. L. Call (Eds.). *Nutrition, National Development and Planning,* Cambridge, Massachusetts, USA and London, England, The MIT Press, 1973. (Much of these proceedings of an International Conference held in 1971, which are fully referenced for those who wish to pursue particular topics, is pertinent to the subject of this chapter.)

Donoso, G. and J. P. Greaves. Food and Nutrution Policy in Developing Countries. *Nutrition Newsletter,* Food and Agriculture Organization of the United Nations, **9,** 26. FAO, Rome (1971).

Ritchie, Jean A. S. *Learning Better Nutrition,* FAO Nutritional Studies No. 20, Rome, Food and Agriculture Organization of the United Nations, 1967.

CHAPTER 24

Nutrition and the United Nations

DONALD S. MCLAREN

This is not an authortative account of the work of these agencies as it is related to nutrition. The agencies that have hitherto been primarily concerned, namely the World Health Organization (WHO), the Food and Agriculture Organization (FAO) and the United Nations Children's Fund (UNICEF) have published their own accounts of their activities and programmes from time to time. A critical appraisal of their achievements and those of such bodies as the Protein Advisory Group (PAG), the World Food Programme (W.F.P.) and more recently the International Bank for Reconstruction and Development (I.B.R.D. or World Bank) has not been made. This would require extensive knowledge of their workings, centrally and in many countries, and a free hand to be fully objective. Here an attempt is made to point out some of the virtues as well as the shortcomings of the U.N. contribution as seen by someone who has on numerous occasions worked for them but only in various temporary capacities.

The greatest virtue of the United Nations in general and its agencies in particular is the ability to act as a 'sounding board' for the whole world. This was perhaps, never better exemplified than in 1974 when conferences on Population and Food held under its auspices focused world attention as never before on these related issues (Chapter 3). This capacity is presumably related to the almost, but not quite, universal representation in these bodies and the ability for all shades of views to be expressed.

Not unrelated is the prestige carried by reports of the technical agencies, in this case WHO and FAO, especially in their technical report series. Nomenclature, classification and methodology advocated by expert groups in these publications receive the imprimatur of the world body and tend to be accepted without question for years by their scientific peers and people at large. A great advantage gained is that in this way unification can be achieved and this can lead to the collection of data all over the world using the same criteria. This is only now beginning to happen for PEM for example and xerophthalmia, but has been in force for the nutritional anaemias for some time.

The converse also has to be true; that is if the imprimatur is laid on a shoddy piece of work, a wrong emphasis, a false concept, the general acceptance is just the same and it may take another decade or longer for the truth to emerge. Not only does it take time for any entrenched ideas to be dislodged but when these are reinforced by action programmes which have been put into operation there is tremendous inertia to be overcome from vested interests. For example, although the tide has begun to turn in the case of the 'Great Protein Fiasco' (Chapter 3) it will take a long time before the trend is completely reversed.

These organizations have the great advantages of acting as 'clearing houses' of information from the world, of being able to call on advice from innumerable experts and they may coordinate research through regional centres as they have done on nutritional anaemias, and malnutrition and infection.

As in the parent body, political considerations have an overriding influence. This may mean that the best available person for the job is not chosen, assistance is divided inequably and certain topics are suppressed.

Certain problems, which would seem to be largely unnecessary but which are entrenched, lie in the nature of the organizations. Conflict of interest is bound to arise when, for example, WHO is strong regionally, FAO strong centrally; WHO and FAO are technical, UNICEF is non-technical; the most powerful division of WHO, PAHO (Pan American Health Organization) is virtually autonomous.

When specialized bodies are set up, only loosely related to the parent organizations, with limited goals, and when a balanced view is not maintained, disastrous results may follow: viz. the Protein Advisory Group (Chapter 3).

In recent years the World Bank has become interested in nutrition, especially in relation to sociological, population and educational aspects. Administratively it comes under the Population and Nutrition Projects Department. The approach is to deal with individual countries, on a rather large-scale and long-term basis, with emphasis on Nutrition rather than on Food. At present actions are mainly of an intervention nature, not limited as far as sector is concerned, i.e. including Health, Education, Agriculture etc. Assistance is given for large-scale feeding and education programmes with a built-in basis for data collection and evaluation. This permits development and continuity with research and training and other inputs. The process of project identification and preparation is gone through before implementation. Components vary considerably in different countries. Project identification is proceeding in Iran and projects are at different stages of preparation in Indonesia, India and Brazil.

REFERENCES

Among many U.N. publications related to Nutrition are the following:
WHO Chronicle, Nutrition: a review of the WHO programme I, **26,** 160 (1972).
UNICEF News, Issue 71, 1972.
PAG Bulletin published quarterly.
FAO Nutrition Newsletter published quarterly.

CHAPTER 25

Role of Private Organizations in Nutrition

E. L. SEVERINGHAUS

Long before governments came to regard it as part of their responsibility to provide for the welfare of their subjects, private individuals and their supporters made efforts to improve the lot of their fellows, at home and abroad, often at great personal sacrifice.

At the present time there are many private agencies with their headquarters mainly in North America and Europe that are concerned in some way or another with nutritional problems. Clearly, in the present context, it is only possible to give some indication of the type of activity these agencies undertake in this field. The mention of organizations by name here is purely for the sake of illustration.

Private organizations with activities in the field of nutrition may be divided into roughly five main categories: (1) General interest and 'academic', (2) General interest and 'service', with sub-divisions into (i) secular and (ii) religious, (3) Confined to nutrition, (4) Religious mission and (5) Food companies.

(1) It is of special interest that some of the most significant contributions towards solving nutritional problems in the community have come not from the U.N. agencies or government or academic institutions but from private foundations like those of Ford and Rockefeller. One thinks naturally of the high-yielding varieties of wheat and rice, the green revolution, and the Nobel Peace prize winner of Norman Borlaug.

Such organizations carry out and assist others to do a great deal of valuable research, train scientists and organize meetings, not only in nutrition of course but in many other areas of applied science.

(2) There are many organizations that have similarly broad interests, that include nutrition, but where the emphasis is on service rather than academic activities. Some of these are secular, like Oxfam, War on Want, Save the Children's Fund in Britain and Care in the United States. Others have religious associations, like World Council of Churches, Catholic Aid and work of the Friends and Quakers, for example. They are especially concerned with relief operations but more and more are becoming involved in longer term measures that aim at combating the problem.

(3) Several organizations are confined in their interests to nutrition. The Nutrition Foundation in the United States and the British Nutrition Foundation, which are supported largely by the food industry, issue publications of scientific value, support research in a limited way and organize conferences.

(4) When all is said and done much of the assistance on the spot by foreigners to developing countries is still being given by religious missions, mostly Christian, both Catholic and Protestant. Hospitals, orphanages, special schools, especially in the remoter places, are often financed and sometimes staffed from North America or Europe. At the present time these positions do not carry the degree of permanence that they used to and it remains to be seen whether the same spirit of dedication will continue as devolution proceeds.

(5) Food companies, like other commerical concerns, if they are of any size, usually carry out research on their own products and frequently assist others in the testing of the wider use of these products. Complete objectivity may not always be maintained under these circumstances. They may provide invaluable assistance to action programmes by formulating products such as vitamins for general use. Their role in the production of protein-rich food mixtures (Chapters 3 and 16) and in 'commerciogenic' malnutrition in infants (Chapters 7 and 8) is a far from happy one.

The most obvious community nutrition problem in the developing countries is the appalling mortality rate of infants and children in the first 5 years of life. This rate varies from 30–50 per cent of those born alive, dead by the end of 5 years (Chapter 8). The recognized causes are malnutrition and infectious diseases. The causal relationship between these two operates reciprocally (Chapter 10). Within the past two decades two types of community approach to this problem have been established. Both have now had widespread trials and both have demonstrated laudable results. The first to be tried is the 'Under Fives Clinics', which began under the guidance of Dr. David Morley, at Ilesha, in Nigeria. The other approach is the 'Mothercraft Centres', initiated by Dr. Kendall King in Haiti. These will be described briefly later on (see also Chapter 15).

Dr. J. George Harrar has recently written,[1] 'We have become increasingly aware of deficiency diseases and their effects upon pregnant mothers, infants, and juveniles and older age groups. We know that juvenile malnutrition can bring about irreversible detrimental effects, both physical and mental, that millions today are doomed to unproductive lives because of their earlier deficient dietary patterns'. Summarizing a 1973 conference on the relations between nutrition and growth and development, Dr. H. N. Munro[2] pointed out the importance of the nutritional status of pregnant women on the growth and development of their children. Thus, babies whose birth weights are significantly below normal still show at 4-years old deficits in height, the maturing of bones and the circumference of their heads.[3] The group at INCAP[4] has demonstrated that adequate supplementation of the diets of pregnant women in Guatemala was followed by larger babies, and significantly fewer babies lost at or before birth. Metcoff and associates[5] have found that babies born with unusually small birth weight show an abnormality in the chemical processes in their white blood cells. These cells remain in immature, large forms, but fail to mature to the smaller, normal types. This disorder of growth is known to occur in many thousands of babies. Furthermore, it has been shown by Winick and associates[6] that reduction in adequate nutrition while the cells of a tissue are being formed leads to permanent handicap. His 'studies on human tissues including brain confirm the importance of malnutrition on cell populations, thus leading to the conclusion that early post-natal malnutrition can play a significant part in limiting human brain development'. The human brain continues to develop new cells during the first 2 years after birth.

To meet these recognized problems, the advantage shared by the 'Under Fives Clinics' and the 'Mothercraft Centres' is an approach both to and through the mothers of the new-born, or of the infants who are in serious difficulties. This is obviously a period in life when a woman is most open to help which includes nutrition education and immunizations of her children. It has been found that at this time the clinic staff is assured of interested attention to the possibility and methods of family planning.

By beginning the use of adequate dietary supplements for children aged 1–5 years real advantages can be obtained. Weight, stature and better bone cortical strength can be achieved. This was based upon cereal, legume and green vegetable foods in common use in India.[7] A confirmatory report[8] includes evidence that the children who received the modest supplemental food showed superior resistance to one of the most dangerous infections, measles. But within the past two decades it has become recognized that delaying adequate nutrition until they are a year old may be disastrous in many infants. This is the reason for the initiation of the Under Fives Clinics and of Mothercraft Centres.

UNDER FIVES CLINICS

The development of the Under Fives Clinics was begun in 1957, by Dr. David C. Morley, at that time a missionary physician serving at Ilesha, in Western Nigeria. The most adequate presentation of these clinics is in his book *Paediatric Priorities in the Developing World*.[9] The clinics are conducted daily in each of a series of villages within the area served by the hospital, where the physician is based. A locally resident woman is trained to be in charge and to manage the details. At frequent intervals a nurse-supervisor travels from the hospital to the village clinics to teach, assist, make decisions for which the local nursing assistant is not prepared, and to determine the need for scheduling a visit by the physician or for moving a seriously ill child to the hospital. On less frequent occasions the physician accompanies the nurse on these visits. The plan is based upon use of indigenous foods when supplemental feeding is in order as the infant grows older.

The aims of these clinics are listed as:

1. The supervision of the health of all children up to the age of 5;
2. The prevention of malnutrition, malaria, measles, pertussis, tuberculosis, smallpox, poliomyelitis, diphtheria and tetanus;
3. The provision of simple treatment for diarrhoea, with or without dehydration, for pneumonia and for the common skin conditions.

Added to these three objectives, the clinics have given opportunities for instruction in birth spacing and therefore in family planning.[10]

The essence of this programme is preventive medicine, conducted by a physician with the assistance of a nurse-supervisor and numerous village assistants, trained for their tasks. Therapy is available when it is needed. Care is made easily available in the villages where people live. Travel of patients to the central hospital is reserved for only those serious illnesses which require it. Costs have been studied carefully. The spread of these clinics to several coutries, operating in many hundreds of villages, led Morley to suggest that the lowest cost is about $3 (U.S.A.) per child per annum. Since the developing countries are said to have approximately $1 per person per annum for all health work, it is obvious that here is an activity for the private agencies. At an earlier date Dr. Morley thought 'that these clinics were suited only to the conditions of church-related hospitals'. But by 1973, 'large numbers of these clinics have now been started by many governments', notably in Africa. This has occurred only following the initiative of private agencies, in establishing the first clinics in a given country.

MOTHERCRAFT CENTRES

The Mothercraft Centres grew from the vision and planning ability of Dr. Kendall W. King. He attributes to Dr. Jose Maria Bengoa, of the World Health Organization, a suggestion in 1955 for the establishment of such centres. In 1958 a group of workers, including Dr. King as the biochemist of the team, carried out an appraisal of the nutrition of Haiti.[11] The following year we undertook an experimental school lunch supplemental feeding in three Haitian schools. Dr. King and his family lived in Haiti for the year while he worked in these communities, and he saw much detail of Haitian peasant life. When we studied our results[12] we became aware of the far more urgent need for attention to malnutrition among the infants and pre-school children. After returning to his post at the Virginia Polytechnic Institute Dr. King and associates carried out some intensive chemical studies of a great variety of Haitian foods. Tests in laboratory animals confirmed the conclusion that simple combinations of Haitian cereals and legumes, in proper proportions, would provide a dependable source of protein for the diets of weanling and growing children.

The next step was to organize in 1964 what was called a 'Mothercraft Centre' in one of the severely disadvantaged villages which had been studied before. Its achievements were reported by Dr. King, with the two physicians, Drs. Beghin and Fourgere, who carried out the supervision of the centre.[13] The most comprehensive discussion of these centres is published in book form.[14] This book has been reviewed, together with the logic presented above, by King.[15]

The basic idea originally was to establish a centre in a village where much serious malnutrition, i.e. kwashiorkor and marasmus, was evident. The physician in charge selected 30 of the most urgent cases for a 3-month period of daily treatment. The mothers of these infants were led through the techniques of nutritional rehabilitation, a few mothers being in attendance each day. When a child is far enough along in recovery his treatment continues by the mother at home. Then another group of 25–30 infants is chosen for the next period.

At first there was a real effort to keep these centres entirely separate from any medical institutional contact, in order to convince the mothers of the importance of nutrition as the responsible factor in saving the child. With few exceptions, all food used was indigenous and procured from the same markets where these mothers purchased family supplies. Similar centres have subsequently been established in Brazil, Colombia, Guatemala and in the Philippines. A recent detailed study of their results[16] in Brazil points out some developmental changes. (See also Chapter 15.) Personal correspondence with Dr. Beghin, who was one of the physicians in the first Haitian centre, has confirmed the necessity of establishing operative connections between the centres and available medical help at hospitals or clinics in the neighbourhood. This is also evident from the experience of Dr. Carroll Behrhorst in a rural situation in Guatemala.

REQUISITE PERSONNEL

The first essential in either plan, obviously, is a paediatrician of competence, who is willing to give a significant portion of his time to supervising the staff and operation of a series of village clinics surrounding any hospital where he is established. The emphasis in Under Fives Clinics is preventive, but there is need for therapy whenever demands arise. The emphasis in Mothercraft Centres is therapeutic, that is rehabilitation of seriously malnourished infants. But the programme becomes secondarily one of preventing recurrences, and of the protection of others in the families, in fact also in the village at large. Without a paediatrician whose vision and commitment fit this specification there is no reason to establish either type of centre. It has been the experience to date that such physicians are found by private agencies, such as mission hospitals or ad hoc community groups. It is hardly to be expected that a government of large size is in a position to secure such a competent and committed doctor to initiate these types of programme.

The second person who is indispensable for either scheme is a trained nurse, who can give her entire time and effort to instructing and supervising the village women who are the actual conductors of the village clinics or centres. Ultimately, even if not at the start, this nurse is ideally a national, selected after standard training, and given special instruction in the details involved.

Both the paediatrician and the nurse-supervisor must have the use of dependable motorized transport in order to facilitate frequent scheduled, as well as emergency, visits to the villages. In the developing countries, where the people live in small villages, the roads are seldom paved. Mothers with their babies must be seen where they live. They cannot be expected to come to a hospital clinic for advice, supervision of nutrition, immunizations, and for treatment of minor illnesses. These are not adequate causes for hospitalization, with its greater cost (Chapter 15).

ESTABLISHING CENTRES

Establishing a centre in any village must be preceded by careful approach to the dominant person or group in the community. Sometimes this is not a woman, in spite of the fact that the operation centres on mothers. If the village head-man is to be approached, he must face the fact that women will be those directly involved in the care of their children. In this process of initial planning with village leaders there should be selection of some building or shelter for the activities. Likewise there must be selection of a young woman who can give much of her time to being available even during those days when the nurse-supervisor is not in attendance. It is this young woman who is directly responsible for the day-to-day operation, and for direct contacts with the mothers. She need not be technically trained except for the special education given by the physician and nurse-supervisor. It is a great advantage if this village woman is literate.

Equipment for the village centres is described in the books referred to.[9,14] For any group planning to establish an Under Fives Clinic there has been a recently published paper-back, *Nutrition in Developing Countries,* by Maurice King and associates.[17] This book is remarkably helpful in the details of establishing, equipping and operating the clinics. It has been 'written in simple English, using a strictly limited vocabulary of only 440 words'. The book will be helpful to physician, nurse and to any other literate participant in the enterprise.

To accomplish maximal effectiveness in optimal nutrition of children continuity of attention is essential. Contrasts between the Under Five Clinics and the Mothercraft Centres must be recognized. In the Mothercraft Centre plan the child and the mother are discharged after 3 months intensive rehabilitative treatment. Experience has demonstrated that the rate of relapse of the malnourished children is far from negligible. Since there is no provision for systematic follow-up work, this is not surprising. On the other hand, the plan of operation of Under Fives Clinics provides for a stout card, in a plastic case, which the mother brings to the clinic as a ticket of admission. On this card is kept the original graphic chart of the child's weight. Whether the mother is literate or not she can see from the graph how her child is growing. Also on this card there are brief notes or signals made by the examining clinic manager, the nurse-supervisor or the doctor, calling attention at subsequent visits to special problems meriting action. The child is expected to be seen periodically at the clinic until the age of 5 years. Experience has shown that the rate of loss of these cards by the mothers is extremely small. The complete record of immunization is seen by the physician at a glance. Furthermore, these graphic record cards are proving very useful in programming efforts at birth spacing and family planning.

In recent years some governments in developing countries have shown genuine interest and willingness to help with starting Mothercraft Centres. Extensive programmes are under way in the Philippines, for example. But even there the beginning was associated with a few individuals in a private agency.[18] Unpublished reports from Dr. R. W. Engel, sent out by the United States Agency for International Development, indicate that the activities of the Mothercraft Centres, chiefly in small villages, have depended upon personnel provided by two private agencies, Catholic Relief Services and Church World Service. Also these reports make it apparent that the Mothercraft Centres are operated as expansions of rural health units.

Recent correspondence from Mrs. Carol Suter revealed a fascinating and encouraging series of steps which led from an intense commitment to the nutritional needs of a particular 'barrio' in 1958, on through local organization, and to the eventual collaboration of the privately supported Nutrition Foundation of the Philippines, and of the Food and Nutrition Research Center, a governmental agency. Nine years later Mrs. Suter participated in the Third Far East Symposium on Nutrition, and learned from Dr. Kendall King more about Mothercraft Centres. Mrs. Suter wrote 'After that time, 1967, we began trying to adapt the Mothercraft Centre concept to the Philippine culture and conditions. The Nutrition Foundation sponsored the Philippine Federation of Nutrition Councils and Related Agencies, which has almost spread like wild fire throughout the land. They have employed many nutritionists who are at work with people in the area of nutrition education and to utilize the materials produced by the Philippine Food and Nutrition Research Center, who have very limited funds for personnel to work in this way'.

EXPERIENCES IN OTHER COUNTRIES

Very few attempts have been reported from India, but one successful Under Fives Clinic programme has been described by Dr. W. A. M. Cutting,[19] connected with a mission hospital. Others are known to have been started, not yet reported in print. Attention should be drawn to an extended discussion of the national effort initiated at the end of 1969 by the Indian government. In a careful evaluation after a year, Alan D. Berg[20] described many of the problems and handicaps of a national governmental effort to improve the nutritional status of children. Although there is recognition of the magnitude of this problem, there was no plan by which to reach the people in the villages where 80 per cent of India's people live. Fortification of bread with amino acids and iron as well as vitamins could be of help to the urban minority only. Furthermore, one conspicuous item in the programme was the production of new commercial products by the associated manufacturers. In a country with such very low family income as is characteristic of India, this leaves the disadvantaged village peasants relatively worse off than before. Much can be learned from the Indian experiment and from this report, but there is no doubt that the approach by private agencies, beginning in small units, must be considered of immediate and ultimate value in meeting even such a tremendous need.

A recent report[21] of a comprehensive community health centre in Hong Kong includes careful attention to the nutrition of pregnant women and nursing mothers, and supervision of infants and growing children. This came from private organizations of churches and their related groups, but the government provided land and some of the operating costs.

One of the most condensed and useful summaries of the *Nutrition Program for Pre-School Children*[22] presents 19 principles which are involved.

Within the United States of America there is still a widespread need both for improvement in nutrition education and for provision of services. For many years attention has been given chiefly to the use of school lunches. These affect children over age 5 years, and usually for only one meal 5 days per week. A review of current progress in the nationally supervised and supported school lunch programme[23] showed that large minority groups and especially those in southern states were very poorly provided for. One reason appears to be local governmental unwillingness to contribute to the costs. Obviously in such situations local private agencies could become actively engaged in establishing the programme. Another recent report[24] finds that the greatest challenge is to increase pupil participation. Incorporating nutrition education has too often been minimal (see Chapter 31).

Under Fives Clinics and Mothercraft Centres fit far more easily into rural communities, with people clustered in small villages. Attempts to accommodate these approaches to urban problems have been few, and fraught with discouraging results in some cases. An encouraging effort has recently been reported[25] by a group affiliated with the Syracuse, New York, University. Their achievements in what they call a 'Family Oriented Child Development Program' will be useful to other groups who attempt urban work.

BOTTLE- VERSUS BREAST-FEEDING

In many developing countries there is a dangerous tendency either to avoid breast-feeding of infants or to cease it prematurely (Chapter 8). This appears to be a trend imitating mothers in western countries. Private agencies can accomplish far more than public ones in counteracting this trend. All those who work in the field of infant nutrition emphasize the value of breast-feeding, even far beyond the period at ages 5–6 months when supplemental feeding is required for the best growth and development of infants. For those who wish for help in mounting local efforts correspondence might well be undertaken with La Leche International, whose headquarters are at 9616 Minneapolis Ave., Franklin Park, Illinois, Zip code 60131, U.S.A.

OTHER FIELDS FOR PRIVATE AGENCIES

The pioneer work on the relationship between iodine deficiency and goitre came from the Himalayan area in India, by McCarrison, three-quarters of a century ago. The need for iodine supplementation is still demonstrable in many areas. Recently this has been confirmed for India, Nepal and Sri Lanka (Ceylon).[26] Unless private agencies and understanding individuals take up the matter, the governments involved cannot be expected to do anything to help their people.

The prevention of blindness, especially in infants, is another very urgent need for private as well as public agencies.* This calls for education in preventive medicine and nutrition. The need is largely one of supplying adequate amounts of vitamin A

*Editor's Note: The Royal Commonwealth Society for the Blind in the United Kingdom and the American Foundation for Overseas Blind in the United States are actively assisting programmes to combat xerophthalmia.

in the diet, or under certain circumstances, by massive oral dosing. Naturally all maternal and infant nutrition work should include this matter. But, even when there are no nutritional clinics or centres, efforts to see that adequate intake of vitamin A occurs might well be the concern of private agencies. A change in public policy may then follow.

The list of opportunities for private efforts in community improvement of nutrition is by no means complete in this chapter. It is hoped that the examples are sufficient to stimulate readers to thinking and action. Adequate nutrition for every pregnant woman and for every child through the first 5 years of life must be considered the crucial concern of the community for nutrition. With the new knowledge and techniques now available in this field, especially with use of indigenous foods, it is possible to hope for a new generation with stronger bodies and with minds more able to cope with a complex world.

REFERENCES

1. Harrar, J. G. *Nutr. Revs., 32,* 97 (1974).
2. Munro, H. N. *Amer. J. Clin. Nutr., 27,* 55 (1974).
3. Fitzhardinge, P. M. and E. M. Steven. *Pediatrics, 49,* 671 (1972).
4a. Lechtig, A., G. Arroyave, J. P. Habicht and M. Behar. *Arch Latinamer. Nutr., 21,* 505 (1971).
4b. Lechtig, A., J. P. Habicht, E. DeLeon, G. Guzman and M. Flores. *Arch. Latinamer. Nut., 22,* 101 (1972).
5. Metcoff, J., J. Wikman-Cogfelt, T. Yoshida, A. Bernal, A. Rosada, P. Yoshida, J. Urrusti, S. Frank, R. Madrazo, L. Velasco and M. Morales. *Pediatrics,* 51, 866 (1973).
6. Sigulem, D. M., J. A. Brasel, E. G. Velasco, P. Rosso and M. Winick. *Amer. J. Clin. Nutr., 26,* 793 (1973).
7. Rajalakshmi, R., S. S. Sail, D. G. Shah and S. K. Ambody. *Brit. J. Nutr., 30,* 77 (1973).
8. Gopalan, C., M. C. Swaminathan, V. K. Krishna Kumari, D. Hanumantha Rao and K. Vijayaragharan. *Amer. J. Clin. Nut., 26,* 563 (1973).
9. Morley, D. C. *Paediatric Priorities in the Developing World,* London, Butterworths, 1973.
10. Morley, D. C. *Trans. Roy. Soc. Trop. Med. and Hyg., 67,* 155 (1973).
11. Sebrell, W. H., Jr., S. C. Smith, E. L. Severinghaus, K. W. King *et al. Amer. J. Clin. Nutr., 7,* 538 (1959).
12. King, K. W., J. Foucauld and E. L. Severinghaus. *Amer. J. Clin. Nutr., 13,* 106 (1963).
13. King, K. W., I. D. Beghin, W. Fougere, G. Dominique, R. Grinker and J. Foucauld. *Arch. Venezolianas Nutr., 18,* 245 (1968).
14. *A Practical Guide to Combating Malnutrition in the Pre-School Child,* New York, Appleton-Century-Crofts, 1970.
15. King, K. W. *Nutr. Revs., 28,* 307 (1970).
16. Beghin, I. D. and F. E. Viteri. *J. Trop. Pediat., 19,* 403 (1973).
17. King, M. H., F. M. A. King, D. C. Morley, H. J. L. Burgess and A. P. Burgess. *Nutrition in Developing Countries,* Nairobi and London, Oxford University Press, 1972.
18. Suter, C. B. *J. Nutr. Educ., 3,* 66 (1971).
19. Cutting, W. A. M. and A. D. Padma Kumari. *J. Christian Med. Assn. India,* 45, 704 (1970).
20. Berg, A. D. *Amer. J. Clin. Nutr., 23,* 1396 (1970).
21. Paterson, E. H. Contact 15, Christian Med. Commission, Geneva (1973).

22. Jelliffe, D. B. and E. F. P. Jelliffe. *Amer. J. Clin. Nutr.,* **25,** 395 (1972).
23. Lukaczer, M. *Nutr. Revs.,* **31,** 385 (1973).
24. National Dairy Council, *Dairy Council Digest,* **45,** Jan–Feb. (1974).
25. Dibble, M. V. and J. R. Lally. *J. Nutr. Educ.,* **5,** 200 (1973).
26. Karmarkar, M. G., M. G. Deo, N. Kochupillai and V. Ramalingaswami. *Amer. J. Clin. Nutr.,* **27,** 96 (1974).

SECTION V

Country Experiences

CHAPTER 26

Nutrition in the Caribbean

ROBERT COOK

THE FOOD AND NUTRITION SITUATION

The English-speaking Caribbean comprises 6 independent states, Jamaica, Trinidad and Tobago, Guyana, Barbados, Bahamas and Grenada, and eleven other territories with varying degrees of self-government. The total population is nearly 5 million. The main ethnic group is of West African origin, but about one-half of the population of Guyana and a substantial minority of the people of Trinidad originate in the Indian sub-continent. While those of African origin were brought to the West Indies between 300–170 years ago, and their languages survive only as remnants in the local dialects of English, those of Indian origin came as indentured labourers more recently, 130–60 years ago, and many retain the ability to understand their original languages, and their food habits and preferences have many similarities with those of that region.

The nutritional problems of the area exhibit certain differences in kind and in degree from those of the great majority of developing countries in Africa, Asia and Latin America. There are even marked differences between those of the English-speaking Caribbean and those of such near Caribbean or Central American neighbours as Haiti, the Dominican Republic or Guatemala. Two of the smaller non-independent states, Bermuda and Cayman Islands, have so prospered from tourism and banking that protein–energy malnutrition of early childhood is a rarity and they can be excluded from further consideration in this chapter. To some extent this has happened also in the Bahamas.

The causes of malnutrition commonly found in other developing countries also prevail in the Caribbean. They include general low level of average income, maldistribution of income, illiteracy, and inadequate availability of health services throughout the countries. However, they are much less severe in degree than in the majority of developing countries. This manifests itself, for example, in lower infant mortality rates than is usual, most of the English-speaking Caribbean having rates of between 30–40 per thousand live births, and 1–4 year rates of between 2–10 per 1000 of that age. However, almost the entire difference between these rates and those of Europe and North America is accounted for by protein–energy malnutrition of early childhood (usually of the marasmic variety and occurring often even under six months of age) and gastroenteritis, or often a combination of both.

However, certain other factors play a major role in malnutrition in this area. They may be conveniently considered under the headings of food supply, food demand and social factors.

Food supply

With considerable difficulty the nations of the Caribbean are struggling to change their plantation economies. From soon after the settlement of these lands by Europeans the basis of the economy was the plantation, producing for the market in Europe and later in North America such crops as sugar, coffee, cocoa, or more recently, bananas and citrus fruits. Above all and longest-lasting has been sugar. So valuable was the land for sugar-cane that it was more profitable to feed the slaves to some extent with imported food, and in particular salted cod as the main animal protein source, than to devote land to growing their food. The imported food was supplemented by starchy roots and fruits (yam, dasheen, sweet potato, breadfruit) grown by the plantation workers on small patches of less arable or sloping ground near the estate. After the abolition of slavery many workers left the estates and made little farms in the hill country, difficult to cultivate and now much fragmented by inheritance. This historical chain of events, rather summarized here, has had a profound effect on the food supply of the peoples.

The pattern of export agriculture has continued, and at the present time most of the countries of the area, with the exception of Guyana, import some 50 per cent of energy supply consumed and somewhat over 50 per cent of protein supply. The main food imports to the region as a whole are wheat and wheat flour, corn (almost the entire supply), some rice, some legumes and a substantial portion of total meat, milk and fish supply. In spite of being in the main a group of islands, the countries of the area are not fortunately situated in regard to fishing, for abundant fish supply requires fishing grounds on the continental shelf, and the only such grounds available are those off Guyana and a few banks near the Central American coast. A typical picture of food availability in the area is given by Table 1, which relates to Jamaica.

The countries have suffered the common fate of all developing countries, with the recent exception of those producing oil, of having their exported primary products priced downwards in relation to the cost of their imports. This applies not only to finished industrial products imported, but now to food also, in spite of cereal prices being relatively stable until 1973. In the case of Jamaica for example, in 1938 the ratio of value of exported agricultural products to food imports was 2 : 1. By 1968 it had become 1 : 1, and now it is even less. The steep rises in world prices of wheat, corn, rice, soya, dried milk powder and other animal products have been a severe blow to the economies of the countries, bringing an imported inflation in cost of living and a foreign exchange problem worsened by the escalation in fuel costs. Some cushioning of the effect has taken place, however, in Trinidad, itself a small oil producer, and very recently in Jamaica, with a rise in the price of bauxite. Sugar prices too were high in 1974, and this also has prevented the wider spread of

Table 1. The relative importance of local production and imports in the availability of the various food groups. From the Food Balance Sheet of Jamaica 1972

Food groups	Weight	Average availability per capita per day									
		Energy (kcal) [a]					Protein—g				
	(g)	Total	Production	%	Import	%	Total	Production	%	Import	%
1. Cereals	253	923	45	5	878	95	28.4	1.1	4	27.3	96
2. Starchy roots and tubers	540	433	433	100	0	0	7.1	7.1	100	0.0	0
3. Sugar and syrups	128	488	425	87	63	13	0.0	0.0	92	0.0	8
4. Pulses, nuts and oilseeds	18	85	76	89	10	11	2.9	2.4	80	0.5	20
5. Vegetables	87	29	24	81	5	19	0.9	0.7	82	0.2	18
6. Fruits	237	83	70	85	13	15	1.4	1.3	91	0.1	9
7. Meats	89	194	105	54	89	46	11.9	6.4	54	5.5	46
8. Eggs	9	13	13	100	0	0	1.0	1.0	100	0.0	0
9. Fish	61	95	14	14	81	86	10.7	2.0	18	8.7	82
10. Milk and products	107	212	145	68	67	32	9.2	4.7	50	4.5	50
11. Oils and fats	40	332	206	62	126	38	0.1	0.1	50	0.0	50
12. Miscellaneous	5	10	1	8	9	90	0.3	0.1	38	0.2	62
13. Alcoholic beverages	79	45	39	86	6	14	0.2	0.2	90	0.0	10
Totals		2945	1597	54	1348	46	74.1	27.1	37	47.0	63

[a] 1 kcal = approx. 4.2 Kjoules

malnutrition which would otherwise have occurred in countries so dependent on food imports. Nevertheless, the experiences of 1973 and 1974 have been traumatic, sharpening considerably the determination of governments to become more self-sufficient in food supply, an achievement which will demand the assistance of nutritionists in several ways discussed below.

Food demand

The pattern of food demand, in the sense of food preferences, is influenced towards the imported by two major factors. The first is the historically determined agricultural pattern outlined above. The second is the influence of social class emulation and advertisement. Porfirio Diaz said of his country, 'Poor Mexico, so far from God, so near to the United States', and the same remark applies to the Caribbean countries. Irrational prejudices against local foods and locally processed foodstuffs are still strong, though fortunately declining, owing to the combined effects of political independence, greater pride in country and culture, and improvement in food technology.

The other aspect of demand, effective demand in the economic sense for the different food groups, is a most important factor. As so much of the food supply is imported, it is therefore purchased. Most of the locally produced component of the food supply goes through the marketing chain, and subsistence agriculture is only a minor portion of total national food supply. Thus on an average some 90 per cent of total food consumed is purchased. The following factors are to be noted:

1. Escalation in food prices in general enriches the North American farmer or food processor far more than the local farmer, since more is imported than locally produced.

2. For that half of the food supply imported the Caribbean consumer, with an *average* per capita income of well under U.S. $1000 per annum, pays more for food than the North American consumer with his far greater average per capita income.

3. The *average* amount of income spent on food is some 50-odd per cent, as compared to 20–30 per cent in Europe and North America. The first quartile of income earners spend some 30–40 per cent of income on food, the lowest quartile spend 80–90 per cent of income on food. Obviously the latter are in no position to withstand inflation in food prices unaccompanied by increased income without suffering nutritional damage.

4. Maximization of food supply therefore is only part of the answer to the problem of undernutrition. The ability of low-income consumers to purchase increased supply is crucial, since it is their young children among whom most of the undernutrition occurs.

The low-income groups purchase a relatively restricted range of food items, some of which supply energy and protein at relatively low cost. An example of typical food patterns as related to income and cost-nutrient value is given in Tables 2, 3 and 4. Here we see which are the main sources of nutrients to the various income groups, and also what is the cost of these items per given quantity of energy or protein.

Table 2. Sources of energy by importance to families in various food expenditure groups[a]

Foods	Food expenditure group			
	Lowest	2nd	3rd	Highest
Dark sugar	1	3	6	11
Flour[b]	2	1	3	5
Rice	3	4	1	1
Oil	4	2	2	2
Green bananas	5	7	7	6
Bread[b]	6	5	5	4
Yam	7	8	8	9
Condensed milk	8	6	4	3
Cornmeal	9	10	9	13
Coconut	10	9	17	14
Margarine	11	16	14	15
Sweet potatoes	12	15	19	—
Refined sugar	—	13	10	7
Butter	—	17	13	12
Beef	20	12	12	8

[a] Approximately quartiles

[b] Flour, sold as flour ('counter flour') as opposed to bread, used more for dumplings than for making bread or pastry

Clearly such matters as trade policy, taxation, price control and subsidies are more important to nutrition in the Caribbean than they are either in the industrialized countries or in the majority of developing countries, where subsistence agriculture and local production play a greater part in food supply. Here again is an important role for the nutritionist, to advise governments as to the nutritional implications of food trade and food price policy.

Social factors

The common problems of urbanization and unemployment, and social and family disruption, afflict the Caribbean to a major extent, for the area is rapidly reaching the position where half of the people dwell in cities and towns of over 20,000 population. In addition there is one important disadvantage that was inherited from the deliberate disruption of family life which was part of the system of plantation slavery. Most births are illegitimate, and not in the sense merely that mother and father are not legally married. A substantial proportion of all births occurs in the context of unions which do not last for much more than a year or two after the birth of the child, and sometimes not even until birth, and in which the mother and father do not live together. This is not to say that most fathers do not support their children and consort, but the support is too often irregular and small in amount, and may cease when the mother, sometimes in an endeavour to gain a more reliable partner, has a baby with another man. The unfortunate results are easily imagined, but those brought up in this kind of family are liable to perpetuate the pattern, whether they be men or women, and so great was the destructive effect of slavery on the family life of the West Africans enslaved that to this day the consequences are felt. It is not for nothing that a famous West Indian sociological work is entitled *My Mother Who Fathered Me*.[1] The West Indian family has been termed 'matriarchal', the West Indian male a butterfly, flitting from flower to flower. Closer examination, however,

Table 3. Sources of protein by importance to families in various food expenditure groups[a]

Foods	Food expenditure group			
	Lowest	2nd	3rd	Highest
Flour	1	1	3	7
Rice	2	5	2	4
Bread	3	2	4	3
Salted cod	4	6	7	6
Yam	5	10	10	10
Condensed milk	6	3	5	5
Green bananas	7	11	14	14
Cornmeal	8	12	12	16
Canned mackerel	9	16	16	15
Chicken	10	4	1	2
Red peas	11	9	11	12
Congo peas	12	15	—	—
Beef	13	8	6	1
Chicken neck and back	14	16	—	—
Salt beef	15	7	9	8
Lamb	—	18	18	9
Egg	—	20	13	13
Pork	17	13	8	11

[a] Approximately quartiles

reveals that this dramatic picture is somewhat exaggerated, and the father contributes more to the nurture of the child, at least the very young child, than he has been given credit for, and women need and respect men more than is generally acknowledged. In summary, while this social malfunction is of some importance in the aetiology of malnutrition, it is mainly so because of the context of harsh poverty in which it takes place.

Table 4. Cost in Jamaican cents[a] per nutrient content of selected foods, retail prices of May 1974

	Cost per 1000 kcal	Cost per 20 g of protein
Dark sugar	5.9	—
Cornmeal	6.7	6.1
Refined sugar	8.9	—
Counter flour	10.3	7.1
Condensed milk (Dawn)	11.0	8.7
Cow peas	15.5	4.4
Dry congo peas	16.4	5.7
Condensed milk (other brands)	18.0	14.3
Green bananas	18.8	29.3
Rice	22.0	22.0
Salt mackerel	26.0	8.6
Dry skim milk	30.6	6.1
Red peas	30.7	9.5
Sweet potatoes	31.8	57.1
Split peas	34.8	10.0
Ripe bananas	35.5	57.1
Macaroni	36.8	23.9
Plantain	41.9	103.2
Green gungo peas	46.6	15.7
Peanuts	46.9	20.3
Yam	48.8	42.6
Sardines	51.4	15.5
Whole milk	52.2	19.5
Cheddar cheese	53.6	16.6
Lactogen (typical powdered infant formula)	58.8	35.5
Irish potato	69.6	57.1
Canned mackerel	77.1	14.6
Goat	86.9	35.1
Mince beef	87.2	32.4
Canned corn beef	90.4	15.4
Salt cod	107.9	9.9
Chicken	125.6	23.5
Beef liver	160.4	21.7
Beef round	167.3	40.1
Eggs	186.9	47.2
King fish	230.4	24.3

[a] Jamaican $1.00 = U.S. $1.10.
1 kcal = 4.2 kjoules

The decline of breast-feeding in this area deserves a prominent mention under the heading of social factors. The practice of exclusively breast-feeding the infant for the first 6 months of life, or longer, and prolonged lactation was very widespread until only 3 decades ago, but has since declined to a level where in urban centres as few as 5 per cent of mothers exclusively breast-feed their children even to the age of 3 months. One trusts that this is a nadir from which there can only be recovery, for along with the lack of relatively cheap, nutritious and compact weaning foods, the decline in breast-feeding, with the gastroenteritis and marasmus which accompany it, is one of the two major immediate causes of protein–energy malnutrition, which in the Caribbean has its peak incidence in the age group 3–24 months.

Nutritional problems other than PEM

Vitamin A deficiency to the extent of causing blindness is extremely rare in the English-speaking Caribbean.* The only deficiency of the B vitamins manifesting itself clinically is riboflavin deficiency, but this must be considered an aspect of generally poor diet rather than a disease against which specific measures could be taken. Scurvy and rickets are virtually unknown. Folic acid deficiency is a contributor, probably seasonal, to nutritional anaemia in some countries (e.g. Barbados) in pregnant women and very young children, but the main cause of nutritional anaemia and of anaemia in general in this area is iron deficiency. The extent of anaemia could reasonably be characterized as that typical of many poor communities anywhere in the world, but without the added burden of such parasitic diseases as malaria, hookworm and schistosomiasis (except in a few areas on the island of St. Lucia in the latter case). Hookworm is prevalent in some country areas, but is not the widespread general problem often met with elsewhere.

One problem peculiar to the Caribbean in regard to its extent and magnitude as a health problem (and as a public health problem inadequately acknowledged) is diabetes mellitus of late onset. Such studies as have been made[2] show a prevalence approaching that of the highest in the world, and the recorded age-adjusted death rates from this disease in the English-speaking Caribbean are at least double those of the rest of the western hemisphere, including the most affluent countries.[3] There is no satisfactory explanation for this unusual problem, although clearly obesity in middle age, also very prevalent particularly among women and in the urban areas, plays some role. Public health action in regard to diabetes has scarcely begun, and it is still widely regarded as a field of action for the private physician or at most the diabetes clinics attached to the main hospitals. Yet there are about 100,000 diabetics in the English-speaking Caribbean, occupying some 10 per cent of hospital beds, often suffering from severe complications. The costs of management and economic losses due to the disease are tentatively believed to exceed $40 million a year in a population of under 5 million. Most diabetics are not diagnosed until they present with complications, and in short the problem, like the patients themselves, is not under control to any great extent. Again this points to a clear role for Caribbean nutritionists in the future.

*Editor's note: It is not uncommon in Haiti and parts of Central America.

PAST AND CURRENT PROGRAMMES TO COMBAT MALNUTRITION

Unable to see much possibility of doing anything about one fundamental cause of the nutrition problems, namely poverty, those working in nutrition and public health in this area have tended to acknowledge its importance but to concentrate on child health programmes and on nutrition education. Nor is it reasonable to think that they were wrong to do so, or that their efforts have made no impact on the problem. On the contrary, it seems likely that certain programmes have contributed significantly to the situation obtaining at present where, in spite of a prevalence of severe malnutrition among the under-fives of between 0.8 and 1.4 per cent, and of moderate malnutrition of between 10–20 per cent, mortality rates are relatively low.

The nutritional state of the West Indies population first attracted official attention in the mid-1930s. The Nutrition Committee of Jamaica, its history an example of the vicissitudes and periodic senescences and rejuvenations typical of nutrition committees, first met in 1937. Early attempts to alleviate the problem included the production of brewer's yeast as a nutritional supplement, but it was not until the late 1940s that any significant progress was made. In the succeeding decade there were two major developments making real contributions to diminishing the problems. The first was the setting up and extension of infant welfare clinics throughout the area, to the extent that although the actual coverage as a percentage of the eligible child population is not adequate, at least such clinics are reasonably accessible to all areas in all the countries, even remote rural areas. Among the services offered at such clinics the steady stream of information on the care and nurture of the infant has undoubtedly had some effect, as surveys of knowledge and attitudes on child feeding in the area clearly show.

The second major development of the 1950s was the inception of distribution programmes of dried skim milk, mostly from overseas aid sources such as UNICEF and USAID. These programmes have been a mixed blessing, for they may have contributed to the decline in breast-feeding and they met with many difficulties and expenses in storage and distribution, but in certain countries there is no doubt that these schemes constituted a major source of high-quality protein to the majority of the population under 5 years, and to many schoolchildren and pregnant mothers also.

Systematic programmes of nutrition education of the public, at clinics, in community groups and through the mass media have been carried out in most of the countries of the region not only by the health ministry, but also by education, agriculture, and community development departments. The second half of the 1960s saw the initiation of Applied Nutrition Programmes in 6 of the countries. These were organized along the lines advocated by WHO, FAO and UNICEF and were assisted by these agencies. They laid their main emphasis on the great captive audience in the schools, on the ground that these were tomorrow's citizens, and it was therefore important to impart to them basic knowledge of nutrition. They incorporated not only education in nutrition but also school gardens and the raising of small livestock. These Applied Nutrition Programmes met with varying success.

They are still active in 3 of the countries, and being extended still in 1, but in the main they were underfinanced and some did not succeed in getting beyond the original pilot areas. Nonetheless, they all made a contribution in heightening awareness of nutritional problems both among the general public and within the civil service, and secondly in giving agriculture, health education and community development departments and agencies the experience of working together for better nutrition.

Many seminars and courses and some widely disseminated publications have served to make most practising members of the medical, nursing and teaching professions reasonably well-informed as to nutrition in its local context. However, nursing and medical curricula are still patterned very much along the lines of courses in the United Kingdom, and attempts to give the subject a systematic instruction more in proportion to its importance have not yet succeeded. Nevertheless, medical and nursing students do get somewhat more instruction in nutrition than is usual in industrialized countries. Teaching of nutrition in teacher-training colleges has only recently begun, and so far in one college only. There is no B.Sc. level training in nutrition or dietetics in the area.

In research, valid contributions to knowledge of the pathology, aetiology, late consequences and management of protein–energy malnutrition have been made by several institutions, and in particular by the Tropical Metabolism Research Unit in the University of the West Indies. Along with this clinical research have gone a number of surveys of special groups or national surveys, including assessments of nutritional status, or knowledge, attitudes and practices concerning food and child care, or of food consumption patterns, or of all of these together. National surveys of the latter kind have been carried out in Barbados, Guyana and St. Lucia with the assistance of the Caribbean Food and Nutrition Institute.

The Caribbean Food and Nutrition Institute is a nutrition project of all the governments of the English-speaking Caribbean, acting in concert. It was established in 1967 and has centres at the University of the West Indies in Jamaica and Trinidad. It is supported also by PAHO/WHO, FAO and UNICEF, and private foundations. It carries out programmes of research, training in nutrition, dissemination of information on food and nutrition. One of its principal activities in the last 2 years has been assistance to governments in appraisal of the national food and nutrition situation and in formulation of national food and nutrition policies. At the time of writing, June 1974, Jamaica, St. Lucia and Guyana are at various stages in the process of formulating such policies.

There are Nutrition Units, headed by well-qualified and experienced West Indian nutritionists, in the Ministries of Health of Jamaica, Trinidad and Tobago, and Barbados. They provide direct advice to their governments, and carry out teaching programmes which are extensive in relation to their resources.

There are nutrition committees in most of the countries of the area. These committees have had their share of the defects which commonly afflict nutrition committees anywhere in the world. They have vicissitudes, periods of activity declining into routine and even suspension, followed by revivals of interest, the whole process depending much on the enthusiasm of individuals. They have a tendency to begin as inter-disciplinary committees, but gradually to lose this characteristic in practice.

The medical members, feeling, as is their wont, that 'doctor knows best', sometimes tend to monopolize the deliberations with a profusion of detailed discussion of medically oriented nutrition activities. The senior agriculturalists and educationists are too shy to interrupt these medical monologues, but do not feel able to participate significantly, and send their deputies, who in turn send their deputies, until representation of these groups ceases. Next to drop out are the Ministry of Health personnel, always somewhat overburdened, until all that remains is a discussion group for medical academics. One is exaggerating the actual history of the committees a little, in order to illustrate what is undoubtedly a tendency or a danger (Chapter 23).

In one or two countries in the area nutrition councils have lately been given a less peripheral place in the government machinery and clearer terms of reference, and put under the responsibility of the Ministry of Economic Development or National Planning Agency, a more realistic and objective location than Health, one feels.

So far there has been little development in food economics and food planning, a relatively new specialty dealing with the interface of agricultural economics and nutrition. Capability in this field is, however, rapidly being developed, particularly in the Caribbean Food and Nutrition Institute but also in government services. Food Balance Sheets for recent years are now available in at least 5 of the countries of the area.

NEWER DEVELOPMENTS IN FOOD AND NUTRITION PROGRAMMES

Nutrition in the national health plan

Most nutritionists with any length of experience could reel off a list of public health nutrition and nutrition education projects which had proved eminently successful in reducing the level of malnutrition among the children of the community. Almost all of these projects would be pilot projects at the level of a single village or at most a province. The ways in which the nutritional status of young children can be improved are clearly mapped out by the reports on these projects and by a number of excellent publications, this one included. But the problem lies in applying these valid solutions on a sufficiently wide national scale to make a significant impact.

The ingenious and devoted individuals responsible for these pilot projects are not numerous. Activities of the kind which they carried out must nevertheless be incorporated into the normal daily work of the country's health service, and the coverage of these services extended as well. The nutritionist working in the public health sector has a major responsibility to help reach this objective. One necessity is nutrition training not only of nursing and medical students, but in-service training to existing staff, and particularly to new or already established cadres of village-level workers. However, programmes of nutrition training for health personnel cannot begin or cannot expand without a clear commitment of the Ministry of Health to the effect that these activities for which they are to be trained have a high degree of priority in the national health policy, and must be carried out in a deliberate and methodical way. To be forever attempting and suggesting to the authorities little bits of the health part of the solution to the problems of malnutrition is more likely in the long run to alienate the recipient and be an obstacle to progress.

Therefore the nutritionist has three responsibilities in this direction. Firstly, he must patiently promote among the political and technical authorities a more informed awareness of the nature of the nutrition problems and the possibilities of solutions. Secondly, he must collaborate in whatever is the machinery of national health planning in that country in order that nutritional objectives may be incorporated. Thirdly, he must assist in determining the norms and procedures relating to these activities in such a way that by virtue of simplicity and economy they can indeed be implemented.

An example of this approach at the Caribbean sub-regional level was the 'Strategy and Plan of Action to Combat Malnutrition and Gastroenteritis Among Children Under Two Years of Age' produced at the specific request of the Caribbean Health Ministers' Conference (Chapter 15). It was devised jointly by experienced government technical personnel from most of the countries, assisted by PAHO/WHO and the University medical faculty. It sets for 1980 goals of reduction of mortality and prevalence of malnutrition, and sets programme targets with target dates in sector by sector. Thus the Ministries of Health have now collectively adopted a fairly comprehensive plan which they can adapt to their own special needs and practicabilities.

National food and nutrition policy

Public health action in nutrition provides results. These results can be obtained in a relatively short time, and these public health actions have a part in any national food and nutrition policy, since the objectives of such a policy must include the significant reduction within a given time period of the prevalence of malnutrition among the most vulnerable groups. However, these actions are only a part, and not the major part, of national food and nutrition policy, since the long-term and permanent solution of the problem lies in the quantity, quality and, above all, the distribution of the nation's food supply. These things must be improved until *all* the people of the country can enjoy levels of food consumption such as will secure them adequate nutrition and dietary well-being.

Put into this larger context a new role can be seen for the nutritionist. Without the assistance of the nutritionist the nature and extent of dietary deficiency cannot be identified, nor can the possible sources with which to make up the shortfall in nutrient intake. If he will interest himself in food balance sheets, familiarize himself with the concept of food demand and food supply and their interactions, with scales of nutrient values in relation to retail cost, with the varying extent of food expenditure in the household budget, then he can work with the economist, the agricultural economist and the sociologist in formulating national food and nutrition policy and programmes for its implementation. If the commitment to, and the infrastructure for, such a complex undertaking are not yet ready, he can at least influence agricultural, social, trade and economic development strategies towards quite specific nutritional objectives. Nutritionists in the Caribbean, aided by the disturbing experiences of 1973's food commodity shortages, are increasingly functioning in this kind of role.

In summary, more traditional activities in the health field cannot be abandoned, but a sustained effort must be made to move from the pilot project level to national implementation. In addition, the nutritionist must play his essential part in the long-term more fundamental solution; the formulation, implementation and evaluation of the national food and nutrition policy.

REFERENCES

1. Clarke, E. *My Mother Who Fathered Me,* London, Allen and Unwin, 1957.
2. Poon-King, T., M. V. Henry and F. Rampersad. *Lancet,* **1,** 155 (1968).
3. Pan American Health Organization. *Health Conditions in the Americas,* Washington, PAHO Scientific Publication No. 207, 1970. See Table V, pp. 34–59.

CHAPTER 27

Nutrition in Ethiopia

Mehari Gebre-Medhin

The nutritional status of a community, particularly in pre-industrial societies, reflects numerous interrelated ecological factors. Thus, settlement patterns, population density, mode of agriculture, national earning capacity, level of education, availability of infrastructure, sanitary standards, social, cultural and political systems are important moulding forces. To appreciate the complex situation responsible for malnutrition in the individual child or in the community and in order to launch effective preventive programmes it is vital to have some understanding of general background realities.

THE ETHIOPIAN SCENE

Situated between 3° and 18° latitude and 33° and 45° longitude, Ethiopia has an area of 1,222,000 km². Although within the tropics, the climate is very much influenced by altitude. Its topography may be roughly described as a block of centrally located highlands accounting for 40 per cent of the total area, surrounded by lowlands with a general elevation of approximately 1000 m. There is a common feature of a high daily range and a low annual range of temperature. Average annual rainfall varies from 60 mm along the Red Sea Coast to 2500 mm in the southwest.

The different climatic regions may be broadly classified as follows: the eastern lowlands with low humidity and only one rainy season (July–September); the south with small rains occurring in two periods; the central highlands with two periods of rainfall (the main one in June–October); the south-eastern highlands where rain falls virtually every month (with a maximum in July–September); the south-west which is very hot and the coastline with sparse rainfall occurring only in the winter.

Over 90 per cent of the population live in rural areas in isolated homesteads, by a subsistence type of agriculture and animal husbandry. It is estimated that more than 2 million of the total population of approximately 24 million are nomads.

The population pyramid is typical of a pre-industrial society with the age group 15 years and below accounting for 46 per cent of the total (Figure 1). The average household is 4.4 persons. Vital rates reflect a harsh environment with a crude birth rate of 42.8 per cent, crude death rate of 19.2 per cent, infant and child mortality of 155 per thousand, and 247 per thousand respectively. The natural rate of population increase is 2.30 per cent.

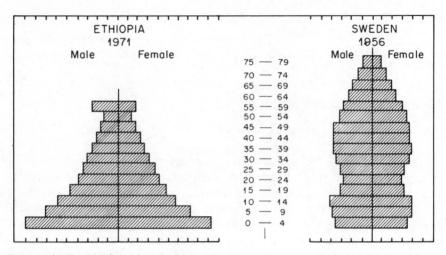

FIGURE 1. Constitution of population. Comparison between Ethiopia and Sweden. Source: CSO, Addis Ababa, and IPPF, London, 1968

Over 90 per cent of the economically active population are farmers, farm labourers or shepherds, and more than 60 per cent of the farmers are tenants. The majority of the peasants cultivate only 20 hectares on an average and the per capita annual income is given as U.S. $75.00. The staple crops vary from area to area, the major ones being 'tef' (*eragrostis abysinnica*) unique to Ethiopia, barley and wheat in the highlands and sorghum and maize in the lowlands. In the southern parts the false banana (enset) is the main crop for a large segment of the population. Cattle are numerous in many regions but are kept mainly for social prestige and make only a modest contribution to the day-to-day diet except among the nomadic tribes, who consume a considerable amount of milk, especially for child rearing.

INFANT FEEDING AND WEANING PRACTICES

Although the practice of infant feeding varies from one area to another, certain common themes can be seen running in all regions of the country. Breast milk, which the newborn infant receives immediately after birth, is the mainstay during the first year of life. In addition to this and often before initiation of breast-feeding, butter, sometimes mixed with water, is given in the belief that this will prevent stomach trouble, rid the infant of intestinal parasites and promote growth.

During the first 2–4 months mainly breast milk is given. However, it is a very widespread practice to give the child either daily or a few times a week a concoction made of butter mixed with water, rue (*Ruta graveolens*) or fenugreek (*Trigonella faenum-graecum*). The leaves or the seeds of rue are boiled for about 10–15 minutes and the water is given to the infant.

There are at least five different ways of preparing fenugreek for infant feeding in Ethiopia. Common for all the processes are thorough boiling, four to five times, either of the whole seeds or the powder from roasted seeds and discarding the boiling water. The infant receives either the supernatant from the last boiling or the cooked fenugreek which is sometimes mixed with emmerwheat.

The pattern of feeding from the 2nd–4th month until the end of the first year is related to the availability of milk or its products, which varies greatly from area to area. This is shown in a striking manner by the results of a dietary survey from different communities in Ethiopia (Table 1).

Table 1. Pattern of cow's milk consumption of children in four Ethiopian communities[a]

Area	No.	% of children on milk	Volume taken ml/day
Addis Ababa	17	28.0	350–430
Ijaji	22	39.2	100–340
Sidamo	9	64.3	100
Begemdir	2	22.2	7

[a] Unpublished data. Children's Nutrition Unit.

In addition to breast milk the infant is given a variety of gruels made either of emmerwheat, corn or barley to which, if available, milk or fenugreek is added. However, emmerwheat alone is the most widely used additional food. Traditionally there are two ways for preparing this for infant feeding in Ethiopia. In the first the emmerwheat is dehusked in a small mortar and then ground lightly on a stone mill before it is soaked overnight. The starchy part is then boiled for 10–15 minutes and given to the child with a little sugar or salt added.

Breast milk, together with the above mentioned additions, is generally continued until about the end of the second year, sometimes even longer. Prolonged breast-feeding is observed in areas where milk is scarce while in communities where milk is relatively plentiful, there is a tendency towards early cessation of breast-feeding (Figure 2). It is evident that surveys of the dietary intake of Ethiopian infants and children, particularly during the weaning period and the subsequent three years, show serious inadequacies in energy as well as protein and other nutrients.

DIETARY PATTERN IN ETHIOPIAN COMMUNITIES

Thanks to the work of the Ethiopian Nutrition Institute (formerly the Children's Nutrition Unit), there is substantial information on dietary intake in representative

312

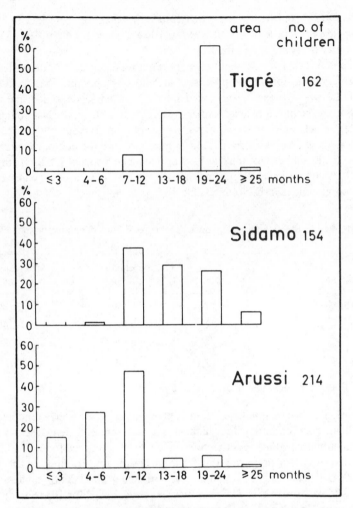

FIGURE 2. Percentage distribution of Ethiopian children in three communities according to duration of breast-feeding. Knutsson and Mellbin. *J. Trop. Ped.* 15, 40 (1969)

parts of the country. A survey from a southern region will be discussed (Figure 3). In this area the false banana, enset (*Ensete ventricosum*) constitutes the staple food. It contains less than 1 g protein per 100 g edible portion and negligible amounts of vitamins. In the age group 6 months–3 years the diet is very unsatisfactory with a energy intake of less than 50 per cent of the WHO-recommended allowance.

The protein intake is slightly better but barely comes up to 60 per cent of recommended figures. Only 30 per cent of the total protein is of animal origin and this is supplied by milk. The intake of vitamin A, thiamine, riboflavin and niacin is unsatisfactory, being between 50–70 per cent of the recommended intake. It is possible that the situation of the infant is slightly better than would seem as breast-feeding, generally continued beyond the age of 6 months, may provide quantities of milk difficult to estimate.

For children above 3 years and for adults the staple diet seems to cover their energy needs adequately. The protein intake was about 65 per cent level of the recommended allowance. The biological value of the protein is very poor with only

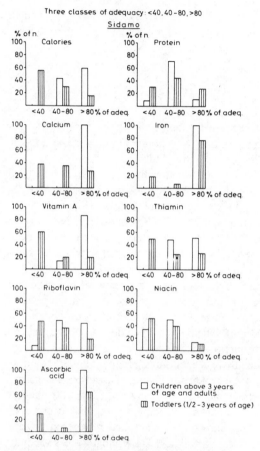

FIGURE 3. Dietary intake in Southern Ethiopia. Percentage distribution of calories and nutrients as related to recommended standards. Selinus, Gobezie and Vahlquist. *Acta Soc. Med. Upsal.* 76, 158 (1971)

20 per cent of the total protein being derived from animal sources. Calcium, iron, vitamin A and ascorbic acid are consumed in abundance. The main source of these nutrients is the kale which is consumed every day in large quantities. On account of the low consumption of cereals and milk, riboflavin and niacin are only on the 75 and 85 per cent level respectively. The consumption of fat was also extremely low, being derived mainly from enset and kale.

These observations, which are very similar to those of many other regions in the country, explain the well-known clinical findings that the nutritional status of the toddler is, in many ways, much worse than that of older children and adults. The monotonous diet of enset and kale shows no seasonal variation. The staple food provides an ample supply of energy but proves inadequate when it concerns the protein needs of the child. The situation is further aggravated by meal patterns which do not recognize the special needs of the rapidly growing infant, the extra demand imposed by infections and infestations and the requirements for catch-up growth in undernourished infants.

FASTING IN ETHIOPIA

The practice of fasting in Ethiopia follows the regulations prescribed by the two major religions in the country, Orthodox Christianity and Islam. Probably close to a total of 20 million observe this tradition.

The Moslem fast, which occurs for one lunar month (Ramadan) each year demands total abstention from foods, including liquids, between dawn and sunset. Eating begins after dusk and there are no restrictions in types or quantities of food consumed. Children under the age of 7 years are exempt and those up to 15 years of age fast only half of the day or merely part of the month. It is believed that Ramadan fasting does not seriously worsen the state of nutrition as satisfactory nutritional compensation can be achieved once the daily fast is over.

Among Orthodox Christians fasting rules have two aspects relating to the time for food consumption and the kinds of food that may be eaten. Thus, a fasting individual is expected to observe total abstention from food until noon, or in some instances until 3.00 p.m. The diet eaten at the end of the fast must not include any foods of animal origin, fish excepted.

Officially, especially in recent times, pregnant and lactating women and children under 8 years are exempt from fasting. However, this often has no more than theoretical importance as it is generally very difficult to acquire non-fasting food during the fast and mothers are reluctant to prepare any dishes from animal sources. The total number of fasting days is estimated at between 150 and 220 per year. The fasting diet, particularly for toddlers, is significantly less adequate in terms of energy and nutrients than the already deficient non-fasting food.

FAMINE IN ETHIOPIA

Accounts of disastrous food shortages in Ethiopian history are well-documented. Since the middle of the 16th century we have numerous records of outbreaks of famine, particularly in the northern provinces. Most of these famines were initiated by disadvantageous climatic changes, sometimes accompanied by plagues of locusts. Undoubtedly both human and animal disease and epidemics were important contributory factors in these disasters.

Ethiopia is currently experiencing the effects of severe drought over the last three to four years. This is believed to have caused the deaths of at least 100,000 people and created havoc in several regions of the country. A Relief and Rehabilitation Commission with wide powers has been established in Addis Ababa and thorough investigations of affected regions have shown that their vulnerability stems from an archaic agricultural and land tenure system, rapid population growth, continuous deterioration of the soil, exacerbated by de-afforestation, lack of infrastructure and heavy bureaucracy. These factors have contributed to the maintenance of a long-standing subsistence level standard of living and grossly sub-optimal nutritional status with the ever-present risk of famine whenever climatic conditions become unfavourable.

CURRENT STATUS OF MALNUTRITION AND DIFICIENCY DISEASES IN ETHIOPIA

Possibly the first evidence of malnutrition in Ethiopia is to be found in the high prevalence of foetal wastage, high stillbirth rate (44 per cent) and high low-birth weight rate (8–13 per cent). There is good evidence to suggest that infants born to low-income mothers with a deficient dietary intake have significantly lower mean birth weight (3.0 kg) when compared to infants of high-income mothers (3.5 kg) with near optimal nutrition. Thus a sizeable proportion of Ethiopian children start extrauterine life in a sub-optimal condition. Although frank cases of nutritional deficiency diseases are rare among pregnant women, preliminary investigations show poor antenatal weight gain and compromised lactation, at least qualitatively, among malnourished mothers. The subsequent state of nutrition of the child is determined by weaning practices and the environment which have been described above. Here only a brief reference will be made to observations from a northern region of the country (Table 2). As is evident from the Table, 83 per cent of the infants under 2 months are judged as

Table 2. Growth categories by 3-months age groupings in a North Ethiopian community[a]

Age (months)	Number of weights	Adequate growth (%)	Latent PEM (%)	Severe PEM (%)
0–2	125	83	17	0
3–5	193	71	27	2
6–8	202	53	42	6
9–11	226	28	68	4
12–14	159	9	83	8
15–17	67	9	86	5
Total	972	44	52	4

[a] Dodge, R. E. and T. Demeke, *Ethiopian Med. J.*, **8**, 53 (1970)

having adequate growth. During the second year 86 per cent show clear signs of malnutrition, while up to 8 per cent will become severely malnourished and often die as a result of intercurrent infections (Figure 4).

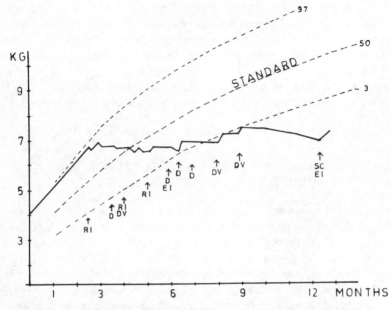

FIGURE 4. Weight development and intercurrent infections in an Ethiopian male infant. RI-respiratory infection, D-diarrhoea, DV-diarrhoea and vomiting, EI-eye inflammation, Sc-scabies. Eksmyr. Mimeographed report. Ethiopian Nutrition Institute, Addis Ababa, 1969

In urban highland Ethiopia, the iron nutrition of infants and children may be regarded as satisfactory. The exceedingly high iron intake derived from 'tef' contributes to the striking rarity of nutritional anaemias among highland Ethiopians. In children between 1–4 years in the Addis Ababa area about 3 per cent have iron-deficiency anaemia while this figure goes up to 9 per cent for a rural highland area. The stress of pregnancy which commonly causes iron-deficiency and megaloblastic anaemias is not a major problem in highland Ethiopia.

Paradoxically, despite abundant sunshine, vitamin-D-deficiency rickets, often in association with an increased morbidity and mortality, is known to be highly prevalent in many parts of Ethiopia. Exposing infants to the rays of the sun is traditionally avoided during the first months of life for fear of the evil eye. In certain areas, the frequency of rickets may be as high as 30 per cent. Peak prevalence occurs between 6–12 months of age. Severe vitamin A deficiency with xerophthalmia also occurs, mostly in conjunction with severe malnutrition of the kwashiorkor type. Frank scurvy is uncommon in spite of what may be considered as very unsatisfactory levels of vitamin C intake.

Goitre occurs in many communities in Ethiopia as is evidenced by Hofvander's findings among children in three communities (Table 3).

Table 3. Prevalence (%) of goitre among Ethiopian children[a]

Age (years)	Addis Ababa[b]	Ijaji[c]	Baco[c]
1–4	1.3	6.9	—
5–9	14.0	37.7	48.0
10–12	30.8	56.9	55.5
Total	8.5	26.9	53.1

[a] Hofvander, Y. *Ethiopian Med. J.*, **8**, 179 (1970)
[b] Central and [c] western Ethiopia.

COMBATING MALNUTRITION IN ETHIOPIA

The formulation and implementation of a community nutrition policy cuts across a wide spectrum of disciplines and requires resources far greater than those allocated to physicians immediately responsible for individual cases of malnutrition. Only when the living standard of the individual family has been raised can lasting nutritional improvement be achieved. However, in many pre-industrial societies the rate of economic development is such that decades will pass before the under-privileged can benefit from such changes. Consequently, it seems logical to design community programmes geared to population groups especially prone to suffer from malnutrition and to encourage a population growth compatible with economic growth.

Nutrition intervention programmes have so far been the responsibility of the Ethiopian Nutrition Institute and its predecessor the Ethio-Swedish Children's Nutrition Unit. Parallel with national endeavours aimed at accelerating general community development through such measures as agrarian reforms, expansion of communications, basic health services and educational facilities, two approaches for nutritional improvement have been tried. Firstly, since extensive field surveys showed lack of good traditional weaning foods to be the main cause of nutritional problems in the pre-school child, the Institute formulated and started marketing an acceptable low-cost weaning food 'Faffa', particularly in urban areas (Tables 4 and 5). (In the Amharic language, Faffa means 'grow big and strong'.)

Secondly, the promotion of 'Faffa' is combined with nutrition and health education with particular emphasis on home-made weaning foods and hygiene. This is done because the Institute realizes that industrially produced supplementary foods reach only a fraction of the needy population and the rest should receive widespread information concerning the proper use of available staples. The weaning-food programme is currently being turned into an independent, self-supporting industrial complex, retaining close links with the mother institute for quality control, product development and preservation of nutritional objectives.

Table 4. Present composition of 'Faffa'

Formula	%
Wheat flour	57.0
Field-pea flour	10.0
Soya flour, non-fat	18.0
Non-fat dry milk	5.0
Sugar	8.0
Salt	1.0
Additives	
Vitamins: A, D, C, B_1, B_2, B_6, B_{12} niacin, folic acid, calcium, D-pantothenate	
Minerals: calcium, iron, iodine and phosphates	

Table 5. 'Faffa' powder: chemical composition per 100 g

Calories	340 (1.42 MJ)	Carbohydrate, total		Thiamine	0.84 mg
Moisture	8 %	including fibre	64.5 g	Riboflavin	0.61 mg
Crude protein =		Fibre	1.0 g	Niacin	9.8 mg
N × 6.25	21.2 g	Ash	4.1 g	Ascorbic acid	31 mg
Fat	2.2 g	Calcium	300 mg		
		Iron	15 mg		

During the past few years, the Institute has expanded its nutrition and health education activities and has been instrumental in large-scale production of teaching kits and training of various cadres of workers in the field of health, agriculture and community development. Future policy will consist of expanding education and training programmes at all levels and preparation of nutrition manuals and other teaching aids in collaboration with various organizations. A nationwide system of rehabilitation units working as integral parts of the basic health services will be established. In addition a programme of continuous food and nutrition survey/surveillance is now under way, through the collaboration of several national institutions. It is hoped that this early warning system will avert further human suffering of the magnitude Ethiopia has recently experienced.

FURTHER READING

Selinus, R., A. Gobezie and B. Vahlquist. *Acta Soc. Med. Upsal.*, **76,** 158 (1971).
Hofvander, Y. *Acta Med. Scand. Suppl.*, **494,** 1 (1968).

Knutsson. K. E. and R. Selinus. *Am. J. Clin. Nutr.,* **23,** 956 (1970).

Knutsson, K. E. and T. Mellbin. *J. Trop. Pediat.,* **15,** 40 (1969).

Selinus, R. *J. Trop. Pediat.,* **16,** 188 (1970).

Hofvander, Y. *Ethiopian Med. J.,* **5,** 21 (1966).

Wickström, B. In *Protein-enriched Cereal Foods for World Needs* (Ed. Max Milner), Minnesota, American Association of Cereal Chemists, 1969.

Hofvander, Y. and R. Eksmyr. *Amer. J. Clin. Nutr.,* **24,** 578 (1971).

Hofvander, Y. *Eth. Med. J.,* **8,** 179 (1970).

Selinus, R., A. Gobezie, K. E. Knuttson and B. Vahlquist. *Amer. J. Clin. Nutr.,* **24,** 365 (1971).

Selinus, R., G. Awalom and A. Gobezie. *Acta Soc. Med. Upsal.,* **76,** 17 (1971).

Gebre-Medhin, M. and B. Vahlquist. *Courrier,* **22,** 12 (1972).

Belew, M., K. Jacobsson, G. Tornell, L. Uppsall, B. Zaar and B. Vahlquist. *J. Trop. Pediat./Environ. Child. Health,* **18,** 246 (1972).

Dodge, R. E. and T. Demeke. *Ethiopian Med. J.,* **8,** 53 (1970).

CHAPTER 28

Nutrition in India

M. C. SWAMINATHAN

Dr. Robert McCarrison, an Army Medical officer, undertook pioneering work during the early part of the 20th century, associating the nutritionally deficient diet of the Indians with their poor physical development and susceptibility to various illnesses, thus laying the foundation for studies on nutrition in India.[1] After his initial interest in endemic goitre, the Indian Research Fund Association (IRFA) with which he was associated, came into existence as a semi-official organization in 1911, supported by funds from the Central Government. His studies on beriberi, which later widened in scope to become the 'Deficiency Disease Inquiry', were started in 1918 at Coonoor, Madras Province, now termed Tamil Nadu. This was the forerunner of the Central Institution, Nutrition Research Laboratory established in 1929. In 1959, this Laboratory was moved to Hyderabad, Andhra Pradesh, and it came to be known as The National Institute of Nutrition in 1969. In 1949, the IRFA took on the name of Indian Council of Medical Research (ICMR) and, guided by the Nutrition Advisory Committee of the ICMR, this Institute has made notable contributions in the field of nutrition.

At the moment 15 States and 2 Union Territories have Nutrition Divisions in their Health Directorates under the charge of health personnel trained in nutrition. Much of the available information on the nutrition status of population groups on an All-India basis is from these State Units.

In recent years, undergraduate and postgraduate medical institutions, Food and Nutrition Departments in Home Science Colleges, and Public Health Training Institutes have introduced Nutrition into their basic curricula. The important role played by the Indian Council of Agricultural Research (ICAR) and its research institutions in initiating the green revolution and increased production of foods in the country is well recognized. The contributions made by the Central Food Technological Research Institute, Council of Scientific and Industrial Research (CSIR) Mysore, in the field of food conservation and more efficient utilization of the country's food resources are of immense value.

GENERAL CONDITIONS

The Indian sub-continent is spread over an area of 3.28 million square miles. The latest census, conducted in 1971, estimated the population in India to be about 548 million, living in over half a million rural villages and more than 2900 towns and cities.[2] The decennial growth rate of the population during the period 1961–1971 was 24.8 per cent. The population in India is relatively young, children under 14 years constituting about 42 per cent and those under 5 years about 15 per cent of the total population.

For administrative purposes India is divided into 21 States and 9 Union Territories. Since rural people form the major segment (80 per cent) of the total population, agriculture is the main occupation and cultivators and agricultural labour together account for about 70 per cent of the working population in India. Out of the total geographical area, about 45 per cent of the land is under cultivation with a mean per capita availability of 0.34 hectares of land for cultivation.

The cultural diversity of the population is indicated by the fact that there are as many as 14 major languages spoken, apart from the numerous dialects associated with these languages and tribal languages. Hindus form the majority and the rest include Muslims, Christians, Sikhs, Buddhists, Jains and many other minor religious groups.

The literacy rate, defined as the capacity to read and write, is 29.5 per cent for the country as a whole. While in the urban areas, for males and females, it is 61 and 42 per cent, the corresponding figures are 34 and 13 per cent respectively for rural areas.

The poor purchasing capacity of the Indian population is apparent as the per capita annual income is estimated to be less than U.S. $100. An indirect assessment[3] based on energy needs and data on expenditure on foods places the proportion of households below the poverty line at between 30–40 per cent total households in the country.

The crude birth rate, which was nearly 50.0 in the beginning of the century, had dropped to 37.2 in 1971.[4] The lowering of the crude death rate was more marked since, from 47.2 in the second decade of this century, it came down to 15.1 in 1971. Between 1911–1918, the infant mortality rate was 204 and in 1969 it was 140. The expectation of life rose from 22–23 years during the early part of the century to about 41–42 years between 1951 to 1961 and currently it is estimated to be 52 years. One significant observation which has relation to nutrition is the finding that the age-specific pre-school child mortality rate has remained more or less stationary over the last 3 or 4 decades at around 12 per thousand and also the proportional mortality rate of the age group below 5 years is still quite high, varying between 30–40 per cent. Infections of the gastro-intestinal and respiratory systems account for most of the morbidity and mortality, particularly among young children, and the underlying factor of malnutrition is fully recognized.

COMMON FOODS OF INDIA

A major share of the income of the country is derived from land produce, the bulk of which is food crops, and subsistence farming has been the mainstay. Though there has been a considerable increase in the production of foodgrains over the past several decades, particularly with the introduction of modern agricultural techniques and the use of better seed varieties, the concomitant increase in the population has offset the balance. In addition, since farming in India is largely dependent on timely and adequate rains, the vagaries of the weather have time and time again contributed to the relative food shortage in the country. The production of food crops during the year 1970–1971 is shown in Table 1.

Table 1. Per capita per day availability of food in India, 1970–1971

Food item	Net food availability[a] per year in thousand metric tonnes	Per capita per day[b] requirements for a balanced diet (g)	Net food availability in g per capita per day
Cereals	81,692	369.5	406.8
Pulses	9333	59.1	46.5
Nuts and oil seeds	1634	9.5[c]	8.2
Roots and tubers	9772	—	48.6
Sugar (gur)	11,565	40.3	57.6
Oils and fats	2358	37.6	11.8
Fruits and vegetables	10,765	269.0[d]	53.6
Milk	21,744	178.4	108.3
Flesh foods (meat)	743		3.8
Eggs	186	35.4	0.9
Fish	1608		8.0

[a]Food Balance Sheet of India, 1970–1971, Directorate of Economics and Statistics, Ministry of Agriculture, Government of India.
[b]Diet Atlas 1971.[12] Population of India 1970–1971 = 550.2 million.
[c]Only groundnuts.
[d]Including roots and tubers.

Cereals form the main item of food in India. The important cereals are wheat, rice, jowar (*Sorghum vulgare*), bajra (*Pennisetum typhoideum*), ragi (*Eleusine coracana*), maize (*Zea mais*) and barley (*Hordeum vulgare*). The conditions of the soil, climate and availability of water invariably determine the type and quantity of cereal produced. By and large, the country can be divided into the wheat-producing north and north-western region, the rice-producing region in the south and east and the millet-producing central region. The less well-known cereals produced termed small millets, are samai (*Panicum miliare*), Italian millet (*Setaria italica*), buckwheat (*Fagopyrum esculentum*) and varagu (*Paspalum scrobiculatum*).

Another important Indian crop is the pulse, which is rich in protein and belongs to the group of legumes. The common pulses are Bengal gram (*Cicer arietinum*), red gram (*Cajanus cajan*), black gram (*Phaseolus mungo*), green gram (*Phaseolus radiatus*) and lentil (*Lens esculenta*). The other varieties are cow gram (*Vigna catiang*), horse gram (*Dolichos biflorus*), pea (*Pisum sativum*) and khesari gram (*Lathyrus sativus*). The term 'gram' refers to the dry seeds in husk and pulse or 'dahl' to the dehusked, split and separated cotyledons. At the moment, soya bean is grown only in limited amounts mainly for use in commercially processed protein-rich foods.

There are many varieties of green leafy vegetables, roots, tubers and other vegetables, including tropical fruits, grown all over the country[5] and their availability depends mostly on the season.

India has quite a large population of cattle and milk is an important foodstuff produce in the country. Cow's and buffalo's milk are the two main types available, but in certain regions goat's milk and even camel's milk are available for consumption. A very large proportion of the milk produced is converted into various products for consumption, like curds (yogurt), a fermented product, buttermilk (diluted curds), butter, ghee (butter fat from which water is removed by heating). Other products are khoa (cream formed after heating of milk), malai (concentrated whole milk turned into a granular solid form) and chana (cheese).

Apart from milk, the other animal foods produced in India are sheep and goat meat, beef, pork and a large variety of fish which are particularly exploited near the coastline as well as from the numerous rivers. Poultry and eggs, both hen and duck eggs are mainly produced in the rural areas. Recently, a number of commercial poultry units have been established and are catering to the needs of urban areas.

India is one of the largest producers of oil seeds such as groundnut, sesame, mustard, coconut. Vegetable fats and oils are used extensively in India as a cooking medium. The commonly produced oils are groundnut oil, mustard oil, sesame oil, safflower oil and coconut oil with some rape seed oil and mahua oil (*Bassia latifolia*). In recent years, hydrogenated oil (*vanaspati*) has come into production and it caters mainly to the urban population. Ghee derived from butter is also used in limited amounts. The sweetening agents produced are jaggery and refined sugar derived from sugar cane.

A number of varieties of spices and condiments which are an essential part of the Indian diet are produced in India and these include chillies, peppers, cardamon, cloves, cummin seeds, mustard etc.

The chemical composition of Indian foodstuffs has been exhaustively investigated by several workers. In 1938, the data collected were first published by the Government of India as 'Health Bulletin No. 23' entitled *The Nutritive Value of Indian Foods and the Planning of Satisfactory Diets,* and the latest revision was published in 1971.[5]

PATTERN OF FOOD CONSUMPTION

In earlier years the major constituents of the Indian diet and their proportions were known but a great deal of knowledge was obtained after the fourth decade of the

20th century. Aykroyd first published his note on results of Diet Surveys in India in 1939 and added more collections in the revised editions in 1945 and 1947.[6]

The publications of ICMR[7] and reports of work done in States by the Nutrition Divisions of the State Health Directorates, now being published annually by the Directorate General of Health Services (DGHS) Government of India, furnish more recent information on diet surveys conducted in the country. The available data on diet surveys are mostly confined to poor-income groups of population, particularly in the rural areas. Some surveys have also been conducted among the middle-income groups in the urban areas. Practically no information is available on the well-to-do segments of the population.

The method adopted for these diet surveys was weighing the raw foods consumed by the whole family before they were cooked. This was undertaken by house-to-house visits over a specified period of time. At first the duration of these surveys extended beyond a week, up to as long as 21 days. Recent research studies[8] have indicated that under the conditions prevailing in the poor rural communities, where the family diet is monotonous, with very little variation from day to day, assessment of the diet even for a single day is expected to give a fairly accurate picture. Apart from the duration of the survey, these studies have also indicated that the laborious process of weighing foods can be conveniently replaced by a questionnaire method.[9]

All the results of the surveys are expressed in terms of 'man value' or 'consumption unit' which is based on energy requirements.[5] In keeping with international procedures, the dietary intakes are increasingly expressed in terms of per capita consumption. In recent years, attention has been directed to the priority needs of vulnerable groups such as children and mothers. For this purpose, family surveys are not useful. Considerable amounts of data on the dietary intake of individuals are being collected by means of the questionnaire method of survey.[10] The assessment is done in terms of cooked foods, using common vessels or containers familiar to the community and these are standardized so that the amounts of cooked foods can be converted to raw foods by appropriate conversion factors. This conversion is essential since the food tables are based on raw foods.

An analysis of the results of diet surveys carried out during the period 1935–1969 indicates practically no change over this period.[11,12] The National Sample Survey data indicate that on an average 10 per cent of the population in India are non-vegetarians. But, due to poor purchasing power, the majority of them subsist mainly on a vegetarian diet with occasional use of meat, eggs, fish etc. Food consumption patterns in India for the period 1960–1969 are given in Table 2.

No matter where they come from, the diet of the poor in India consists mainly of cereals with very little intake of other foods. It is of interest to note that the dietary patterns conform to the patterns of food production in the country (see Table 1). This is due to the fact that the mainstay of agriculture and food production in the country is subsistence farming with emphasis on production of food grains and most of the available data on food consumption relate to the poor rural masses.

The few studies available on the higher income groups, particularly in the urban areas, show that with increasing income the diet becomes more diversified, with the inclusion of more expensive protective foods like milk, flesh foods and increased use of fats and sugar.[13] In the very high-income groups these intakes are expected to exceed their requirements.

It is difficult to quantitate the extent of changes in food habits over the years. The widespread use of wheat in the rice-eating southern parts of India after the Second World War has been noted. In recent years, processed foods, particularly when they are available in a convenient form, as for example bread, are increasingly popular.

Table 2. Food consumption pattern of India (1960–1969) (g per person per day)

	Mean intake	Recommended balanced diet
Total cereals	434	370
Pulses	34	70
Leafy vegetables	21	110
Other vegetables	71	125
Fruits	10	37
Fats and oils	12	38
Milk and milk products	69	180
Meat, fish and eggs	14	35
Sugar and jaggery	19	40
Condiments	18	—
Calories	1985 (8.34 MJ)	2400 (10.08 MJ)
Proteins	55g	44g

From reference 12

This may be attributable to the influences of urbanization and industrialization. The percentage of expenditure on food to the total monthly expenditure among families in India in general is between 60–70 per cent.[12] With increasing income the amount spent on food grains becomes less, but rises on items like fat, milk, sugar and animal foods.

The mean intake of energy per person per day in India is 1985 Calories (8.34 MJ) as against a recommended allowance of 2400 (10.08MJ). But the intake of protein derived mostly from vegetable sources is 55 g which is more than the recommended figure of 44 g. The intake of animal proteins on an average is 6 g. With the possible exception of iron, all the other nutrients are consumed in amounts far less than the recommended values and particular mention should be made of vitamin A and riboflavin.[12]

Infants and pre-school children

In their survey of protein malnutrition in South India Rao *et al.*[14] were the first to initiate large-scale investigations on the diets of infants and pre-school children.

Undertaken on a total sample of 3664 children under 5 years of age, it was confined to the poor socio-economic groups in both rural and urban areas of the four Southern States of India. More recently, under the auspices of ICMR a collaborative study on the nutritional problems of pre-school children was undertaken in 1966 in six centres, representative of the country as a whole and which included rural and urban areas. Results of these investigations were more or less similar with minor variations attributable to location.[12,15]

In general, prolonged breast-feeding was the rule in all the regions. Usually this was started within 2 or 3 days after delivery and continued into the second or third year or even longer. Owing to the commonly held belief that there would be no milk during the first few days after birth, the babies were given a variety of foods like water with or without sugar, glucose, cow's milk, honey, dates etc. Breast-feeding was usually done on demand and not according to any time schedule.

During the first 6 months of life a steady rise in the intake of breast milk is observed. After this age, there is a gradual fall. It was noted that even mothers belonging to the poor-income groups secrete as much as 400 ml of breast milk after 18 months of lactation. No qualitative differences in the content of proximate principles and sulphur-containing amino acids have been observed in the breast milk of mothers belonging to poor socio-economic and western counterparts.[16] Between the ages of one and two more rural children were on breast milk. Pregnancy was the most common cause for the stoppage of breast milk to the child. The children were weaned off the breast by 18–24 months. Supplements were usually started around 12–18 months of age and these usually were milk and/or cereal foods in the form of cooked rice, wheat or millets either as *rotis* or soft cooked as porridges prepared with broken cereals. In certain communities processed-milk products such as infant milk powder and condensed milk were used, in dilutions far in excess of the recommended levels. The mean intake of foods by pre-school children is given in Table 3.

Pregnant and lactating women

The available data among low-income groups of families indicate that the diets of pregnant and lactating women are not very different from the usual diets generally consumed by women in the community.[12] As such they are grossly deficient in protective foods like milk, pulse and leafy vegetables and even the staple cereals are consumed in amounts much less than the recommended allowances. The mean energy intake of pregnant and lactating women varies from 1400–1800 kcal (5.88–7.56 MJ). The intake of protein, iron and calcium is 40 g, 18 mg and 200 mg respectively. Many of the nutritious foods are avoided during pregnancy. Though this is attributed to customs and traditions, it is partly due to the belief that consumption of nutritious foods during pregnancy will increase the size of the baby and may lead to complications at the time of delivery. During the lactation period, it is customary to include a variety of nutritious foods, especially during the first 40 days after delivery. This is done mainly with the idea of making sufficient quantities of breast milk available for the nursing infant.

Table 3. Diet and nutrient intake of pre-school children (per child per day)

Foodstuffs (g)	Intake	Recommended allowances	
		Vegetarian	Non-vegetarian
Cereals	147	175	175
Pulses	16	55	45
Milk	80	275	200
Oils and fats	4	23	23
Leafy vegetables	4	63	63
Other vegetables	14	40	40
Sugar and jaggery	5	35	35
Flesh foods	4	—	30
Fruits	7	50	50
Snacks	5	—	—
Nutrients			
Protein (g)	19.5	19.3	
Energy (kcal)	758 (3.18 MJ)	1275 (5.36 MJ)	
Vitamin A (I.U.)	572	1050	
Iron (mg)	8.6	17.5	
Calcium (mg)	230	450	

From reference 12

School children

Only very few isolated reports are available on the dietary intake of school children.[12] However, it is generally observed that the dietary pattern more or less reflects the prevailing situation in the community. Inadequacies with regard to energy, vitamin A, reiboflavin, iron and calcium are usually noted in this group.

Industrial workers

Information on the dietary intake of industrial workers is very meagre.[12] The general observation is that the diet of workers consists of a little more cereal than that of the rest of the community and inadequate intake of protective foods still persists, with the result that the nutrients derived mainly from cereals like protein, iron and calcium are consumed by this group in greater amount. Yet the mean energy intake, which is around 3000 kcal (12.6 MJ), does not always meet the increased requirements of these workers.

NUTRITIONAL DEFICIENCY DISORDERS OF INDIA

In India, clinical nutrition surveys of a limited nature have been conducted as early as 1914 onwards. With the establishment of State Nutrition Divisions in several States in the third decade, surveys were being regularly undertaken. Realizing that no standard procedures were adopted by the various agencies, the ICMR in 1948 introduced standard methods and schedules for collection of data. Most of the available data pertained to school children and very few were related to community studies.

The results of these surveys[17] indicate that conditions in the Indian community favoured the occurrence of widespread malnutrition in all age and sex groups, reflecting the poor dietary intake. Children predominantly exhibited signs of deficiency of vitamins A and B Complex. Anaemia was prevalent among women of child-bearing age. Gross underweight was a feature in all age and sex groups. In general, the poorer sections of the community, particularly the vulnerable segments, usually suffer most from malnutrition. As will be seen in later sections, no substantial change has occurred over the years, and even today malnutrition continues to be one of the major public health problems in the country.

Growth and physical development in Indian children

In the past, the cultural diversity prevailing in India provided ample opportunities for anthropologists to conduct somatometric studies. The differences observed in the measurements in different segments of the population were invariably attributed to racial and genetic factors. Later, with the realization that malnutrition was widely prevalent in the country, attention was directed to the field of growth and physical development of children, mainly through isolated studies by health workers on school children. Though considerable amounts of data were available over the last 3 or 4 decades on heights and weights of school children, there were marked differences in the methodology of collection of these data.[17] In comparison with the rice diets of South Indian children, the association of better growth with wheat diets of North Indian children was observed, but there was no conclusive evidence of this relationship. The urban child was found to have better growth performance than a rural child. One significant finding in all these studies was the poor growth of Indian children as compared to their western counterparts and poor nutrition was invariably attributed to be the main cause for this difference.

Since growth deficiency was observed to be a cardinal sign of PEM, attention was then directed to pre-school children. But unlike the school children, who were easily available, it was very difficult to collect information on the growth of pre-school children and many studies were confined to hospital situations. A few studies undertaken in the community have provided valuable information on the various factors that may affect growth of infant and pre-school children.[18] Both cross-section and longitudinal studies[15,19] are available and most of them pertain to low socio-economic groups of population.

The results of these studies conformed to the classical pattern of growth observed in all the developing regions. In comparison with western standards, the birth weights were lower, but up to the age of 6 months the rate of growth of infants was more or less similar, the curves being parallel with but lower than those of the western counterparts for both height and weight. After 6 months, there is a lag period extending over the entire pre-school age period and the curve actually flattens out. This is explained by the observation that breast-milk intake of children up to 6 months of age is adequate to meet the nutritional needs of the infants but thereafter it is insufficient and practically nil or inadequate supplements are provided during the rest of the period of infancy. This feature extends beyond the weaning period up to about 5 years of age. Another factor which contributes, is the occurrence of repeated episodes of infections. The extreme nature of growth deficiency during this period of life is obvious when it is seen that the growth curves for height and weight of pre-school children belonging to low socio-economic groups in India are below the 10th percentile curve of western children.[14]

These investigations clearly brought out the need for the extensive use of growth charts in the early detection of Protein–Energy Malnutrition (PEM).

In spite of the fact that birth weights are taken as a matter of routine in most of the hospitals in the country, much of the data remains unutilized. Very few centres have recorded their observations on birth weights of Indian children. Apart from socio-economic differences in birth weights, these investigations have clearly pointed out that the definition of pre-maturity laid down by the Expert Committee of WHO (less than 2500 g) may not be applicable to Indian conditions. This is also supported by similar observations in other developing nations. Shantha and Tasker,[20] analysing data on birth weights totalling 10,756 (5656 males, 5100 females) new-born babies from 20 hospitals in India, representing 10 States, conclude that for Indian new-borns, the limit of pre-maturity was 2250 g or less, the mean birth weights for male and female babies being 2788 and 2707 respectively. Nearly 60 per cent of the babies had birth weights of more than 2500 g.

One of the biggest problems faced is the accurate determination of dates of birth. The system of registration of births has not yet developed to the desired level. Experience has shown the usefulness of local calendars indicating festivals, fairs and major events in the area in assessing dates of birth, especially of pre-school children, with a fair degree of accuracy. However, this method is not found to be of use in the older age group of school children and school records are most unreliable.

The lack of local reference standards for the growth and physical development of children has been one of the main handicaps for a proper interpretation of the data collected. In order to meet this long-felt need, the ICMR sponsored a nationwide cross-sectional study, with the object of constructing a reference standard for growth and physical development of Indian infants and children from birth to 21 years. These data were collected by trained workers in 7 units located in different regions of the country but using uniform and standardized procedures. A total of 127,866 children were examined (69,804 males, 58,062 females). The data were analysed according to sex, socio-economic status, religion and residence (rural/urban). This compilation[21] provides a good reference manual for nutrition workers in India.

Recently, another study[22] was undertaken on 9000 children belonging to the really well-to-do segment of the population in India. Children of both sexes between the ages of 5–16 years attending 14 public schools in different parts of the country were surveyed. These children were all healthy and subsisting on a more than adequate diet.

These two major surveys clearly indicated that children belonging to the well-to-do sections who have no nutrition or other constraints grow as well as their western counterparts. However, one interesting feature was that around the age of 12 years in females and 14 years in males Indian children begin to lag behind the western counterparts. The reason for this is not clear.

In contrast, the poor growth of children belonging to the low socio-economic groups is evidence by the fact that the 50th percentile for heights and weights of this group corresponds to the 5th percentile of the well-to-do children. In fact, only the 95th percentile for heights and weights of the children from low-income groups corresponds to the 50th percentile of the well-to-do group of children.

The relationship between malnutrition and puberty has also been investigated. Though there were common wide variations, distinct socio-economic differences were observed. In boys the earliest age of onset of puberty was 13.4 years and 14.2 years in the highest and lowest income groups respectively. Among girls the onset of menstruation was at the ages of 13.0 years and 14.0 years in the highest and lowest income groups respectively.

With the increasing realization that physical growth of children is a reliable and good index of community nutrition and health, a variety of anthropometric measurements are being taken on children. Apart from the simple measurements of height and weight, others include head circumference, arm and calf circumference, skin-fold measurements at various sites in the body, namely triceps region, biceps region, subscapular region etc. In addition, a number of indices have been suggested, based on these various measurements, for the assessment of nutritional status.[23] Some of these, such as the ratio of head and chest circumferences, weight by height ratio, Wt/Ht^2 have been shown to have a good correlation with the nutritional status and these are valuable in identifying early cases of PEM and in grading them.

Protein–energy malnutrition

By far the most important public health nutritional problem in India is protein–energy malnutrition (PEM) which is mainly confined to pre-school children belonging to low-income groups. The occurrence of PEM has been well-documented over the last 3 decades. The first phase consisted mostly of reports of clinical studies in major hospitals and research institutions in the country. Gopalan and Ramalingaswami[24] have highlighted these studies in their review.

In India the peak prevalence of kwashiorkor is between the ages of 1–2 years but that for marasmus is earlier. Acute infections particularly measles and gastroenteritis, are usually precipitating causes. Evidence that the experience of malnutrition during the early period of life may have permanent effects on both the physical and mental development of surviving children is still under investigation.

With increasing knowledge that a proper combination of cereals, pulses and other protein-rich foods from vegetable sources is as effective as skim milk, various regimes based on these alternate sources of food have been extensively used with equal success.[25] Feeding trials[26] in the community confirmed the usefulness of these foods of vegetable origin in the improvement of the protein–energy status of pre-school children as determined by growth studies. With these developments the second phase of assessment of the problem of PEM in the community began. Rao *et al.*[14] in their study of about 5000 pre-school children of low socio-economic groups of families in South India estimate the prevalence of kwashiorkor and marasmus to be about 1 and 2 per cent respectively, giving a total of about 3 per cent prevalence for PEM. The recent collaborative studies of ICMR also confirm these estimates.[15] Though there are minor regional variations in the different parts of the country, the fact remains that PEM is a problem among the low-income group of pre-school children all over India. If body weights alone are considered,[15] the problem of PEM assumes greater dimensions. The estimates for the milder forms Grade I and Grade II will be around 79 per cent and that for Grade III 18 per cent.

The causation for PEM as determined by these surveys as well as through follow-up studies in the community points to three main factors: poor purchasing power of the community with consequent inadequate intake of diet; infections and infestations contributed by poor environmental and personal hygiene; ignorance of the nutritional needs of children, associated with faulty notions and beliefs regarding diet and illness. The observation that in a community under the same influences only a certain proportion of the children develop PEM has been explained as due to differences in level of intelligence and capacity of mothers for child care.[27]

Reaching the pre-school child has always been one of the major bottlenecks in implementing programmes for this vulnerable segment. In this connection the experiences of organizing centres of various types like nutrition clinics, nutrition rehabilitation centres and day-care centres in many countries has been good. In India one of the earliest attempts was by Dr Achar in Madras City where a chain of MCH Centres provided a link with the Paediatric Department of the main Hospital. Similar experience in certain rural areas of the country were also good.[37] The essential features of these centres were utilization of locally available foods, men and material resources, health and nutrition education of the mothers and community through active participation and training of health workers.

In the choice of supplements for the management of PEM, since milk is a scarce and expensive commodity, alternative sources were looked for. Recent information on the dietary intake of pre-school children has clearly indicated that energy deficiency or rather 'food gap' was more important and that protein deficiency, even accounting for the poor quality of proteins derived from vegetable sources, was not a significant feature.[28] It has been observed that while the proportion of pre-school children subsisting on an energy-deficient diet was more than 90 per cent, those with both energy and protein deficiency formed about 35 per cent. But bulk of food is a factor which has to be reckoned with and it has been demonstrated that instead of the normal practice of feeding children in 2 or 3 meals, increasing the frequency of meals at sufficient intervals would be desirable. Another aspect which deserves to be emphasized is that the diets based on cereals and pulses are invariably deficient in other nutrients like vitamins and minerals, particularly vitamin A, iron and calcium. The inclusion of foods rich in these nutrients is a must for the improvement of nutritional status of pre-school children in India.

Vitamin A deficiency

The occurrence of ocular manifestations due to vitamin A deficiency in children has been noted by earlier workers, particularly in the rice-eating belt of southern and eastern parts of the country. A very high prevalence of vitamin A deficiency with xerosis of the conjunctiva and night blindness, even as much as 50 per cent has been reported among children by some workers. However, estimates based on xerosis of the conjunctiva are subject to a lot of observor errors which are subjective in nature. Many had wrongly attributed the dark pigmentation of the conjunctiva observed in children to vitamin A deficiency. The current estimates based on recent surveys undertaken by many experienced workers indicate that the prevalence of vitamin A deficiency is about 3–8 per cent among pre-school children[15] and about 10–15 per cent in school children. Thus, an overall prevalence rate of about 10 per cent in children is observed in India.

In general, vitamin A deficiency is observed to be less prevalent in female children as compared with males. Though signs of vitamin A deficiency are not common in adults, its occurrence during pregnancy is not rare. Earlier, many workers considered dryness of skin and phrynoderma as signs of vitamin A deficiency, but recent evidence is against any such specific association.

Though some doubts have been raised as to the significance of Bitot's spots as a sign of vitamin A deficiency, from the experience of Indian workers it can be categorically stated that it is definitely one of the signs of vitamin A deficiency in young children. However, a small proportion of children usually of older age who manifest the sign of Bitot's spots over a long period do not always respond to administration of vitamin A. This is possibly due to irreversible changes in the conjunctiva.

Children belonging to poor socio-economic groups do not manifest signs of deficiency of vitamin A as long as they are breast-fed. After the age of one year clinical evidences of vitamin A deficiency occur and this is observed to increase with age.

Regular intake of green leaves has been shown to improve the serum vitamin A level even in as short a period as 15 days in pre-school children. It is realized that nutrition education in the community is a difficult and long-drawn process and can serve only as a long-term measure. For several years after the Second World War, with the help of International Agencies like UNICEF, supplements of vitamins A and D in capsule form as well as skim milk fortified with vitamin A were distributed through health centres.* This has not had the desired effect of reducing the

---

*Editor's note: See Chapter 3 for skim milk and xerophthalmia.

prevalence of vitamin A deficiency for the reason that regular intake of these supplements was not possible, due to the difficulties encountered in reaching the pre-school children. In view of the serious consequences of vitamin A deficiency, leading to blindness among children, the need for an effective measure for prevention was found necessary as an immediate preventive measure. Since vitamin A can be stored in the liver for long periods, the administration of a massive dose so as to form a depot seemed a possible solution.

A series of preliminary investigations[29] on experimental animals and pre-school children indicated that oral administration of a large dose of oil-soluble solution of vitamin A can maintain the level of serum vitamin A for periods of more than 6 months. Hepatic storage in animals was also better with the oil preparation.

A study[30,31] undertaken in the rural areas around Hyderabad where 1800 pre-school children received an annual dose of 300,000 units oil preparation of vitamin A, taken orally, showed over a period of 4 years that 84 per cent of these children were protected from vitamin A deficiency. This effect was marked in the younger age group of 1–2 years. It was also observed that the water-soluble preparation of the same dose produced signs of hypervitaminosis A in many cases. The subsequent use of oil preparation produced toxic effects only on a small proportion of children (4 per cent) and even these were mild in nature. Based on this experience the Department of Family Planning, Government of India, launched a Prophylaxis Programme for prevention of vitamin A deficiency and blindness in pre-school children in several regions where this deficiency was prevalent.

Nutritional anaemia

Several studies[32] carried out in India indicate that nutritional anaemia is widespread among women of child-bearing age and children, especially from the low-income groups which form the major segment of the population. Though the results of these studies bring out the fact that iron deficiency is the most important form of anaemia in India, deficiencies of folic acid and vitamin B_{12} cannot be ignored.

A few isolated community studies, on the basis of haemoglobin estimations in the blood, indicate that more than 20 per cent of the community suffer from anaemia and this was confined mostly to women of child-bearing age, particularly during pregnancy, and growing children. The results of the collaborative studies on a large number of pre-school children mentioned earlier showed that more than 50 per cent of pre-school children surveyed had haemoglobin levels less than 10.8 per cent.[15]

Haemoglobin estimation carried out in various parts of the country especially among pregnant women attending health centres indicates that more than 50 per cent of these women have haemoglobin levels below 10 per cent. In contrast, anaemia among nursing mothers is not so much of a problem. However, in areas where there was widespread occurrence of hook worm infestation anaemia was prevalent in all age and sex groups and the prevalence among male members of the community was also observed.

Dietary assessment among low socio-economic groups reveals that the mean intake of iron through food is around 20 mg per adult per day. This amount of intake is considered to be marginal from the point of view of requirement for the population. The intake of pre-school children is estimated to be about 6 mg per day. Cereals being the main constituent of the diet of Indian communities, the relationship between anaemia and high intake of cereals with its high level of phytates has been investigated through several studies.It has also been observed that the presence of adequate amounts of both vitamin C and calcium favours absorption of iron, even in the presence of phytates. Another significant finding is the loss of substantial amounts of iron through sweat, and this has relevance in tropical areas like India, but it has also been observed that the loss of iron through sweat is less among anaemic subjects. Estimates are also now available on the loss of iron in women during menstrural periods and during childbirth. All these studies[33] have helped in the better understanding of the problem of anaemia in relation to the public health needs of the vulnerable segments of the population and a national programme for the prevention of anaemia in women and children is now being implemented in the country.

Deficiency of B complex vitamins

The most common manifestation is angular stomatitis with or without changes in the tongue like glossitis, hypertrophic and atrophic papillae of the tongue. These manifestations are prevalent to a greater extent in the vulnerable groups of children, pregnant and lactating mothers. Unlike many other nutritional diseases it is also observed among adult males and seasonal occurrence is not unknown. The overall prevalence rate in the community is about 20 per cent.

Many cases respond best with the administration of B Complex groups of vitamins indicating thereby that deficiency of other vitamins of the B Complex group may also be important. The prevention of riboflavin deficiency through improvements in the poor Indian diet is beset with problems since foods rich in riboflavin, such as milk and foods of animal origin, are relatively expensive.

Hand-pounding of rice, which was advocated earlier to prevent losses in B vitamins, is no longer used since in every part of the country rice mills are now available. However, another method to preserve these vitamins, namely parboiling, is still practised and consumption of parboiled rice is prevalent in a few regions of the country.

During the third and fourth decade of the present century, beriberi was reported to be endemic in the northern region of the State of Andra Pradesh in South India.[1] This was attributed to the extensive use of highly polished or milled rice and faulty cooking practices such as excessive washing of rice and straining the water after cooking rice with excess water. Where parboiled rice was consumed in certain other parts of South India like Kerala, beriberi was not encountered. At the present moment beriberi is no longer prevalent in the previously endemic areas. The reason for this change, though not clear, is stated to be the enactment of laws for under-milling and improvement in the technology of milling, and increased standards of living with resultant diversification of diets. However, with the continued prevalence of faulty cooking practices associated with marginal deficiency of thiamine in the diet, it is possible that sub-clinical states of deficiency of the vitamins do exist in the rice-eating belts of South India.

Pellagra, the classical syndrome due to deficiency of nicotinic acid, occurs sporadically and is reported from every part of India, where it is related to the excessive consumption of jowar (*Sorghum vulgare*), especially during certain lean seasons of the year.

Situated as it is in an area where jowar is the staple diet of the region, the National Institute of Nutrition, Hyderabad, Andhra Pradesh, has done some pioneering studies to show the relationship between jowar consumption and pellagra. Clinical and experimental studies indicated that pellagra may be due to a state of amino-acid imbalance. Jowar as such is not deficient in tryptophan or nicotinic acid, but is rich in leucine. Studies indicate that a high level of the essential amino-acid leucine present in jowar, as well as the relatively low level of isoleucine, another amino-acid, may be responsible for the prevalence of pellagra in a jowar-eating population. This was later confirmed by the observation that the use of opaque 2 maize which has a low leucine content was capable of preventing the development of pellagra in experimental animals and subjects subsisting on jowar.[34]

On an analysis of a large number of varieties of jowar, it was found that certain strains have low leucine content. This observation may pave the way for the public health approach to the problem of prevention of pellagra in the country.

Deficiency of vitamin C

Nutrition workers in India have always been intrigued by the observation that in spite of the low level of intake of vitamin C in the average Indian diet, clinical manifestations of vitamin C deficiency are not widely prevalent. The cooking practices in the country favour considerable loss of this vitamin. However, recent studies tend to indicate biochemical evidences of deficiency of vitamin C. It is also possible that the suggested requirements and allowances may be higher than necessary.[34]

Vitamin D deficiency

The average Indian diet does not contain a sufficient amount of vitamin D-rich foods. The general availability of sunshine is responsible for the belief that vitamin D deficiency is not a public health problem in the country. The obvious clinical features of rickets occur among children in the community but in very few numbers, especially in urban areas. In the northern regions of the country, rickets and osteomalacia are reported to be much more common than elsewhere. Many of the studies on vitamin D deficiency relate to hospital cases. As such, the public health implications of vitamin D deficiency in India are still not fully known.

Endemic goitre

Recent data on the prevalence of goitre in the neighbourhood of the Himalayan ranges indicate that on an average the prevalence is about 25 per cent, ranging from

3 per cent to over 60 per cent. On this basis, it can be estimated that in the entire endemic area goitre would now account for about 25 million cases.[35]

The efficacy of iodization of salt has been demonstrated under Indian conditions through a pilot study.[36] The average estimated daily intake of salt per person in India is 15 g. Based upon local needs of the endemic regions in the country, the Ministry of Health has prescribed that the level of iodization of salt in India should be 1 in 40,000 with potassium iodate. In India modified techniques of spray and dry mixing methods are utilized for the purpose.

The National Goitre Control Programme has been in operation in the country since the late 1950s, under the direct control of the DGHS, Ministry of Health, Government of India. In areas where the prevalence of goitre is 10 per cent or more, after issuing ban orders for the entry of non-iodized salt, iodized salt is supplied on a priority basis. The iodized salt is produced at three locations in the country with plants donated by UNICEF. Currently there is much variation in the distribution of the allocation, ranging from 40–90 per cent, depending on the area. Some of the reasons for underutilization are deficiencies in the regular and timely placement of indents for the salt by salt traders nominated for the purpose in the different regions, inadequacies in rail transport and ineffectiveness of the ban order for the entry of non-iodized salt.

DISORDERS DUE TO TOXINS IN FOOD (Chapter 12)

Fluorosis

In certain parts of Andhra Pradesh widespread prevalence of mottling of permanent teeth in children was reported,[1] in areas where the fluorine content of water was in the range of 5–11 parts per million, much in excess of the permissible limit of 1 p.p.m. Loss of lustre in the enamel, chalkiness, brown pigmentation and pitting of teeth were also seen. These changes are commonly found in the central upper incisors. In the older age groups bones and tendons show the characteristic changes with deposition of fluoride compounds. Extensive new bone formation, exostosis, ossification of ligaments and tendons and interosseous membranes finally lead to limitation of movement, particularly of the spine. Neurrological manifestations due to pressure may occur.

The disorder has now been reported from other parts of the country, as in Punjab, Rajasthan and Kerala. The occurrence of genuvalgum (knock knees) in young adults in the endemic area of Nalgonda District of Andhra Pradesh is reported to be of recent origin. This has been attributed to the rise in the level of subsoil water as a result of the construction of an irrigation dam in the area with consequent alterations in the trace element content of the soil and water. In this connection the role of molybdenum is being investigated.[37] Use of paddy husk carbon digested with alkali and treatment with alum for the removal of fluorine in water, a relatively inexpensive method, is already available. The villagers use water from scattered wells and, for reasons of cost, community supply of treated water was not feasible. The recent availability of canal waters from reservoirs in the area provides opportunities for alternate supply of water with low levels of fluorine.

The Central Public Health Engineering Research Institute, Nagpur, has now developed defluorinating units both for homes, as well as for large-scale purposes, using sodium aluminate and alum. These are currently being tested in the State of Rajasthan. It has also been reported that certain rocks known as Serpentine, containing one or both of the minerals Crysotile and Antigorite, formed a weak defluorinating agent.

Human lathyrism

'Lathyrism', associated with excessive consumption of the pulse *Lathyrus sativus* (khesari dal) as a staple food, is known to occur sporadically in several parts of India, particularly among the lower socio-economic groups. It is one of the important public health problems of the States of Madhya Pradesh and Uttar Pradesh and occurs as an endemic disorder particularly in the districts of Rawa, Satna in Madhya Pradesh and adjoining areas of Uttar Pradesh. In these areas about 2–4 per cent of the population are affected by the disease.[38]

Lathyrism is characterized by progressive spastic paralysis of the lower limbs and is irreversible. Young adults of both sexes are susceptible to the disease. The poor agro-economic condition prevailing in these areas is responsible for the high intake of the pulse as a staple, since the soil, climate and agricultural situation are not very suitable for other crops to be grown. The pulse is a hardy crop, is able to withstand drought conditions and does not need much care. Moreover, it is customary for the farmers to give wages in kind to the agriculture labourers and this pulse crop comes in handy.

Recently, the isolation of a water-soluble neurotoxin from the pulse, identified as B—N—Oxalyl Amino Alanine (BOAA), which is capable of producing paralytic syndromes in chicks and monkeys, has renewed interest in the problem of lathyrism.[39] The steeping of pulse in hot water for a short period of an hour and repeated washing thereafter with excess cold water has been shown to remove 90–95 per cent of the toxin. As an outcome of this, the well-known process of parboiling has been advocated for removal of the toxin on a commercial basis. However, in both these methods a considerable loss of the water-soluble vitamins cannot be prevented, though in the latter process the loss is minimized.

In the endemic areas wide variations were noted in the prevalence of lathyrism. Analysis of over 600 samples from different areas showed that the toxin content varied from 0.1–2.3 per cent on dry weight basis. A promising preventive approach to the problem of lathyrism would thus be for the selective propagation of low-toxin strains of pulse, and this is being attempted, with the collaboration of the Indian Council of Agricultural Research. The widespread use of the cheap khesari dal as an adulterant in Bengal gram flour is well-known in the country. The isolation of neurotoxin BOAA and the development of simple methods for its detection have now proved useful in checking this type of adulteration.

Epidemic dropsy

As recently as 1973 outbreaks of this disease were reported from the Southern State of Andhra Pradesh where groundnut oil and sesame oil only are consumed.

The onset of the disease may be sudden or insidious and the early symptoms and signs include nausea, loss of appetite, loose bowels and irregular fever. Oedema is confined to the lower extremities but later extends to the other parts of the body. The skin is hypereamic with vascular mottling and petechial rash. Right heart failure is common and glaucoma also occurs. The disorder, however, has a low mortality rate. No specific treatment is available and what is done is mainly palliative. This toxic condition is due either to adulteration or accidental contamination of edible oils with Argemone oil, from the seeds of the plant *Argemone mexicana* which is a wild crop resembling mustard seeds. Available information indicates that the alkaloid Sanguinarine, present in the seed and in the oil, is responsible for the toxic manifestations.[38]

It is obvious that the approach to the problem of argemone toxicity is prevention of adulteration or contamination. Thus, an important aspect from the public health point of view is detection and the fixation of safe limits of contamination of edible oils with argemone oil. It has been suggested that the permissible contamination would be 0.004 per cent of the oil.

Aflatoxin[38]

The toxin present in cattle feed can pass into the milk and this is of importance in view of the fact that in developing countries like India, large-scale, groundnut-based supplementary feeding programmes are in operation. The observation that in experimental animals the effect of the toxin is more marked under conditions of lowered protein intake, has relevance to developing countries. A survey of the fungus contamination of groundnuts in different parts of the country showed that apart from conditions which favour access of the fungi to the kernel, such as type of harvesting, damage to the pods, storage etc., the climatic variables like humidity and temperature are also important factors for the survival of the mould and production of toxin. The recognition of certain varieties of groundnut (U.S. 26 Tanganyika) resistant to the production of toxin is of practical importance, as a selective cultivation of such varieties would be capable of minimizing the problem of aflatoxin. So far the role of aflatoxin in hepatic disorders like infantile childhood cirrhosis and malignancy has not been definitely demonstrated.

PROGRAMMES FOR THE PREVENTION OF MALNUTRITION IN INDIA

The control of malnutrition requires a coordinated approach by various agencies, such as Food and Agriculture, Health, Education, Social Welfare and Community Development. The efforts to combat deficiencies in nutrition in India are briefly considered below.

Production of food

In the last decade, with the use of improved agricultural technology, a considerable augmentation of food grain production has been achieved. While a beginning has been made as regards cereals, the continued and intense effort is also likely to bring in good results with other necessary foods. Emphasis is not only placed on increasing the yields but also in upgrading the nutritional quality of foods. The coordinated programmes, especially between ICMR and ICAR and other related agencies, are a step in this direction. A further development is the increased utilization of foods which hitherto have not been fully exploited like oil seeds, soya bean, etc. The augmentation of production of milk and milk substitutes from vegetable sources (Miltone using defatted groundnut) is receiving support. The extensive use of food technology for the prevention of losses and conservation of foods, as for example improved storage and milling methods and control of contamination, particularly by fungi, are important developments. The development of nutritious formulations and recipes for both large-scale and home processing, with the use of local food resources, is proving valuable for the supplementary feeding programmes. The agro-economic conditions and food habits do not permit the fortification of staple foods with required nutrients though there has been a limited attempt to fortify wheatflour with calcium. However, salt as a vehicle for fortification of a nutrient like iron is still being investigated and promises hope, apart from the already available iodized salt, for the prevention of goitre.

Supplementary feeding programmes

These programmes provide ample opportunities for health and nutrition education. The major supplementary feeding programmes now being implemented are detailed below.

1. *Mid-day meal programme*

This is being implemented by the Ministry of Education; it caters for the primary school children in the age group 6–11 years and has been in operation for nearly a decade. In some areas use is made of central kitchens. At present, the CARE organization provides the food as free aid and it is shipped up to the nearest port, the rest of the cost being borne by the Government. The food supplied to children is usually corn soya meal (CSM) cooked with butter oil or soya bean oil; but other types like milk, toned milk, Balahar etc. are also used. The meal is expected to cover one-third of the daily needs of the child and provides about 400 calories (1.68 MJ) and 15 g of protein. The feeding is undertaken for a period of 200 days in a year. The present coverage of children under the programme is about 12 million and an additional 4 million are to be covered in the next 5 years.

2. *Special nutrition programme*

Implemented in 1970 by the Department of Social Welfare, this programme caters to pre-school children and pregnant and lactating women of tribal areas and slums of cities with over 100,000 population. In the feeding centres, voluntary workers in the area are responsible for the collection, storage and distribution of the supplements. In the cities, convenient foods like bread, buns etc. are mainly used. In tribal areas, locally available foods are cooked and distributed. The supplements give 300 and 500 calories (1.26 and 2.1 MJ) and 10–15 g and 10–25 g of protein for children and women respectively. The feeding is undertaken for a period of 300 days in a year. The present coverage of beneficiaries is about 4 million and an additional 6 million have been planned for the next 5 years.

3. *Applied nutrition programme*

This is being implemented by the Community Development (C.D.) Department with the help of International Agencies—UNICEF, FAO, WHO—in the rural areas, in selected villages of certain blocks of C.D. (a unit composed of 80–100 thousand population). The basic objectives of this programme are to demonstrate to the community that nutritious foods could be grown with local resources to meet nutritional needs, particularly those of the vulnerable groups. In this process, their economic condition can also be improved by marketing the surplus produce. In the initial stages the various inputs necessary are provided free of cost. The foods grown are vegetables, and fruits, through school gardens, community gardens and kitchen gardens; and poultry and eggs obtained by breeding non-indigenous varieties of birds with high yield under deep-litter system, using nutritious formula feeds. Increase in the production of fish is achieved through better methods of breeding and exploitation. A certain proportion of the foods produced is utilized in demonstration feeding programmes for children and mothers. An important aspect is the training of personnel and the health and nutrition education of the community. From the year 1961 until now 1081 blocks have been covered and in the next 5 years 700 further blocks will be added.

4. *Prophylaxis against blindness in children caused by vitamin A deficiency*

This is implemented by the Department of Family Planning, Ministry of Health. Children between the ages of 1–6 years are fed an oral dose of 200,000 I.U. of vitamin A solution in oil once every 6 months up to the age of 6 years. This was initiated in 1970 in areas where vitamin A deficiency was a serious problem and is being extended to other areas, based upon recent information on the prevalence of this nutritional deficiency. The vitamin A is being distributed through the existing health agencies in the rural and urban areas as a preventive measure. The target number of beneficiaries up to the current year was 12 million and during the next 5 years is expected to reach 60 million.

5. *Prophylaxis against nutritional anaemia*

This programme is organized on similar lines to the vitamin A programme, but both the vulnerable groups of women and pre-school children derive the benefits of a daily supply of tablets of iron and folic acid varying in size and colour. Large tablets meant for women contain 180 mg of ferrous sulphate and 500 μg of folic acid. The small tablets for children contain 50 mg of iron and 100 μg of folic acid. The expected coverage up to the current year was 18 million and in the next 5 years is estimated to go up to 60 million beneficiaries.

The total cost of all these supplementary feeding programmes is estimated to be about Rs. 4050 million for the next 5 years and works out to about 4–5 U.S. cents per beneficiary.

NUTRITION EDUCATION, TRAINING AND RESEARCH

Ignorance and lack of knowledge about nutritional needs, widely prevalent in the country, emphasized the importance of nutrition education and training at all levels. Various types of orientation courses are now available for all categories of personnel implementing the programmes. Nutrition education of the community, though a stupendous task for a country like India, is being attempted through all available media and channels. In addition, courses leading to certificates, diplomas and degrees in public health nutrition are being conducted by certain institutes in the country. Research studies in the field of nutrition with emphasis on applied aspects are also being encouraged in suitable centres.

There is need for a coordinated approach to the problem of nutrition by the various agencies implementing the programmes. With the emergence of this concept, it is proposed to implement a programme of integrated packages of services to the vulnerable groups. These services will include supplementary feeding, health care both curative and preventive, family planning, safe drinking water and nutrition and health education.

REFERENCES

1. Patwardhan, V. N. *Nutrition in India,* 2nd. edition Indian Journal of Medical Sciences, Bombay, 1961.
2. *Pocket Book of Population Statistics,* Registrar General and Census Commissioner, India, 1972.
3. Dandekar, V. M. and N. Rath. *Poverty in India.* Indian School of Political Economy, Bombay, 1971.
4. *Pocket Book of Health Statistics,* Central Bureau of Health Intelligence, DGHS, Ministry of Health & Family Planning, Government of India, 1973.
5. *Nutritive Value of Indian Foods,* National Institute of Nutrition ICMR, 1971.
6. Aykroyd, W. R. IRFA, Special Report Series No. 3, 1939, 1945, 1947.
7. ICMR, Report of Diet Surveys in India—Special Report No. 20, 1951, and Supplement Special Report No. 25, 1953.
8. Tasker, A. D., M. C. Swaminathan and S. Madhavan. Diet Surveys by weighment method—a comparison of random day, three day and seven day period, *Indian J. Med. Res.,* **55,** 90 (1967).
9. Madhavan, S. and M. C. Swaminathan. A comparative study of two methods of diet survey, *Indian J. Med. Res.,* **54,** 480 (1966).
10. Pasricha, S. An assessment of reliability of the oral questionnaire method of diet survey as applied to Indian communities, *Indian J. Med. Res.,* **47,** 207 (1959).

343

11. Pandit, C. G. and K. S. Rao. *Nutrition in India,* I.C.M.R., 1946–1958, 1960.
12. *Diet Atlas of India.* National Institute of Nutrition, ICMR, 1971.
13. Thiammayamma, B. V. S., K. Satyanarayana, P. Rao and M. C. Swaminathan. Effect of socio-economic differences on the dietary intake of urban population of Hyderabad, *Indian J. Nutr. Dietet.,* **10,** 8 (1973)
14. Rao, K., M. C. Swaminathan, S. Swarup and V. N. Patwardhan. Protein malnutrition in South India, *Bull. Wld. Hlth. Org.,* **20,** 603 (1959).
15. Studies on Pre-school Children, Report of the Working Party of the ICMR, 1973.
16. Belavaday, B. Studies on Human Lactation, A Review. ICMR Special Report Series No 45, 1963.
17. Review of Nutrition Surveys conducted in India, Special Report Series No. 36, ICMR, 1961.
18. Swaminathan, M. C., K. K. Jyothi, R. Singh, S. Madhavan and C. Gopalan. A semi-longitudinal study of growth of Indian children and the related factors, *Indian Paediat.,* **1,** 255 (1964).
19. Datta Banik, N. D., R. Krishna, S. I. S. Manu, L. Raj and A. D. Tasker. A longitudinal study of physical growth of children from birth to 5 years of age in Delhi, *Indian J. Med. Res.,* **58,** 135 (1970).
20. Madhavan, S. and A. D. Tasker. Birth weight of Indian babies born in hospitals, *Indian J. of Paediat.,* **36,** 257 (1969).
21. ICMR. Growth and Physical Development of Indian Infants and Children, Technical Report Series No. 18, 1972.
22. Vijaraghavan, K., D. Singh and M. C. Swaminathan. Heights and weights of well-nourished Indian school children, *Indian J. Med. Res.,* **59,** 648 (1971).
23. Visweswara Rao, K. and D. Singh. An evaluation of the relationship between nutritional status and anthropometric measurements. *Amer. J. Clin. Nutr.,* **23,** 83 (1970).
24. Gopalan, C. and V. Ramalingaswami. Kwashiorkor in India. *Indian J. Med. Res.,* **43,** 751 (1965).
25. Narasinga Rao, B. S. A Decade of Progress 1961–1970, National Institute of Nutrition. *ICMR.,* 1970, p. 54.
26. Ganapati, R., M. C. Swaminathan, A. D. Tasker and K. Someswara Rao. Feeding trials with vegetable protein foods. *Indian J. Med. Res.,* **49,** 306 (1961).
27. Srikantia, S. G. and C. Y. Sastry. Effect of maternal attributes on malnutrition in children, *Proc. First Asian Congr. Nutr., 1971,* Hyderabad, 1972, p. 584.
28. Narasinga Rao, B. S., K. Visweswara Rao and A. Nadami Naidu. Calorie and protein adequacy of the dietaries of pre-school children in India, *J. Nutr. Dietet.,* **6,** 238 (1969).
29. Srikantia, S. G. and Vinedini Reddy. Effect of a single massive dose of vitamin A on serum and liver levels of vitamin, *Amer. J. Clin. Nutr.,* **23,** 114 (1970).
30. Swaminathan, M. C., T. P. Susheela and B. V. S. Thimmayamma. Field prophylactic trial with a single annual oral massive dose of vitamin A., *Amer. J. Clin. Nutr.,* **23,** 119 (1970).
31. Swaminathan, M. C. Prevention of vitamin deficiency by administration of massive dose of vitamin A, *Proc. First Asian Congr. Nutr., Hyderabad,* 1972, p. 695.
32. Nutritional anaemia, *Proc. of Nutr. Soc. India,* **2,** 4 (1965).
33. Apte, S. V. Studies on iron metabolism, decade of progress 1961–1970, *National*
34. Nutrition Research, Indian Golden Jubliee Symposium, *Amer. J. Clin. Nutr.,* **23,** 1 (1970).
35. National Goitre Control Project, DGHS, Government of India (unpublished).
36. Sooch, S. S. and V. Ramalingaswami. Preliminary report of an experiment in the Kangra Valley for the prevention of Himalayan endemic goitre with iodised salt, *Bull. Wld. Hlth. Org.,* **32,** 299 (1965).
37. Annual Report of the National Institute of Nutrition for the year 1973, ICMR, India.
38. Nagarajan, V. Toxins in foods, Decade of Progress 1961–1970, *National Institute of*

Nutrition, Hyderabad, 1970, p. 20.
39. Sarma, P. S. and G. Padmanaban. In *Toxic Constituents in Plant Foodstuffs* (ed. Irwin E. Leiner), New York, Academic Press, 1969, p. 267.

CHAPTER 29

Nutrition in the Philippines

CONRADO R. PASCUAL

Present nutrition work in the country has reached a height wherein every Filipino is made aware of the importance of the right kind and amount of food in daily living. It is also at a stage at which each and every community worker learns how his discipline relates to the total effort of improving his clientele's nutritional status. Local nutrition scientists are also at a point whereby researches are made relevant to the country's nutrition needs and problems. The progress that has been made so far has met full administrative support and recognition that nutrition has been given the governmental priority it deserves.

HISTORY OF NUTRITION

Nutrition studies in the Philippines had their beginning as early as the American occupation in 1900. Isolated individual studies on foods and nutrition were undertaken by the Americans, Germans and other foreign nationals who came to the Philippines, as well as by local scientists. Among these studies were those on composition of body fluids, the nutritive value of local foods and their processing, food intake of Filipinos in some urban and rural areas and certain physiological problems related to nutrition noted in early reviews made by leading local scientists.[1-5] These scientific investigations were given impetus in 1933 with the formal organization of the National Research Council of the Philippines (NRCP). The Council gave Filipino workers the necessary funding and facilities for research, although still on a limited scale. A certain degree of awareness of the importance of nutrition was manifested by the creation of a nutrition section under the NRCP. This section, whose function was essentially educational, however, was severely undermanned and its activities were consequently limited. Fortunately, some types of nutrition education activities were undertaken by other sectors and organizations.[6]

The sporadic nature of such undertakings did not gain much headway until after the Second World War. At about this time, the Philippine Association of Nutrition (PAN) was born out of the interest of a group of local nutrition workers in the food and nutrition problems of the country. The Association sought to elevate the standards of nutrition of the people, stimulate researches and propagate the newer knowledge of this important branch of science.[7] It was through PAN that government authorities were convinced of the need to set up a specific agency to take charge of the food and nutrition activities of the country. On 4 October, 1947 by virtue of Section 30 of the Executive Order No. 924, the Institute of Nutrition (IN) was established under the Office of the President of the Philippines.

The seed of coordination and cooperation in community nutrition work was sown in the Philippines when the Institute of Nutrition Board was created in 1948 with the perspective of an integrated approach to the solution of nutrition problems. The Board was composed of persons of diverse experience who could view the problems of nutrition from the points of view of health, agriculture, labour, economics and finance, social welfare, etc.

On its opening to the public in 1948, the Institute set up a nutritional biochemistry laboratory to provide tools for community nutrition work. Food analyses were undertaken, data of which were published in a handbook *Food Composition Tables* for use by nutrition and allied workers. The IN also developed the Basic Six Food Groups to serve as a guide in planning adequate meals. Since beriberi was one of the leading deficiency diseases at that time, the IN launched the Rice Enrichment Program. A systematic programme of nutrition education, information and training was also conducted to help combat ignorance of fundamental nutrition facts, to develop an appreciation of the importance of attaining facts, to develop an appreciation of the importance of attaining good health through proper nutrition and to educate the public on the wise choice of foods.

In 1950, the IN was transferred from the Office of the President to the Department of Health. However, the increasing recognition of the need for more studies in food and nutrition shifted the IN to the National Science Development Board, as a research arm under one of its agencies by virtue of the Science Act of 1958. It was then renamed the Food and Nutrition Research Center (FNRC). The personnel of the IN and that of the Food Technology Division of the Institute of Science and Technology formed the nucleus of the Research Center.

The original five divisions of the Center were reduced to four with the transfer of the Rice Enrichment Division back to the Department of Health. Again, in 1974 by virtue of Presidential Decree No. 233 (IPS), the FNRC was elevated into a commission level and is now an agency directly under the NSDB. Its research activities in the basic and applied science of food and nutrition have been expanded and can be categorized as follows.

Nutrition research*

Some local foods and mixed diets are evaluated through availability, digestibility and toxicity studies as well as through their effects on growth and reproduction. Normal nutrient levels and the nutrient requirements of Filipinos have been established for use as bases in recommendeding nutrient allowances and in evaluating nutrition survey data. In turn, these recommendations and evaluations are used by

*Editor's note: The work of the International Rice Research Institute at Los Banos is referred to in Chapter 25.

various agencies as bases for national food plans. A table on standard heights and weights has been recently developed as a tool in evaluating the nutritional status of Filipinos.

Food research

Analysis of local foods for nutritive value is given priority. Data obtained have been used in the preparation of food composition tables, in the evaluation of diets and in the formulation of some agricultural programmes in the country. Food formulations are continually developed to come out with low-cost nutrient-packed products. At present, studies are geared to high-protein food supplements from local materials for use in supplementary feeding of infants and young children.

Medical and applied nutrition

Studies on dietary intake and energy cost of different occupational activities and institutional feeding, standardization of native recipes and development of food plans and guides are conducted. Community nutrition education programmes are evaluated for their effectiveness as measures for promoting good nutrition. Also being studied is the relationship between food and disease, including measures to prevent and correct nutritional disturbances. The FNRC has conducted a nationwide nutrition survey on a regional basis (1958–1969). The survey results provided the rationale in formulating the *Philippine Food and Nutrition Program*. This survey identified the scope of the problem in terms of population groups affected and specific nutritional deficiencies. The FNRC has recently launched the first of a series of food consumption surveys that will ultimately cover the entire country. This survey will be carried out periodically to monitor the Filipino people's dietary habits.

In addition to its research activities, the FNRC has at the same time retained 'service' functions such as technical consultation and laboratory analyses for both government and private sectors.

The Food and Nutrition Research Center has provided leadership in the country's fight against malnutrition. It has stimulated the interest of and action from all those who should be concerned in the national nutrition effort.

THE COUNTRY'S MALNUTRITION PROBLEM

The nationwide nutrition survey conducted by the Food and Nutrition Research Center shows glaring deficiencies in the typical Filipino meal of 'rice and fish'. Table 1 suggests the nutritional problems in the country.

Except for cereals and 'other fruits and vegetables' intake of all other foods is below the daily recommended food allowances. In terms of nutrients (Table 2), the typical diet is lacking in energy value. It is estimated that about two-thirds of all households in the country eat energy deficient meals. In spite of a more than sufficient intake of cereals (Table 1), the diet is lacking in energy value because of low consumption of all other foods. While the protein intake (93.5 per cent adequate) is almost satisfactory, the energy lack does not allow the use of protein for its more important function of body-building, and instead it is expensively used for energy purposes. Such lack results in rampant protein–energy malnutrition and nutritional dwarfism particularly among pre-school children.[8]

Table 1. Mean daily per capita food intake compared to recommended daily allowances[a]

Food groups	RDA	Intake (g)	% Adequacy
Cereals	325	335	103
Starchy roots and tubers	60	52	87
Sugars and syrups	28	18	64
Dried beans, nuts and seeds	16	7	44
Leafy and yellow vegetables	55	18	33
Vitamin C-rich fruits	55	23	42
Other fruits and vegetables	90	92	102
Meat, poultry and fish	87	76	87
Eggs	13	4	31
Milk and milk products	90	24	27
Fats and oils	30	8	27

[a] Results of the nine regional nutrition surveys conducted in the Philippines by the Food and Nutrition Research Center, National Science Development Board, unpublished.

The energy consumption pattern shows that 11 per cent of the energy intake is derived from protein food sources, 10 per cent from fat and 79 per cent from carbohydrate foods. The recommended pattern is for 11 per cent of energy to come from protein, 21 per cent from fat and 68 per cent from carbohydrates.[9] To close the energy gap (deficient by 16.6 per cent), the corrective measures lie in increasing the proportion of both fat and protein, particularly animal protein. Thus, a more generous consumption of fish, meat, eggs and milk and most especially fats and oils is needed. Incidentally, the increase in fat intake will help to correct the existing vitamin A deficiency which is also one of our major nutrition problems.

About a quarter of the population have deficient/low blood vitamin A level. Leafy green vegetables which are good sources of carotene (precursor of vitamin A) are not eaten in sufficient amounts (only 33 per cent adequate, Table 1). In the rural areas, butter or animal fat seldom appear in the diet so that preformed vitamin A is hardly present. The carotene obtained from leafy vegetables is poorly converted to vitamin A because the amount of dietary fat is not sufficient to make this possible.

Iron deficiency constitutes one of our major nutritional problems although dietary data (Table 2) do not show this. Blood analysis and clinical diagnosis showed that the 1–6 years age group, the pregnant and the lactating mothers are the vulnerable groups seriously affected by nutritional anaemia. There is rampant anaemia, in spite of a supposedly high iron intake as revealed in the dietary survey, due to the fact that the source of iron in our diet is mostly from plant foods. Iron from plant foods is not easily absorbed or made available to the body. Furthermore, in the presence of a high cereal intake, the utilization of iron is further decreased. Another reason for anaemia is intestinal parasitism. Ninety-three per cent of our children have ascaris. For adults, the overall incidence of parasitism is 87 per cent. Sixty-seven per cent of deaths from the country's ten major causes of deaths are from infections.

Table 2. Mean daily per capita nutrient intake compared to recommended daily allowances (RDA) in *Nine Regions of the Philippines*, 1958–1969[a]

	RDA	Intake	% Adequacy
Calories [b]	2003	1671	83.4
Protein (g)	49.4	46.2	93.5
Calcium (g)	0.57	0.34	59.6
Iron (g)	10	9	90.0
Vitamin A (I.U.)	4006	1812	44.6
Thiamine (mg)	1.02	0.73	71.6
Riboflavin (mg)	1.02	0.47	46.1
Niacin (mg)	13	14	107.7
Ascorbic acid (mg)	69	67	97.1

[a] Results of the nine regional nutrition surveys conducted in the Philippines by the Food and Nutrition Research Center, National Science Development Board, unpublished.

[b] 1 Calorie = approx. 4.2 joules.

The major causes of malnutrition in the country have been traced to lack of knowledge of food values and a low food supply aggravated by a high birth rate and low income.

COORDINATION: A BOLD APPROACH TO THE MALNUTRITION PROBLEM IN THE PHILIPPINES

As an initial step towards synchronizing activities, the Food and Nutrition Research Center initiated the organization of intra-agency committees for nutrition within the Departments of Health, Agriculture, Education and National Defense.[10] The organization of these intra-agency committees paved the way for the formal creation of the National Coordinating Committee on Food and Nutrition (NCCFN) in June, 1960 by the FNRC. Member agencies included the major government agencies represented by the respective chairmen of intra-agencies together with representatives of other allied agencies and organizations. These representatives were from the intermediate level (supervisory) which placed them in a position of being able to deal directly with the policy-making authorities in their offices while at the same time capable of reaching their workers in direct contact with the communities. Member agencies adopted the scheme of self-finance in carrying out activities agreed upon by the Committee.

NCCFN activity: The regional post nutrition survey conferences

The Food and Nutrition Research Center conducted regional conferences to bring back to the local people results of the nutrition survey conducted in the area. The first regional post nutrition survey conference started in November, 1960. By 1968, all ten regions of the country were covered. This was a total NCCFN undertaking, member agencies participated in the conferences by sending regional and provincial personnel to deliberate on the survey results and plan local programmes.

The conferences served as a meeting ground for various disciplines from the administrative, supervisory and working levels. Participation in the conference committed each one to carry over the philosophy of coordination down to the local level: the barrio (village). Each participant also served to sensitize the local people and their leaders to the need for action programmes in nutrition.

As an offshoot of the regional conferences, local coordinating councils on nutrition at various geographical levels were subsequently organized. One member agency, Nutrition Foundation of the Philippines, was made largely responsible for the organization of local machinery for action.

Meanwhile, at about the same time, significant developments were taking place at the national level.[11] From the original ten-member agency representatives, the Committee expanded to involve more agencies which signified an interest in joining. Thus, three Committees evolved to coordinate activities within their sphere; Food Research, Nutrition Research and Applied Nutrition. With the expansion to about 45 representatives from a total of 40 agencies/organizations came the change of the name of 'Committee' to 'Council'.

The National Council is credited for the ideas of group thinking and planning which gave birth to many of the country's nutrition projects. The blueprint for the Philippine Applied Nutrition Project under the Department of Education and Culture was drawn from NCCFN deliberations.[12] The encouraging experience in the pilot area motivated other provinces to implement an ANP, even if only on a self-help basis.[13]

Ten years after NCCFN was formally established, the President of the Republic, through Executive Order 285 dated January 21, 1971, authorized the National Food and Agriculture Council* (NFAC) to coordinate all nutrition activities. This gave way to a merger between NFAC and NCCFN, providing the latter with an op-

---

*NFAC was organised on 6 May, 1969 to coordinate the production of rice, corn, feed grain, livestock and fruits and vegetables.

portunity to influence the formulation of the country's food and nutrition policies based on the widespread incidence of malnutrition. The machinery established by NCCFN and its experiences in planning and implementing nutrition programmes have been very useful indeed in directing NFAC's seemingly difficult task of coordinating nutrition activities of agencies engaged in nutrition work.

THE PHILIPPINE FOOD AND NUTRITION PROGRAMME

As an initial step towards the development of a nationwide coordinated programme on food and nutrition, NFAC created a working committee composed of NCCFN member agencies 'to review the country's malnutrition problems; make an inventory of activities and agencies undertaking them: and to draft a 4-Year National Plan on Food and Nutrition'.

Specifically, the objectives of the PFNP were formulated on a basis of existing malnutrition problems. The improvement of the nutritional status of vulnerable groups (pregnant women and lactating mothers, pre-school and school children) comes as a major objective. Goals have been set on increasing food supply, promotion of good nutrition, intensification of relevant food and nutrition researches as well as family planning and establishment of income-generating activities to complete the total development approach through good nutrition. Lending valuable support and cooperation are bilateral and international agencies such as UNICEF, USAID, WHO and FAO.

Sectoral projects

In building up the Programme, nutrition activities were grouped into four major sectoral activities. Responsibility for implementing a sectoral project remains with the particular agency which by nature of its function should be most rightly concerned therein. Thus, the sectoral activity on Nutrition Training is led by the Department of Education and Culture (DEC); Community Nutrition Education is under the Bureau of Agriculture Extension (BAEx) of the Department of Agriculture and Natural Resources (DANR); Food Production falls within the Bureau of Agricultural Extension and Bureau of Plant Industry (also of the DANR), Supplementary Feeding and Nutrition Rehabilitation (establishment of Malnutrition Wards) are led by the Department of Health.

The Food and Nutrition Research Center is responsible for the training of professional nutrition workers. It offers a three-month voluntary training course for graduates of medicine, nutrition, food technology and chemistry in specialized fields of nutrition and food research and activities.

Community nutrition education, which is the lead function of the Bureau of Agricultural Extension, enjoins the participation of various members of the community, from mothers to youths, in cooperative endeavours such as attending the homemakers' course, cooking demonstrations, and community assemblies. The community is organized into a Rural Improvement Club (association of village women), 4-H Club (youth) and Farmers' Club. Such local organizations serve as the machinery for implementing the various activities. Nutrition education in the schools centres on motivating school children to intensify food production and observe proper nutrition through demonstrations of meal planning, and the selection, preparation and preservation of food. Lessons on food and nutrition are integrated in all classroom subjects at all levels.

Family planning is one aspect taken up in all nutrition education activities. Population education is also given in the schools.

As an expedient measure to improve the nutritional status of the vulnerable groups and, more importantly, as an approach to nutrition education, feeding centres are operated with the Department of Health taking the lead. With mothers of the malnourished children actively participating in the preparation of suitable foods, the centre serves as a demonstration site whereby the community learns one way of combating its own nutrition problems. A close link between the nutrition education activities and the supplementary feeding programme, is readily apparent, bringing the home extension workers and rural health personnel into direct cooperation. Many other government and private agencies and organizations are actually involved in feeding operations with the local health staff coordinating such activities.

Nutrition rehabilitation wards are established in local hospitals to take care of severely malnourished children. The ward also serves as a training site for health personnel on the recognition of signs and symptoms of malnutrition and on the rehabilitation of the malnourished child through diet therapy and nutrition education of mothers.

Supporting activities

The conduct of relevant food and nutrition researches is a supportive activity of the PFNP. This is the primary responsibility of the Food and Nutrition Research Center which coordinates the country's research activities on food and nutrition.

The Mass Communication Program on Food and Nutrition has been designed to provide the communication support to the Nutrition Program. The strategy formulated utilizes the interpersonal link established by community workers with the target group and the use of print and broadcast media in disseminating research-based, accurate and consistent nutrition information. Again the FNRC, through the Interdepartmental Committee on Nutrition Communication, has been given the responsibility of coordinating the development, production and distribution of information materials.

Organizational machinery

At the national level, the Secretary of Agriculture serves as the Chairman of the National Food and Agriculture Council. He is assisted by the Executive Director, who directs implementation of the nutrition programme. A Secretariat composed of technical personnel prepares all the necessary working documents in consultation with cooperating agencies.

Several committees have been created at the *national level* to facilitate implementation. These include: 1. A Policy Committee composed of the Secretariats of the Department of Agriculture and Natural Resources, Department of Education and Culture, Department of Health, Department of Social Welfare and the Chairman of the National Science Development Board. This Committee formulates national policies on food and nutrition and ensures their implementation.

2. A Management Committee composed of heads or their representatives, of all agencies cooperating under the programme. This Committee outlines common agreements on strategies and programme targets as well as preparing guidelines for the operation of the programme. It meets once a month regularly and as the need arises.

3. An Inter-agency Action Team for Nutrition (INTACT) composed of members from cooperating agencies. This group develops evaluation instruments for determining progress in programme implementation. In the field, it institutes spot decisions for improved coordination and programme implementation. Members maintain a periodic schedule of field visits. The members, also sitting in the Management Committee, serve as the liaison between the Provisional Nutrition Councils and the Management Committee.

4. An Interdepartmental Committee on Nutrition Communication (ICNC) composed of representatives from cooperating agencies who are directly involved in the development and production of information materials. The ICNC takes charge of coordinating the development, production and dissemination of information materials for consistency of nutrition information.

At the *provincial level*, NFAC designates a Chairman who is a food production man. He serves as the overall coordinator of the six NFAC-coordinated programmes, in the province (rice and corn, feedtrains, poultry and livestock, fisheries, fruits and vegetables, and nutrition, which is the latest addition). At the same level can be found the Provincial Nutrition Council, composed of heads of the provincial offices of national agencies. Members also include representatives from the Office of the Provincial Administrator as well as those from private, religious and civic organizations. The Chairman of the Council, who is elected from among its members, at the same time serves as the Provincial Program Officer for Nutrition. Assisting the Program Officer are Project officers on each of the major sectoral activities. The Project Officer is designated from the lead agency implementing the specific activity. Together, the officers constitute the Provincial Program Staff. At the *municipal and barrio levels,* the same set-up is duplicated. Nutrition councils at these levels are responsible for planning and implementing food and nutrition activities in their areas.

The Nutrition Foundation of the Philippines, a private agency and another cooperator, is responsible for breaking the ground for the scheme by spearheading the organization of the provincial nutrition councils. As part of its commitment, NFP nutritionists see to it that the Councils are viable organizations that actively implement the programme.

At the *barrio level,* the organisation of a team of workers helps ensure the availability of technical manpower to oversee implementation of the programme.

Agency contribution in terms of personnel deployment puts together the home management technician (BAEx), farm management technician (BAEx), rural health physician, nurse or midwife (Department of Health), Home Economics and Agriculture teachers (Department of Education). It is through this team that the Program is able to reach the grass-roots level. These personnel make up the barrio team as a concrete demonstration of coordination in action in the solution of local nutrition problems.

Concentration of resources

A gradual expansion scheme covering ten provinces* every year was initially adopted to make an effective demonstration of the feasibility of the team approach in programme implementation. Ten barrios† are selected from each province as demonstration areas for the integrated, intersectoral approach. In each of these, a complete team is assigned to look after programme implementation. The programme is envisioned to radiate from here to adjoining barrios and municipalities.

Currently, the programme is covering 967 barrios in 21 provinces. The modest success experienced during the past three years has brought new dimensions to the programme. By the middle of 1974, 20 more provinces located in various parts of the country had launched the coordinated scheme. Many more provinces than can now be covered by present logistics have signified interest through their respective governors. It is envisioned that the remaining 30 provinces will be served by the programme in the very near future.

Evaluation

Periodic visits to the provinces are conducted by members of the INTACT group. Strengths and weaknesses of the programme are noted and these are immediately brought to the attention of the Management Committee should there be need for any action at the national level. Otherwise, local problems are encouraged to be resolved in the area concerned. The Provincial Program Staff also monitor the implementation of the programme. They hold monthly meetings and undertake quarterly team evaluation apart from the monthly visits to each programme barrio by the respective project officers. Results of these visits are used as bases for planning course of action, and the programme has been continually enriched by experiences gained in the field. Although the programme continues to show the promise of the coordinated scheme, some barriers remain that need to be overcome, primarily that of funding.

*Programme provinces are selected on the following bases: extent of malnutrition problem in the province; desire of the province to undertake such a programme; support of the provincial government in terms of financial, material and technical resources; availability of field technicians; presence of an established food and nutrition activity.

†Programme barrios are selected by the Provincial Nutrition Council on the basis of the following criteria: expressed need and desire by the community; willingness of the community to participate in the programme; possibility of food production; presence of a programme organization and ongoing activities in food and nutrition.

CONCLUSION

The fact that nutrition should be a top priority in the nation's development has been given a most concrete recognition. The President has recently signed a Decree creating the Nutrition Center of the Philippines, a supportive private organization that will mobilize the necessary resources for the country's nutrition programme. The same Decree established the National Nutrition Council, the government nutrition-coordinating body at the highest level. The elevation of the Council to this level has placed the Philippine Food and Nutrition Program in a position where it can now maximize its spread and impact.

REFERENCES

1. Concepcion, I. Development of nutrition work in the Philippines, *Bull. Nat. Res. Counc. (Philippines)*, **5**, 503 (1935).
2. Concepcion, I. Recent programs in nutrition, *Philippine Women's Magazine,* **9**(3), 3 (1938).
3. Salcedo, J. Jr. and D. L. Bocobo. Progress of nutrition work in the Philippines, *Nutr. News,* **7**(1), (1954).
4. Intengan, C. L., A. M. Manguera and D. B. Aguillon. Forty year review of nutrition progress in the Philippines, *Philippine J. Nutr.,* **15,** (3), July–September (1962).
5. Intengan, C. L. Progress report of nutrition in the Philippines, *Third Far East Symp. Nutr.,* Manila, Philippines, February 14–21, 1967.
6. Pascual, C. R., F. Herrera and D. B. Aguillon. The Nutrition Education Program in the Philippines, *Philippine J. Nutr.,* **16,** 12 (1963).
7. Inciong, M. B. The Philippine Association of Nutrition, *Philippine J. Nutr.,* **15** (2), April–June (1962).
8. Jayme, J. B. Profile of malnutrition and ill-health in the Philippines. *FNRC Publication No. 143,* Revised June 15, 1974. Mimeo.
9. Intengan, C. L. What is the protein gap? *Philippine J. Nutr.,* **25,** January–March, 7 (1972).
10. Pascual, C. R. A. coordinated approach toward a more effective community nutrition programme, *Proc. the Sixth Intern. Congr. Nutr.,* Edinburgh, Scotland, August 9–15, 1963, p. 175.
11. National Coordinating Council on Food and Nutrition. Report of Activities of NCCFN, 1965–1967, Manila, 1969.
12. Bureau of Public Schools, The Applied Nutrition Project, An International Brochure, 1966–1967.
13. Suter, C. B. Strengthening cooperation and coordination in community nutrition work in Isabela, *Philippine J. Nutr.,* **20** April–June, 1967.

CHAPTER 30

Nutrition in the United Kingdom

DOROTHY F. HOLLINGSWORTH AND FREDA S. PATTON

BEFORE THE SECOND WORLD WAR

The dietary problems that faced Britain a century ago were different from those against which we contend now. A lack of appreciation of the relationship between the food a person eats and his or her ability to live in health and to work must have been at least partly responsible for the semi-starvation during the early part of the 19th century in prisons, institutions and schools, which is vividly described in the literature of the time. A first step towards improvement was the setting up in 1843 of a Royal Commission to inquire into 'the state of the large towns and populous districts with reference to the causes of disease and into the best means of promoting and securing the public health . . .'; this led to the appointment of the first Medical Officer of Health in Liverpool in 1847, and to the Public Health Act of 1848, which carried a regulation which made compulsory the appointment of Medical Officers of Health throughout the country.

Socially aware people grew increasingly concerned at the poor living conditions and poverty in working-class districts in England. One result of this was the efforts of a number of charities to provide some food, perhaps only a bowl of soup during the winter months, for poor children at school. Seebohm Rowntree in York and Charles Booth in London were struggling to make known the evils of poverty, but no great public notice was taken of their efforts until the Director-General of the Army Medical Service reported that the Inspector of Recruiting was having great difficulty in finding suffieient men of satisfactory physique for service in the South African War.

These difficulties led to the appointment of the inter-departmental committee on physical deterioration, the report of which, published in 1904, still makes fascinating, though horrifying, reading.[1] The committee attempted to identify the causes of poor physique and ill health in the working class. With modern nutritional knowledge, it is fairly easy to incriminate food shortage and ill balance of diet caused by sheer poverty. Several witnesses mentioned lack of cooking skills among working-class women and one medical witness deplored the fact that the poor ate white bread and drank tea instead of, as was claimed for former times, living on oatmeal and milk. The report led indirectly to the Education (Provision of Meals)

Act of 1906 which gave local education authorities power to provide meals free or at reduced charge for necessitous children. Thus, it had far-reaching importance for nutrition in the community.

At much the same time there was concern about the teaching of cooking in schools and the demand for teachers of cookery exceeded the supply. At the end of the century the first inspectors of needlework and of cookery and laundry were appointed by the Board of Education and in 1902 the establishment of women inspectors was increased so that by 1904 seven had been appointed. This impetus to women's education was the result, at least in part, of the disturbing findings about the physical condition of men being recruited to fight at the end of Queen Victoria's reign. The report on physical deterioration was the starting point in the long chain of legislation leading to the present national school meals service and widespread teaching of home economics, not only to girls but also in some instances to boys.

The year 1906 was also memorable for the first national conference on infant mortality, which was held in London under the presidency of the head of the local government board at a time when the infant mortality rate was 138 per 1000 live births (compared with the present rate of less than 20),[2] and for the publication of *Infant Mortality, a Social Problem,* by George Newman.[3] These influences led to the infant welfare movement through which mothers were taught improved methods of child care, including infant feeding.

By 1912, the existence and importance of 'accessory food factors' had been established by Frederick Gowland Hopkins and others, and in that year Casimir Funk described deficiency diseases which he concluded were caused by lack of substances in the diet that he called 'vitamines'.

The First World War broke out before the importance of the discovery of vitamins was appreciated, and in August 1914 neither side understood that the successful solution of food problems would play a big part in determining victory. Nevertheless, in late 1916 a Royal Society committee of physiologists drew up the first estimate of the food resources and requirements of Britain, and the first Ministry of Food was formed. At first scientific advice was not sought but the Royal Society Food (War) Committee protested and pressed hard for the introduction of measures that now seem commonplace. After May 1917, with new direction at the Ministry, changes were made in the national diet in accordance with scientific knowledge, with the result that Britain ended the war in a better nutritional position than the rest of combatant Europe.[4]

Advance in applied nutrition seems to have been accelerated by wars. The South African War revealed the poor physique of large sections of the population; the 1914–1918 war brought the first application of scientific findings to the problem of feeding the nation; and the spread of disease across post-war continental Europe offered opportunities of studying the causes of various diseases of dietetic origin, particularly rickets.

It took another catastrophe in the shape of the economic depression and unemployment of the 1930s to cause the authorities to consider how sufficient food, which by that time was known scientifically to be necessary for health, could be provided at a cost within the means of the whole population. Dietary surveys made in the 1930s revealed diets among the unemployed of comparable quality to the poverty diets of the late 19th century. There was growing understanding that gross poverty is a worldwide limitation to good nutrition. In 1931 the Minister of Health set up an advisory committee of physiologists to advise him 'on the practical application of modern advances in the knowledge of nutrition'.[5] The British Medical Association[6] reported the recommendations of their Committee on Nutrition on the minimum cost of an adequate diet. In 1935 the National Birthday Trust began an experiment in the Rhondda Valley, which showed that the combined stillbirth and infant mortality rate of the children born to a group of mothers whose diet had been supplemented was 58 per 1000 compared with 85 per 1000 for the group whose diet was not supplemented. In 1936 John Boyd Orr published *Food Health and Income,* which showed that the average diet of the poorest section of the population, comprising $4\frac{1}{2}$ million people, was deficient in every constituent examined; over one-fifth of the children in Britain were estimated to belong to that group.[7]

In earlier years undernutrition could be directly traced to the failure of harvests, but in the 1930s the reverse was true: not shortage, but the inability of the farmer to sell his produce was the first of a sequence of events that led to economic depression. The first proposal to expand the market for food came from Australia. Experiments were in progress in Britain and America for the disposal of surplus milk and other foods, not by the then accepted method of destruction but by giving them away in the form of relief to the unemployed or for the feeding of school children. The principle of the 'marriage of health and agriculture' was first enunciated by an Australian, F. L. McDougall (who later became Deputy Director of the Food and Agriculture Organization of the United Nations) and was put before the League of Nations in 1935 by Viscount Bruce, at that time Australian High Commissioner. The result was the establishment of the League of Nations Mixed Committee on the Relation of Nutrition to Health, Agriculture and Economic Policy, the final report of which can be studied with profit today.[8]

Thus, when a fourth catastrophe struck Britain in 1939 the government was fitted to apply the nutritional and economic experience of the previous 40 years. Many of the problems which had to be faced then have still, perhaps for other reasons, to be tackled today. Thus, it is of both historical interest and present relevance to consider how Britain was fed in wartime.[9]

WARTIME NUTRITION POLICY

Plans for rationing and distribution of foods based on the experience of the First World War had been drawn up before the outbreak of war in 1939, and early in 1940 the Scientific Adviser of the newly established second Ministry of Food prepared a notable document 'on certain nutritional aspects of the food position', in which he reviewed the pre-war nutritional situation of the United Kingdom and the likely effects on it of the restrictions of war, particularly on the poorer groups of the population. It is clear from the official documents on food prepared at the time that the nutritional advisers of the government, supported by Lord Woolton at the

Ministry of Food, set out from the beginning of the war to maintain and improve the nutritional value of the diet. The first official indication of the influence of J. C. Drummond (the first Scientific Adviser of the Ministry of Food) on food policy appeared in May 1940 in the Ministry's import programme for the second year of war, which carried an appendix, *A Survey of Wartime Nutrition,* in which was stated in detailed and quantitative form a nutritional strategy for the Ministry. This was probably the first attempt made jointly by economists, statisticians and nutritional scientists to provide a practical basis for a national nutrition policy. Such plans have subsequently become almost commonplace, but the British wartime plan was a prototype. The plan contained estimates of the nutritional requirements of the total population and the nutritional value of expected imports and home production of foods. In it the need for sufficient food energy to meet the national human energy expenditure was emphasized.

The measures which were planned and put into effect included steps to increase the supply of milk and milk products, particularly for expectant and nursing mothers, infants and children; to provide orange juice and cod liver oil or vitamin A and D tablets for the same groups; to expand the school meals service; to increase the national supplies of vitamins of the B complex by raising the extraction rate of flour; to fortify flour with calcium carbonate; and to increase the production and consumption of carrots and green vegetables. These measures were superimposed on a general system of rationing of carcase meat, bacon, fats, sugar, preserves, sweets and tea, and of allocation of eggs and milk a 'points' rationing scheme under which non-perishable foods, mainly canned and dried, too scarce to ration, could be bought against special coupons. There was also a system of generous allowances to factory and works canteens in which nourishing meals, which were not rationed, were obtained. Throughout the war bread, flour and potatoes were not rationed and this ready supply of these important energy sources in the British diet ensured that the rationing system was not too restrictive for those with particularly large energy requirements. After the end of the war, when there was a severe world cereal shortage, flour, bread and flour confectionery were also rationed and, because of a poor potato crop, the distribution of potatoes had to be controlled during the winter 1947–1948. Wartime food policy included measures to increase British agricultural production, including the intensive cultivation of vegetables in small plots and gardens. As a result of great effort the energy value of home-produced foods was increased from about 900 kcal (3.8 MJ) per head per day (or about 30 per cent of the total supply) before the war to 1200 kcal (5.0 MJ) (or 40 per cent of the total) in 1943 and 1944 (compared with about half the total of about 3100 kcal (13.0 MJ) per head per day in 1974). Import programmes were reviewed so that priority could be given to foods with the greatest energy density. Space was saved by importing boneless meat and 'telescoped' carcases and such unfamiliar foods as dried eggs and dried milk.[4]

The introduction of unfamiliar foods and the need to change food habits led to the instigation of a national food advice service, based on the Ministry of Food, which included on its staff home economists and dietitians, and operated through some 50 centres in the larger towns. Part of its task was to teach the people how to use unfamiliar foods, such as dried eggs and dried milk, and how to compensate for the shortage of vitamin C from fresh fruits by eating raw vegetable salads or by cooking green vegetables conservatively. This relatively simple aim led to a widespread programme of cookery instruction and of education in nutrition by means of leaflets, posters, lectures and radio talks and extensive advertising in the national press, and practical cookery demonstrations. Though the focal point of this effort was the Ministry of Food, the programme had the cooperation of the Ministries of Health and Education and of many voluntary organizations. It became a truly national one because of the enthusiastic and trained support of countless home economics teachers, dietitians, school meal organizers, hospital caterers and public health workers who all demonstrated that simple nutrition could be both taught and practised. An important aid to teaching was the Ministry of Food's booklet, *Manual of Nutrition,* first published in 1945. It became an immediate bestseller and, so far, has run to seven editions.[10]

During the war hospitals experienced many new catering problems, and to advise on hospital diet and feeding arrangements in 1944 the Ministry of Health appointed two dieticians. In the same year the King Edward's Hospital Fund for London appointed one dietician to provide a similar service for voluntary hospitals within the London area, and a second in the following year. Later, the Ministry of Health increased its staff of advisory dieticians. Thus began a new valuable advisory service which continued with the institution of the National Health Service.

In 1947 the American Public Health Association recognized the British wartime achievement in national nutrition by giving the Lasker Group Award to the British Ministries of Food and Health 'For the unprecedented program of food distribution in Great Britain, with resulting improvement in the health of the people'.

In considering in retrospect this story of success at least two points should be understood. The first was that the 1939–1945 war gave the British government a unique opportunity to impose a nutritionally sound food policy because the government owned most of the food supply at some point in the chain of food distribution, and took advantage of that opportunity. The second point is made in the history of the second Ministry of Food by Hammond[11] who reached the view that 'it was only possible for scientists to influence food policy if they were behind the scenes and privy to the innermost counsels of the Ministries of Food and Agriculture' and that the employment in these Ministeries of appropriate scientists, who could exert 'steady pressure from within', was more effective than pronouncements from outside.

After the end of the war the national diet suffered through the abrupt ending of the 'lend-lease' arrangements with the USA and the consequent need to switch purchases of food from dollar to non-dollar sources. However, after a few years of somewhat precarious food supply, food rationing came quietly to an end in 1954. Since then part of the national nutritional policy has been retained. For example, in 1974 there were still controls over the nutritional composition of bread and margarine. After some changes in the various welfare provisions young school children were still entitled to free school milk and all school children to subsidized or free school meals, according to income. Subsidized milk was no longer available for expectant mothers and pre-school children, though there was special 'welfare' provision of vitamins A, C and D. At the time of rapid inflation general subsidies were introduced on some important foods.

TRENDS IN FOOD CONSUMPTION IN THE 20th CENTURY

The long-term trends in the consumption of foods can be summarized in terms of their nutritional value.[12,13] The total amount of food energy available in the average diet rose between the beginning of the century and the years following the Second World War. Since then it has hardly varied, though the amount of energy expended by the population has almost certainly decreased. No national statistics on the incidence of obesity exist, but there is a general impression that it is increasing. Any increase is probably associated with decreased physical activity and many public health authorities are expressing concern about this (Chapters 9 and 19). The consumption of total carbohydrate rose slightly during and after the war, but since 1970 has been gradually falling. The consumption of sucrose, as opposed to that of total carbohydrate, has shown a different trend. Except for decreased consumption during both world wars and in the early 1920s when prices were high, the consumption of sucrose rose until 1958, since when there has been a slight fall. From the beginning of the century till the early 1960s the consumption of fat rose, and then became almost constant. During the same interval of time the percentage of food energy derived from fat rose from just over 30 per cent to 42 per cent, while that from carbohydrate fell from 56 per cent to 47 per cent (mainly because of constantly decreasing consumption of flour and bread). The consumption of protein has not changed much, though in recent years the proportion from animal sources has increased. Protein usually provides 11–12 per cent of the food energy. In recent years there has been a steady rise in alcohol consumption from an amount equivalent to less than 100 kcal (418 kJ) per head per day in 1955 to an equivalent of over 140 kcal (586 kJ) in 1972. These changes resemble those occurring in other affluent societies and are the cause of concern among public health authorities.

PRESENT-DAY DEVELOPMENTS IN COMMUNITY NUTRITION

Since the end of food rationing and control there has been no publicly agreed policy for nutrition or nutrition education and, because of this, there has been an increasing demand by local authorities and by the general public for advice on current nutritional problems.

People have come to realize that obesity in babies, in school children and in adults has increased and that it is unhealthy; that there has been an increase in the number of deaths from coronary heart disease; that there has been an increase in the incidence of dental caries; that the steep and steady increase in food prices makes it necessary to budget for food more carefully; and they realize that in terms of good health it is important to learn about the nutritional value of the food they eat. The problems of Commonwealth immigrants in adapting to different foods and environments are becoming recognized. One of the most urgent problems is that osteomalacia among Asian women and rickets among Asian children has been reported from many parts of the country, and research is in progress into the cause of this and the ways of dealing with it.*

Shopping facilities have changed. In the 1940s and 1950s most people used small family shops where they were able to receive some advice and assessment of the foods they bought through personal contact with the shopkeeper. These have largely been replaced by the supermarkets which offer a wide variety of both new and familiar foods. Food manufacturers advertising in all the media have persuaded people to try new products, thus creating a demand for simple advice about the nutritional effects of modern food processing, the quality of food and comparative nutritional values. People are beginning to question the value of food now available and its effect on health.

The evaluation of nutritional intakes, the composition of foods, and research studies involving dietary changes are continuously assessed and monitored by appropriately qualified professional and scientific staff in government departments and research institutions.[14-16] This work is directly applicable to nutrition in the community.

Some local authorities, under the guidance of Medical Officers of Health, became aware that they needed professional help with nutrition problems and with the giving of nutrition advice and in 1946 C. Fraser Brockington (1946), then County Medical Officer of Health for Warwickshire, recommended the creation of posts for dieticians 'from which can be surveyed the whole dietetic field, including the mass of the people, old and young, healthy and diseased, at home or in hospital, school, factory or workshop'.[17] Yet 20 years later, R. C. Wofinden, Professor of Public Health at the University of Bristol, and Medical Officer of Health for the City and County of Bristol (where a nutritionist had been working since 1949), pointed out with Margaret Chapman[18] that not more than five local authorities were employing dieticians, saying that: 'In this country sufficient food is available for everyone to be adequately fed; nevertheless, malnutrition as manifest by, for example, obesity, anaemia, dental decay, still exists because essential nutrients are not taken in the correct proportion. This failure to eat the right foods for promoting good health often presents a greater problem than an overall insufficiency because it involves bringing the individual or the community to understand and accept the advantages of choosing one food rather than another. The work of a dietician in a Department of Public Health is, therefore, directed towards promoting this better understanding of food values so that through wise choice and consumption of foods, nutritional standards are raised, thereby preventing disease and improving health'.

In 1974 23 dietitians and nutritionists were working in the community in the United Kingdom (8 in Scotland). Some were in part-time employment. Most appointments had been made to local authority or county Health Departments, and a few were appointed to Social Service Directorates and Health Education Departments. About half of these appointments were made between 1969 and

*Editor's note: See reference 15.

1974. The group of community dietitians working in the United Kingdom in prepared 'Notes for guidance for dietitians working in the community.[19] These notes state clearly that the main aims of community work are to promote health and to prevent disease by promoting improved nutrition in the population at large. Working in conjunction with community physicians, the nursing and health education services, the dietician should advise on nutritional problems, provide the necessary educational material and diet sheets and participate fully in health education campaigns. In the Social Services and Education Services she has a responsibility to advise on nutritional requirements in community feeding centres, residential homes and schools, and to advise on dietary modifications for the elderly and any specially vulnerable groups.

Nutrition advice in the community health service has traditionally been offered by a variety of professional people which includes doctors, dentists, district nurses, school nurses, health visitors, midwives, and health education officers; dieticians in the hospital service have seized every opportunity that ocurs for working in the community.

The dietitian or nutritionist in the community works in conjunction with and through her colleagues by giving them her specialist knowledge. Even where appointments had been made to do a specific job, those occupying such posts have expanded their work wherever there was a need. The work is largely of an educational nature and requires a close liaison with those working in health education in the use of visual aids and the production of leaflets and other material. The pattern of good or bad eating habits is established early in life and liaison with home economics and science teachers in schools as a sustained and continuous programme of education is offered by some dieticians. Home economics teachers instruct pupils from the age of 11 onwards in the basic elements of sound nutrition, and through practical lessons on choosing, buying, cooking and serving nutritious meals they introduce the foundations of good family eating habits.

Free choice of foods coupled with affluence have led to malnutrition in the form of overnutrition. The problem of obesity is tackled in the community in various ways: in child health clinics; in schools; by group therapy (including physical exercise classes), which is a service offered through general medical practitioners by some authorities. Other group therapy classes to help obese adults, set up by commercial organizations and popular magazines, have also played a part in promoting good eating habits. The long-term success of all forms of weight-reduction programmes is, however, acknowledged to be low. The difficulty of achieving and maintaining weight loss requires further study (Chapter 20).

Dietitians, nutritionists and home economists are consulted about the provision of meals to the elderly in their homes (the Meals on Wheels service) and in residential and day-care centres. Such professional people are employed by commercial food firms and organizations and by public relations firms and they are involved in journalism. In the course of their work they are also promoting good nutrition.

Since 1 April 1974 the National Health Service in England and Wales has been reorganized.[20] In Scotland and Northern Ireland this occurred in 1973. The United Kingdom had been divided into a number of Regional Health Authorities and each

Region has within it a number of Area Health Authorities, each serving a population of approximately half a million people. Each Area Health Authority has within it one or more districts, based on a District General Hospital. The dietetic service, it is expected, will operate at district level and will be coordinated by a district dietitian so that the nutrition advice in the district will be provided by dietitians working in hospitals and in the community. The community health care planning teams which are being set up in each district will have access to the district dietician in planning nutrition projects and surveys.

Other attempts have been made to widen the knowledge of nutrition in the community. In 1947 the Royal Society of Health started a course for caterers and catering and other students entitled 'Nutrition in Relation to Catering and Cooking'. Some courses were run as day courses and others at adult evening education centres. In 1974 there were 23 centres in the United Kingdom which offered this certificate and diploma course aimed at promoting good nutrition.

In 1954 the U.K. Federation for Education in Home Economics was founded. This is a coordinating body which represents the professional interests of those engaged in all aspects of education in home economics in its widest sense. The Federation is a collective member of the International Federation for Home Economics which seeks new and better ways of dealing with problems throughout the world, including teaching nutrition.

It is not easy to assess either the volume or the individual quality of this diverse array of education in nutrition known to be in progress in 1974. Nor is it possible to measure its effectiveness. There is a professional opinion that the general public's knowledge on nutritional matters is confused, very elementary or wrong. There is, however, also the impression to be gained from scrutiny of articles in the popular and specialist women's press and radio and television programmes that there is a demand for knowledge. An important factor in the increasing awareness is the publication, particularly by the Department of Health and Social Security, of various reports on health and social subjects.[13,21,22] The last of these, on diet and coronary heart disease, is a particularly important condensation of strongly held and sometimes conflicting views on a subject which is of profound public concern.

We have attempted to describe the progress that has been made during the last 100 years, and it is our belief that much of this progress can be attributed to the enthusiastic work of individuals who seized opportunities as they arose to promote better nutrition throughout the community.

REFERENCES

1. Great Britain, Parliament. *Report of the Inter-Departmental Committee on Physical Deterioration*, London, H.M. Stationery Office, 1904.
2. Aykroyd, W. R. Nutrition and mortality in infancy and early childhood: past and present relationships, *Amer. J. clin. Nutr.*, **24**, 480 (1971).
3. Newman, G. *Infant Mortality, a Social Problem*, London, Methuen, 1906.
4. Drummond, J. C. and A. Wilbraham. *The Englishman's Food*, 2nd Edn. prep. by Dorothy Hollingsworth, London, Jonathan Cape, 1958.

366

5. Ministry of Health. *Advisory Committee on Nutrition: First Report*, London, H.M. Stationery Office, 1937.
6. British Medical Association. *Report of Committee on Nutrition* , London, British Medical Association, 1933.
7. Orr, J. B. *Food Health and Income: Report on a Survey of Adequacy of Diet in Relation to Income*, London, Macmillan, 1936.
8. League of Nations. *Nutrition. Final Report of the Mixed Committee of the League of Nations on the relation of nutrition to health, agriculture and economic policy*, Geneva, 1937.
9. Ministry of Food. *How Britain was fed in war time, Food control 1939–1945*, London, H.M. Stationery Office, 1946.
10. Ministry of Agriculture, Fisheries and Food. *Manual of Nutrition*, 7th Ed., London, H.M. Stationery Office, 1970.
11. Hammond, J. R. *Food. Volume 1. The growth of policy*, London, H.M. Stationery Office and Longmans, Green, 1951, pp. 96, 222.
12. Greaves, J. P. and D. F. Hollingsworth. Trends in food consumption in the United Kingdom, *Wld. Rev. Nutr. Dietet.*, **6,** 34 (1966).
13. Department of Health and Social Security. Diet and coronary heart disease. Report of the Advisory Panel of the Committee on Medical Aspects of Food Policy (Nutrition) on Diet in relation to Cardiovascular and Cerebrovascular Disease, *Reports on Health and Social Subjects*, No. 7, London, H.M. Stationery Office, 1974.
14. Marr, J. W. Individual dietary surveys: purposes and methods, *Wld. Rev. Nutr. Dietet.*, **13,** 105 (1971)
15. Hollingsworth, D. and M. Russell (Eds.). *Nutritional Problems in a Changing World*, London, Applied Science Publishers, 1973.
16. Marr, Jean W. and W. T. C. Berry. Income, secular change and family food consumption levels: a review of the National Food Survey, 1955–1971, *Nutrition, Lond.*, **28,** 39 (1974).
17. Brockington, C. F. The dietitian in the public health service, *Proc. Nutr. Soc.*, **4,** 278 (1946).
18. Wofinden, R. C. and M. Chapman. The case for, and the work of, a community dietitian, *Proc. Nutr. Soc.*, **27,** 24 (1968).
19. British Dietetic Association. Notes for guidance for dietitians working in the community, *Nutrition, Lond.*, **28,** 110 (1974).
20. Great Britain, Parliament. *National Health Service Reorganisation, England*, (Cmnd. 5055), London, H.M. Stationery Office, 1972.
21. Department of Health and Social Security. A nutrition survey of the elderly: Report by the Panel on Nutrition of the Elderly, *Reports on Health and Social Subjects*, No. 3, London, H.M. Stationery Office, 1972.
22. Department of Health and Social Security. First Report by the Sub-Committee on Nutritional Surveillance.·*Reports on Health and Social Subjects*, No. 6, London, H.M. Stationery Office, 1973.

RECOMMENDED READING

Burn, J. L. Nutrition and public health, *Nutrition, Lond.*, **6,** 20 (1952).
Burnett, J. *Plenty and Want: a Social History of Diet in England from 1815 to the Present Day*, London, Thomas Nelson, 1966 (also published in Pelican Books, London, 1968).
Exton-Smith, A. N. and B. R. Stanton. *Report of an Investigation into the Dietary of Elderly Women Living Alone*, King Edward's Hospital Fund for London, 1965.
Exton-Smith, A. N., B. R. Stanton and A. C. M. Windsor. *Nutrition of Housebound Old*

People, King Edward's Hospital Fund for London, 1972.

Reid, J. J. A. Public health interest in nutrition, *Nutrition, Lond.,* **20,** 144 (1966).

Stanton, B. R. *Meals for the Elderly,* King Edward's Hospital Fund for London, 1971.

Stanton, B. R. and A. N. Exton-Smith. *A Longitudinal Study of the Dietary of Elderly Women,* King Edward's Hospital Fund for London, 1970.

Titmus, R. M. *Problems of Social Policy,* London, H. M. Stationery Office and Longmans, Green, 1950.

CHAPTER 31

Nutrition in the United States of America

A. E. SCHAEFER

LEGISLATIVE MANDATE

The partnership for Health Amendment of 1967 of the United States Congress included instructions to the Secretary of Health, Education and Welfare (HEW) to 'Conduct a comprehensive survey to determine the prevalence of malnutrition and other related hunger problems among low income populations across the Nation . . . and to submit a preliminary report within 6 months of the signing of the bill'. The bill was signed 5 December 1967. By 1 February 1968 the 'Nutrition Program of Health Services and Mental Health Administration' (formerly the Interdepartmental Committee on Nutrition for National Defense — ICNND) was selected by HEW to be responsible for organizing and directing the National Nutrition Survey.

The first subject was examined in May 1968 and the last subject in May 1970. The plan of operation,[1-3] selection of States random sample, methodology and guidelines for interpretation of the findings were reviewed and discussed before the 'Select Committee on Nutrition and Human Needs', of the U.S. Senate — Testimony Part 3, 22–29 January 1969.

SURVEY SAMPLE

Ten states were judgmentally selected to provide geographic representation of major regions of the country to reflect broad diversity of economic, ethnic and socio-cultural composition, high-risk vulnerable groups such as migrant workers, to include areas where infant and maternal mortality rates were above the national average and to include some states wherein participation in food donation and welfare programmes were rated poor. The ten states were: Texas, South Carolina, Louisiana, West Virginia, Kentucky, New York, Massachusetts, Michigan, Washington and California. For each state a random selection was made from the Bureau of Census enumeration districts wherein the largest percentage of families were living below the Department of Health, Education and Welfare's poverty index.* The sampling frame represented 25 per cent of the population drawn from the

* Poverty index for an urban family of four, with a male as head, had an income of less than $3335 per year, or $2345 for a farm family.

lowest income quartile based on the 1960 census data. Approximately 100 enumeration districts were selected per state with 20 households randomly selected from each enumeration district. For California and New York 200 enumeration districts were selected.

Demographic data were obtained on over 24,000 families containing over 86,000 individuals. Evaluation of nutritional status by biochemical assessment involved 40,847 individuals which included 7800 pre-school children (0–5 years of age).

The data are biased by nature of the sample and do not represent the entire population within a state nor certainly the United States as a whole. The data do describe one-fourth of each of the ten states' population. Furthermore, the characteristics of the sampled population groups (income, housing, education, age, sex, family composition, ethnic origin, participation in feeding and/or welfare programmes) enable one to predict the kinds of problems to be expected in population groups with similar characteristics.

METHODOLOGY

The methodology employed was indeed virtually identical to those used in the International surveys of the ICNND[4] in 33 developing countries during the period of 1956–1967, and the nutrition surveys of the Navajo Indians 1955, in Alaska 1957, and in the Montana Indians in 1961. Basically, five types of data were obtained: (i) general household socio-economic health data; (ii) medical and dental examinations; (iii) anthropometric measurements including wrist-bone X-ray; (iv) biochemical analysis of blood and urine, for the purpose of objectively identifying the percentage of the population at nutritional health risk and (v) dietary, i.e. food composition surveys.

Numerous other studies besides the Ten-State Survey were launched in various vulnerable population groups throughout the U.S. These studies, although usually done in populations with greater overall poverty problems, revealed the same kinds of nutrition problems found but usually at a much higher prevalence and of more severe nature.

PROBLEMS IDENTIFIED

The families that formed the bulk of the sample studies were the working poor, had limited education, lived under crowded housing conditions, were most frequently members of minority groups, had a low participation in the food donation or food stamp or welfare programmes, and received very limited medical and dental services.

The *real* poor studied were primarily from Texas, South Carolina, Louisiana, West Virginia and Kentucky. For example, the percentage of families studied per state, with annual incomes of less than half the Poverty Index Ratio (PIR) (less than

$1660.00 per year for an urban family of 4) were: 38 per cent South Carolina, 24 per cent Kentucky, and 19 per cent Texas, versus only approximately 4 per cent from California, Massachusetts and New York. Likewise the number of families studied that had incomes twice or more than the PIR ($6669.00 for urban family of 4) were: 53 per cent New York, 41 per cent California, 44 per cent Massachusetts, 42 per cent Washington, versus only 5.3 per cent for South Carolina, 10 per cent Texas and 15 per cent for Kentucky (Table 1).

Table 1. Per cent distribution of families by poverty index ratio

Poverty index ratio	Annual income urban family 4 members $	Texas	L.A.	So. Carol.	Kent.	W.Va.	Mich.	N.Y.	N.Y. City	Mass.	Wash.	Calif.
0–0.25	834	a	a	12.6	a	2.0	a	a	0	0.8	2.2	0.7
0.26–0.50	1668	19.0	16.1	25.2	23.7	14.0	13.8	4.3	2.3	2.9	4.5	3.2
0.51–1.00	3334	41.8	30.3	37.9	34.1	27.0	18.6	13.7	25.9	17.4	20.1	16.9
1.10–1.50	5002	18.6	15.5	13.9	19.5	20.1	17.5	14.8	28.5	21.7	16.7	22.4
1.51–2.00	6669	10.6	11.7	5.1	7.9	12.7	13.9	13.7	14.8	13.3	14.3	15.5[a]
2.10–2.5	8337	10.0	26.4	2.6	14.8	8.7	36.2	53.5	10.3	12.0	11.3	10.1
2.51 +	8338			2.7		15.5			18.2	31.9	30.9	31.2
Mean PIR		1.1	1.4	0.8	1.2	1.4	1.8	1.9	1.6	1.9	1.8	1.9

[a] For these States PIR of 0–.50 combined and PIR of 2 + combined.

BIOCHEMICAL AND DIETARY FINDINGS

Assessment of nutritional status of population groups by nutrient intake and biochemical analysis of nutrient levels in serum and urine enables one to identify the percentage of the population studied as being at nutritional 'risk' or even 'severe risk'. The use of the term 'unacceptable' blood or urine values is indicative of nutritional risk and 'deficient' levels as 'severe risk'. The biochemical profile of the entire populations studied in the ten states is given in Table 2. Interpretation of the biochemical data was based on the ICNND guidelines for interpretation[4] as modified and expanded by the Nutrition Program Advisory Committee, which had membership from the Food and Nutrition Board, Committee on Nutrition of the American Academy of Pediatrics and the Food and Nutrition Council of the American Medical Association.[3] The dietary guidelines likewise are similar to those used by the ICNND, adjusted for age, sex and pregnancy.

Anaemia

The prevalence of individuals with a haemoglobin value classified as 'unacceptable' varied from approximately 40 per cent in South Carolina and Louisiana to 10

Table 2. Biochemical findings; percentage of population at risk; 'unacceptable tissue nutrient levels'

	Haemoglobin	Vit. A	Vit. C	Serum albumin	Riboflavin	Thiamine
Texas	20	17	12	16	21	10
So. Carolina	38	10	3	7	30	9
Louisiana	42	8	14	14	15	11
Kentucky	18	9	8	3	10	6
West Virginia	13	8	8	1	10	12
Michigan	19	4	1	4	13	6
New York	10	—	2	4	4	4
N.Y. City	16	3	1	1	9	11
Massachusetts	9	10	6	8	7	4
Washington	10	23	2	5	11	6
California	10	1	3	2	7	5

per cent for Washington, California, Massachusetts and New York. However, in the latter states the prevalence in blacks was over 20 per cent. Individuals from families with an income of less than half the PIR ($1616.00 per year, family of 4) usually had twice the number of 'unacceptable' haemoglobin values than individuals from families with an income of twice the PIR (see Table 3).

Table 3. Haemoglobin values and percentage of unacceptable males and females by poverty index ratio

State		Females			Males		
		Income <0.5	Levels 1–1.5	PIR[a] 2+	Income <0.5	Levels 1–1.5	PIR 2+
So. Carolina	Hb gms, mean	11.9	12.2	12.8	12.5	12.3	13.3
	% 'low' values	38	31	19	45	40	38
Washington	Hb gms, mean	13.2	13.2	13.5	14.0	13.9	14.5
	% 'low' values	9	8	5	17	16	9

[a] Poverty Income Ratio.

Since anaemia can be caused by a deficiency of several nutrients, special studies were conducted for us by the U.S. Army Medical Research and Nutrition Laboratory at Fitzsimonds General Hospital. All blood samples identified as 'unacceptable' reference the haemoglobin values were analysed for serum iron, iron-binding capacity, transferrin saturation index, serum folic acid and red blood cell folates. In addition, these samples were matched from so-called normal haemoglobin levels. In the state of Washington *all samples* collected were analysed for serum iron and folate. 'Deficient' levels of folic acid based on red blood cell folate values were noted in from 10 per cent of samples from West Virginia to 52 per cent of those from Michigan. A comparison of folate and iron data in populations from South Carolina and Washington is given in Table 4.

Table 4. Folate and iron status

State	Per cent population 'deficient levels' R.B.C. folate	transferrin sat.
South Carolina	27	52
Washington	21	28

Serum iron or transferrin saturation index data revealed that the major cause of anaemia is iron deficiency. In Washington 28 per cent of all the serum samples analysed had 'unacceptable levels of transferrin saturation', indicative of an iron deficiency. Mild — yes, but still indicative of suboptimal iron nutrition. However, much of the anaemia may also have been complicated by suboptimal folate levels. Thus, a prevention programme should also consider folic acid intake and utilization as well as iron. The data revealed that the prevalence of 'low' haemoglobin, potential risk of anaemia, was virtually as high in males (especially teenage males) as in females. Since males do not suffer the blood loss that females do the assumption has been that the iron requirement for males is much less. There is no argument with this point. However, serum iron values and transferrin saturation index levels in males clearly implicate an insufficiency of dietary utilizable iron for males as well as females. Likewise, in those individuals with 'low' haemoglobin nearly one-third of the males as well as the females had evidence of folic acid deficiency as indicated by red blood cell folate levels. In fact, there was consistently a higher prevalence in males. The definition of 'low' haemoglobin for the male of 15 years of age and over was less than 14 gm of haemoglobin, whereas for the female the level was 12 gm. If we apply the female standard, of course, the prevalence of 'low' haemoglobin in the male is reduced. However, perhaps the female level should really be raised to 14 gm.

Recently we had the opportunity of reviewing the findings of the Central American surveys by the ICNND (Interdepartmental Committee of Nutrition for National Defense) and INCAP (Institute of Nutrition for Central America and Panama) for 1965–1967. Based on nearly 20,000 blood samples analysed for haemoglobin, red blood cell counts, serum iron, folate, and vitamin B_{12}, the haemoglobin values indicative of a risk of anaemia are indeed very similar to the guides used for the U.S. survey, with the exception that the female level used for the U.S. data is apparently too low and should be 13 gm of haemoglobin per 100 ml of blood — unless we take the position that somehow the U.S. female is different from the Central American female and does not require an equivalent level of haemoglobin (see Table 5). We also noted a higher prevalence of anaemia in the black population groups regardless of where they resided.

Table 5. Haemoglobin — mean values, gms/100 ml by ethnic group and age

Age (yrs)	U.S. Males			U.S. Females			Central America[a]	
	White	Negro	Spanish American	White	Negro	Spanish American	Males	Females
2–5	12.2	11.4	12.1	12.2	11.4	12.1	12.7	12.7
13–16	14.2	13.0	13.7	13.3	12.1	12.7	13.9	13.6
17–44	15.2	14.2	14.8	13.3	12.3	12.7	15.4	13.6
60+	14.6	13.4	14.0	13.6	12.5	13.2	14.6	13.9

[a] Central America and Panama Nutrition Survey

Dietary intake data substantiate the poor iron status (Table 6). Regardless of income status, a very high percentage of infants, teenagers and pregnant mothers consumed less than two-thirds of the level of dietary iron as recommended by the Food and Nutrition Board (R.D.A.).

Table 6. Dietary intake of iron percentage consuming <2/3 R.D.A.

Age (yrs)	Sex	High income	Low income
2–3		77	85
12–14	M	41	48
	F	62	67
60 +	M	15	18
	F	25	41
Pregnant		61	68

Vitamin A

The high prevalence of 'unacceptable' serum vitamin A levels in children 0–16 years of age in seven of the ten states and especially in pre-school children should be of vital concern. The pre-clinical period, that is where blood concentration is being depleted and prior to appearance of overt physical lesions, of vitamin A deficiency is usually prolonged due to liver storage. However, the subsequent stage, ('deficient') of continued depletion can lead to overt disease in a short time and proceed with disastrous rapidity leading to xeropthalmia and blindness in children. Fortunately, no child was diagnosed as having severe eye lesions. In the first five states studied, Texas, Louisiana, Kentucky, Massachusetts and New York, clinical physical lesions associated with vitamin A deficiency were noted, follicular hyperkeratosis in 1 per cent of children under six years of age. Bitot's spots, an eye lesion, associated with but not always specifically due to vitamin A deficiency, was seen in 23 subjects. Twenty of these were found in Texas where a high prevalence of 'unacceptable' vitamin A values was noted.

The vast majority of the 'unacceptable' and 'deficient' levels of vitamin A were contributed by the 0–5 year-old age groups. In Texas 40 per cent of all pre-school children had values of less than 20 mcg and 80 per cent less than 30 mcg; in South Carolina 26 per cent of the pre-school children had less than 20 mcg; 34 per cent less than 22 mcg and 45 per cent less than 25 mcg. In the black population of Michigan and Kentucky 20 per cent had unacceptable levels of vitamin A.

The dietary intake data for the first five states indicated that 20–40 per cent of the groups studied consumed less than two-thirds of the recommended dietary allowance.* It must be remembered that in the early stages of the surveys (Texas, Louisiana, Michigan, Kentucky and New York State) the vast majority of skim milk powder (distributed by U.S.D.A. in the Food Distribution Program) had not been enriched with vitamins A and D. The Department of Agriculture, in November 1968, issued a directive requiring the enrichment of all skim milk distributed through their food donation programme with vitamins A and D. While the Nutrition Survey was in progress numerous research investigators not only substantiated the survey findings with reference to vitamin A but identified an even more serious problem in selected poverty population groups.

Sandstead[5] and coworkers of Vanderbilt University reported that 96 per cent of 101 pre-school children attending two nurseries in Nashville, Tennessee had vitamin A serum values of less than 20 mcg. High,[5] from Meharry University, reported that of 178 pre-school children studied in the Bluffton and Hilton Health Areas of South Carolina, 30 per cent had less than 20 mcg and 8 per cent less than 10 mcg. Hepner, of the Community Pediatric Center, University of Maryland, Baltimore,[5] reported that 14.5 per cent of 4–5 year-olds had less than 15 mcg. Unglaub,[5] of Tulane University, found a prevalence of 16–35 per cent in 900 Head Start children studied in Alabama, Louisiana and Mississippi with levels of less than

* Recommended allowance: 1500 International Units vitamin A for infants, 2000 International Units for 1–6 year-olds, 2500 International Units for 6–12 year-olds and 3500 International Units for adults.

20 mcg. Chase,[6] of the University of Colorado Medical Center, reported prevalence of 20 per cent in 300 pre-school migrant children in 1969, with serum levels of less than 20 mcg. Zee,[7] of St. Judes Children Research Hospital, Memphis, Tennessee, reported a prevalence in pre-school children of 44 per cent with less than 20 mcg.

Table 7. Serum vitamin A distribution and mean values

mcg per 100 ml	Per cent prevalence less than [a]				Mean value mcg per 100 ml
	10	20	25	30	
Texas	2.0	17	Na[b]	41	31.6
South Carolina	0.6	10	22	36	34.1
Louisiana	0.9	8	Na	15	47.2
Kentucky	3.6	9	19	31	40.1
West Virginia	0	8	18	28	37.7
Michigan	0.1	4	16	24	40.4
New York City	1.5	3	9	13	44.9
Massachusetts	1.0	10	17	25	44.4
Washington	6.0	23	36	38	31.1
California	0.1	1	3	6	57.8

[a] <10 mcg per 100 ml: 'deficient' — severe risk group.
   <20 mcg per 100 ml: 'unacceptable level' — moderate risk group.
[b] Values not available.

While the physical-clinical evidence did not suggest a severe medical problem, the biochemical findings do indicate a *serious degree of risk* that warranted preventive action.

Vitamin C

The prevalence of 'unacceptable' serum vitamin C values (less than 0.2 mg per 100 ml serum) varied greatly between states. Five of the ten states, Texas, Louisiana, Kentucky, West Virginia and Massachussetts, had a prevalence of from 6–14 per cent, whereas in the other states and New York City the prevalence was 3 per cent or less. Dietary data analysed for the first five states provide a partial answer. Approximately 27 per cent of the households in Texas and Louisiana had a mean intake of less than 21 mg of vitamin C or 70 per cent of the intake considered 'acceptable'. The 30 mg per day level of vitamin C standard applied to the dietary intake data is an austere level, since it is less than 50 per cent of the Food and Nutrition Board's 'recommended dietary allowance'.

Serum Albumin Measure of Protein Nutrition

Texas and Louisiana had the highest prevalence of 'unacceptable' serum albumin levels, 16 and 14 per cent respectively, with 8 per cent in Massachusetts and 7 per cent in South Carolina. The rates for unacceptable serum albumin values were in general highest in the aged. This could very well be related to the higher prevalence of chronic disease. Dietary data suggest that less than acceptable levels of protein intake did occur, but to a lower degree than for the other nutrients studied (Table 8).

Table 8. Protein intake percentage consuming <2/3 R.D.A.

Age (yrs)	High income-states	Low income-states
2–3	1	3
12–14	4	11
60+	14	23
Pregnant	13	27

Riboflavin

The pattern of 'unacceptable' urinary riboflavin values was in general similar to the vitamin A results. In seven of the states 10 per cent or more had 'unacceptable riboflavin values'. The dietary data indicate that 10–30 per cent of the surveyed population groups consumed less than two-thirds of the recommended standard for riboflavin.

PHYSICAL FINDINGS IN PRE-SCHOOL CHILDREN

A variety of physical lesions usually associated with nutritional deficits, were found at a relatively low level of prevalence. However, the 'rare case' of overt marasmus or kwashiorkor was found. Although in our physical examination forms the physician was not asked to diagnose marasmus or kwashiorkor, follow-up studies on eleven children revealed varying degrees of mild to severe caloric deficiency; four cases were severe and required hospitalization. In the opinion of my staff, the prevalence of more than one case identified in the random poulation sample was cause for concern. Why didn't the parents, neighbours or relatives recognize the failure to thrive?

Evidence of rickets is defined by such symptoms as bowed legs, beading of the ribs, and bossing of the skull varied from 0.3–5.0 per cent of the children under six years of age examined.

Follicular hyperkoratosis on the arms was noted in 2.7 per cent of the Spanish American children in Texas, 2.9 per cent of the black, and 2.5 per cent of the white children of the high-income states. Bitot's spots usually associated with vitamin A deficiency were infrequent, yet 24 cases were reported in children under age 10. Cheilosis usually associated with riboflavin deficiency was found in 0.6 to 4.1 per cent of the children. Tongue lesions such as filiform papillary atrophy were noted in approximately 5 per cent of the children.

ANTHROPOMETRIC FINDINGS (completed on 62,532 people)

Height Retardation (Table 9)

Growth retardation as evaluated by height in comparison to the growth of normal children as reflected by the Stuart–Meredith norms was noted in all ethnic groups and irrespective of whether the children were from the high- or low-income states.

Table 9. Height retardation (percentage below the 15th centile of Stuart–Meredith Standard)

	Percentage of children			
	Male		Female	
Age (yrs)	White	Black	White	Black
2	42	46	46	37
4	39	34	44	36
6	37	30	38	32
8	45	36	39	25

The percentage of children below the 15th centile of height at two years and four years of age ranged from 34–46 per cent, dependent upon sex and ethnic origin. The Spanish American children from Texas, data we omitted from the official Ten-State Survey report,[1] revealed that the average height followed the 16th centile curve and by age 4 revealed a retardation in growth rate of 6–9 months. The effect of income on growth was noted. For some groups the children from families with an annual income of greater than approximately $5000 for a family of four were advanced as much as *a year* in height over the children from families with an income of less than $5000.

Weight Retardation (Table 10)

For the 2, 4 or 6 year-olds, 22–35 per cent of the children by sex and ethnic origin were below the 15th centile of standard weight. The Texas Spanish American children exhibited a greater retardation in weight.

Table 10. Weight retardation (percentage below 15th centile for weight of Stuart-Meredith Standard)

| Age (yrs) | Percentage of Children | | | |
| | Male | | Female | |
	White	Black	White	Black
2	26	34	31	27
4	22	22	33	33
6	27	27	35	37
8	39	32	32	31
10	34	45	20	27

Obesity (Table 11)

Unfortunately, the data regarding obesity in children have not been completely analysed; however, the basic data is in the survey data bank at the U.S. Center for Disease Control. Based on the Seltzer–Mayer[8] minimum triceps fat-fold thickness (18 mm for 12 year-old male, 22 mm for 12-year old female, etc.) the percentage of obese adolescents (12 years of age) varied from 11–39 per cent in white males (average of 18.3 per cent) and 9–19 per cent in white females (average 10 per cent).

Table 11. Percentage obese[a]

| Age (Mid-point yrs.) | Percentage of individuals | | | |
| | Male | | Female | |
	White	Black	White	Black
12	18.3	9.8	10.0	9.0
14	18.8	12.5	15.3	18.6
16	29.0	13.0	11.7	11.1
21	15.1	8.3	16.6	18.1
30	21.0	12.0	25.9	36.4

[a] Obesity defined as triceps fat-fold above 18.6 mm for males, and 25.1 mm for females (Seltzer and Mayer)[8]

Black women had the highest prevalence of obesity, exceeding 50 per cent in the 45–55 year age group, white women were not far behind, namely, 40 per cent were obese in the same age group.

Pregnant and Lactating Females — Biochemical and Dietary Data

The vast majority of the data collected on the pregnant and lactating females have not been analysed by the Center for Disease Control of HEW. The data available on haemoglobin and serum albumin (Table 12) indicate nutrition

Table 12. Biochemical findings in pregnant and lactating females by ethnic group

	Haemoglobin g/100 ml		Serum albumin g/100 ml	
	<10	<11	<10	<11
White, %				
Low-income states	0	13.6	10.0	10.0
High-income states	1.0	7.9	8.5	17.0
Black, %				
Low-income states	13.8	37.6	13.6	21.2
High-income states	4.9	19.6	4.0	12.0
Spanish-American, %				
Low-income states	10.0	13.3	10.7	21.4
High-income states	6.1	20.4	5.0	10.0

problems, especially in the black pregnant females; however, in all ethnic groups irrespective of whether they reside in the low- or high-income state the prevalence of 'low' serum albumin levels is reason for concern.

DISCUSSION

The primary causes for the types of malnutrition noted are indeed multiple in nature:

1. Poverty: lack of sufficient income to provide a well-balanced, nutritionally optimum diet.

2. Lack of knowledge regarding what foods and how much is required to ensure optimum nutrition.

3. Lack of health and dental care with little if any guidance or assistance in the prevention of nutritional problems.

4. Lack of or ignorance of fortified or enriched foods.

5. Meagre or non-existence of sound nutrition education for pregnant mothers, pre-school children, adolescents and *for the providers of health care.*

6. The change in food consumption patterns, further complicated by the enormous variety of foods available in the market.

7. Low participation at the time of the survey (less than 20 per cent of the really needy families) in the food donation, food stamp or welfare programmes.

The fundamental *causes* of malnutrition are really not different for the populations we studied in the U.S. from those noted in many other countries, wherein basically the same techniques of assessment were applied. The kinds of nutrition problems noted were in general much less severe; however, for the need to ensure optimum nutrition for growth and development of children, there can be no compromise nor satisfaction in waiting for more severe symptoms to develop.

Following the Congressional legislative mandate, to investigate malnutrition in the U.S.A., the United States Senate authorized and established a Select Committee on Nutrition and Human Needs in 1968. This has provided an opportunity for scientists, legislators, government employees, the poor and industry to testify and assist in structuring legislative support for improvement of nutrition, health, housing and education needs of the less fortunate of our country.

This congressional interest and the Ten-State Nutrition Survey stimulated the assembly of the First White House Conference on Food, Nutrition and Human Needs. Even though the bureaucracy stymied many of the recommendations for action, much good was accomplished. For example, the Department of Agriculture *with* Congressional urging truly revamped an unimaginative, ineffective food donation programme. The Food and Drug Administration has introduced a new system of nutrition labelling directed towards an updated consumer education programme. The Department of Agriculture took action in requiring the fortification of dried skim milk with vitamins A and D and an improved cereal enrichment with iron, lysine, thiamine, riboflavin, niacin, and vitamin A was evaluated in selected test areas in the United States.

EVALUATION OF PROGRAMMES TO COMBAT MALNUTRITION

Zee and collaborators reported in 1969 the results of a nutrition health survey of black pre-school children living in a poverty area in Memphis, Tennessee.[7] The median family income was $1838.00 with a household size of 6.8 members. In January 1969, through agreements with the Tennessee and U.S. Department of Agriculture, the Memphis and Shelby County Health Departments and the Model Cities Program, fifty health aids and three nurse practitioners from the Nutrition Clinic of St. Jude's Children Research Hospital identified the needy families for the federal supplementary feeding programme. The programme was directed to all children six years and under, pregnant women and mothers less than one year postpartum of poor families. A nutrition survey was conducted in January 1969 of three hundred children randomly selected from 2427 black children of poverty families (Table 13).

Table 13. Effect of applied nutrition program, Memphis, Tennessee

| | Per cent of pre-school children | |
	1969	1972
Height		
Below 25th centile	50	29[a]
Weight		
Below 25th centile	50	39[a]
Haemoglobin		
<10gm/100 ml	28	11[a]
Plasma		
<20 mcg/100 ml	44	26[a]

[a] p = <0.01.

Half of the children were below the 25th centile for height and weight standards. Bone age assessed by wrist bone X-ray was less than 75 per cent of the chronological age and in 11 per cent of the children bone age was less than 50 per cent of the chronological age.

Anaemia was common; 28 per cent of children less than three years of age had haemoglobin values of less than 10 gms/100 ml, and 25 per cent of children older than three years had haemoglobin below 11 gms/100 ml. Forty-four per cent of the children had serum vitamin A values below 20 mcg/100 ml.

A resurvey in 1972,[9] of 250 pre-school children randomly selected from the same population group studied in 1969 revealed a significant improvement. The results clearly indicate that nutritional assistance programmes produced improvements among impoverished populations. Median income changed very little over the three-year period, still being less than $1900.00 per year in 1972. Such programmes need to be continued to break the cycle of nutritional poverty.

Hepner[5] of the Community Pediatric Center, Baltimore, Maryland, recently shared with the authors his appraisal of nutritional statue in children before and after participation in intervention programmes supervised by the Community Pediatric Center in conjunction with a model cities programme (Table 14). An iron-enriched milk formula was furnished to all newborns through age 9 months. Nearly 1000 infants were studied, with and without the iron supplement. The prevalence of haemoglobin levels below 10 gms per cent was reduced from 55 to 2.5 per cent. In a second study of nutrition surveillance as a tool for programme planning and evaluation in a Child and Youth Project, 5284 Baltimore inner city children were studied over a four-year period. Public support for free school meals rose from 127 in 1967 to 3700 per day by 1971. Meals began in 1969 for grades kindergarten and 1 and 2, in 1970 for grades 3 and 4 and in 1971 for grades 5 and 6. The tremendous improvement of nutritional health is illustrated by the reduction in low haemoglobins, serum albumin and vitamin A levels and in the number of children below the third centile in skin-fold thickness.

Table 14. Child and youth project, Baltimore, Maryland

	Infants Iron-enriched formula	9 Months of age none
Mean 1 hb gm/100 ml	11.6	10.1
Hb less than 10 gm/100 ml per cent of children	2.5	55.0

Child youth and model cities project (5284 children)

	Per cent of 5 year-olds	
	1967	1971
Hb 11 gms/100 ml	25	6
Serum albumin 3.7 gms/100 ml	47	0
Vitamin A 20 mcg/100 ml	24	8
Skin-fold thickness third centile	68	28

SUMMARY

The Ten-State Nutrition Survey, conducted in 1968–1970, clearly established that various types of malnutrition exist in the populations studied — namely in the people living in the lower quartile of income areas in these states. A consistent pattern of nutrition problems emerged which identified the population groups at a nutritional health risk or even at severe risk. The problems identified are much more prevalent in the poor, minority groups: migrant workers, blacks, and Appalachian whites. Physical growth retardation in pre-school age children in conjunction with retardation of bone age as measured by wrist bone X-ray, biochemical evidence of 'unacceptable' and 'deficient' levels of numerous nutrients and the dietary findings, provide evidence of the nutrition–health risk in some of our pre-school children.

The findings clearly indicate that of the populations studied a substantial number of children were indeed malnourished. Evidence of retarded growth was apparent in children from low-income families. Relative to what would be expected for a well-nourished population as a whole, twice as many black children and three times as many white children in families living in poverty were below the 15th centile for accepted American standards of height. As family income increased, the children were taller, heavier, had a greater head circumference, had more advanced skeletal maturity, more advanced dental maturity and had higher haemoglobin values. Boys 7 through 12 years of age with normal haemoglobin levels averaged 3 to 4 cm taller than those with low haemoglobin values.

384

Obesity is a serious problem of malnutrition. The data base provided an opportunity to evaluate parent–child relationships. There were 21,000 possible parent–child comparisons, 30,000 sibling comparisons and 2000 spouse comparisons. Two obese parents provide a 40 per cent probability of having an obese child. Children of obese parents are three times as fat as are progeny of lean parents.

REFERENCES

1. U.S. Department of Health Education and Welfare, *Ten-state Nutrition Survey* 1968–1970, HEW pub. No. (HSM) 72–8134, 1972.
2. Schaefer, A. E. The national nutrition survey, *J. am. diet. Ass.*, **54,** No. 5 (1969).
3. O'Neal, R. M., O. C. Johnson and A. E. Schaefer, Guidelines for classification and interpretation of group blood and urine data collected as part of the national nutrition survey. *Pediat. Res.*, **4,** p. 103 (1970).
4. Interdepartmental Committee on Nutrition for National Defense; *Manual for Nutrition Surveys*, 2nd edn., U.S. Govt. Print., Wash., D. C. 1963.
5. Personal communication.
6. Chase, H. P., V. Kumar, J. M. Dodds, H. E. Sauberlich, R. M. Hunter, R. S. Brocton and V. Spalding. Nutritional Status of Pre-school Mexican-American Migrant Farm Children, *Am. J. Dis. Child.,* **122,** p. 316 (1971).
7. Zee, P., T. Walters and C. Mitchell. Nutrition and poverty in pre-school children, *J. amer. med. Ass.,* **213,** No. 5, p. 739 (1970).
8. Seltzer, C. C. and J. Mayer. A simple criterion of obesity, post grad Med 38, A p. 101 (1965).
9. Zee, P. and A. G. Kafatos. Nutrition and federal food-assistance programs: A survey of impoverished pre-school blacks in Memphis, Tennessee, *Fed. Proc.,* **32,** No. 3 (1973).

Index

388